Antibiotic Resistance in Bacteria

Scientific Editor: *Naomi Datta*

	PAGE			PAGE
Introduction	*Naomi Datta*	1	Self defence in antibiotic-producing organisms	
			E Cundliffe	61
Resistance of the antibiotic target site	*P E Reynolds*	3	Drug resistance in gram-negative aerobic bacilli	
			B Rowe & E J Threlfall	68
Antibiotic resistance resulting from decreased drug accumulation	*I Chopra*	11	Antibiotic resistance in *Staphylococcus aureus* and streptococci	*R W Lacey*	77
β-Lactamases	*A A Medeiros*	18		
Aminoglycoside resistance	*I Phillips & K Shannon*	28	Drug resistance in mycobacteria	*D A Mitchison*	84
Bacterial resistance to chloramphenicol	*W V Shaw*	36	Antibiotic-resistant bacteria in animal husbandry		
			A H Linton	91
Bacterial resistance to antifolate chemotherapeutic agents mediated by plasmids	*J T Smith & S G B Amyes*	42	Counteracting antibiotic resistance: new drugs		
			R B Sykes & D P Bonner	96
Inducible erythromycin resistance in bacteria	*B Weisblum*	47	Impact on therapy	*H P Lambert*	102
Genetics and evolution of antibiotic resistance	*J R Saunders*	54		

Notes on Contributors	107
Index	110

Professor Naomi Datta chaired the committee, which included Professor E F Gale, Professor F W O'Grady and Professor I Phillips, that planned this number of *British Medical Bulletin*. We are grateful to them for their help, and particularly to Professor Datta, who acted as Scientific Editor for the number.

British Medical Bulletin is published by Churchill Livingstone for the British Council, 10 Spring Gardens, London SW1A 2BN.

KA 0051782 8

Encyclopaedia of occupational health and safety

3rd edition (completely revised and updated)

An indispensable reference work for all those concerned with protecting workers' safety and health—entrepreneurs, trade unionists, works safety and health committees—presented objectively and systematically, even for those with little or no specialised medical or technical knowledge. In the light of recent developments all entries have been brought up-to-date in order to take account of progress and trends in industrial toxicology and cancerology, wider adoption of epidemiological methods, studies of the immune response, widespread concern for improving the working environment, increasing workers' participation and strengthening preventive standards and legislation. The accent is on the safety precautions to be taken against the main hazards encountered in each branch of industry.
ISBN 92-2-103289-2 (2 volumes) £78.00

Accident prevention

A Workers' Education Manual, 2nd (revised) edition

Every year millions of workers throughout the world are victims of occupational accidents which cause permanent or temporary disability. This up-to-date edition discusses the causes and efects of accidents and goes on to give the basic principles of prevention, after having taken accunt of recent developments. It explains how safety is promoted and which kinds of authorities, institutions and bodies are responsible for it.
ISBN 92-2-103392-9 £5.00

Deterrence and compensation: Legal liability in occupational safety and health

By Felice Morgenstern

This study examines the manner in which penal and civil liability contribute to the prevention of occupational accidents and diseases and to the compensation of their victims. It surveys the law and practice of countries with different legal systems with respect to the civil and criminal liability of manufacturers, suppliers, employers, supervisors and workers. It will be of particular interest to those interested in this subject especially those with responsibilities for drawing up and implementing legislation.
ISBN 92-2-103010-5 £5.00

INTERNATIONAL LABOUR OFFICE

Branch Office
96-98 Marsham Street
LONDON SW1P 4LY
Tel: 01-828 6401

BOOKS

THE MEDICAL AND SCIENTIFIC BOOKSHOP

large stock of Textbooks and new editions on all branches of Medicine, Surgery and their allied subjects.

Catalogue post free on request.

MEDICAL AND SCIENTIFIC LIBRARY

Annual subscription from £9.50
(Available in the UK only)
Prospectus post free on request

H. K. LEWIS & CO. LTD.
136 Gower Street, London WC1E 6BS
01-387 4282

TO ADVERTISE IN THIS PUBLICATION

Please contact
Sheila Devereux at:

Longman Group Ltd
6th Floor
Westgate House
The High
Harlow
Essex CM20 1NE
Tel: (0279) 442601

British Medical Bulletin (1984) Vol. 40, No. 1, pp. 1–2

INTRODUCTION

NAOMI DATTA   MD FRCPath

Department of Bacteriology
Royal Postgraduate Medical School
London

Infections caused by resistant bacteria have been a fact of life ever since effective antibacterial drugs became available in medicine. In most cases, the resistance is apparently acquired rather than intrinsic, the infecting organisms belonging to species that were characteristically sensitive to the particular drug at the time of its development and first medical use. Many 'opportunistic' infections, however, have been and are caused by intrinsically resistant bacteria. Obviously, resistant bacteria are of great clinical and economic importance; if they had never made their appearance, treatment of infections would be relatively easy and there would have been no call for the enormous investment of time, money and ingenuity which goes into the discovery and development of new antibacterial drugs.

The rapidity with which resistance often appears after introduction of a new drug is astonishing. Their very short generation time allows bacteria to undergo evolutionary changes easily seen within one human generation. Not only have the bacteria evolved over the last 30 years, but also our concepts of their genetics and biochemistry have greatly changed.

My own introduction to the study of antibiotic resistance was in 1957 when I came to work in the same department as D A Mitchison and the late Mary Barber, each concerned with different aspects of the subject. Mary's primary interest was in the practical, clinical aspects of resistance and the prevention of its spread but she was very much aware of the necessity for understanding its basis. At that time, when the study of microbial genetics was in its infancy, there were two conflicting views on the basis of acquired drug resistance in bacteria—one that it resulted from mutation with subsequent selection of initially small numbers of resistant mutants, the other that all cells in a culture could adapt to the presence of an antibiotic by adjustment in the enzyme reactions necessary for cell growth. (More about this almost-forgotten controversy can be found in the 1953 Symposium.[1])

Papers in this Bulletin describe the great advances that have since been made in understanding the mechanisms, both genetic and biochemical, by which bacteria have become resistant. In many cases, neither of the explanations proposed in the 1950s is the right one. Resistance in bacteria pathogenic for man and animals has most frequently resulted from the acquisition of new DNA, encoding genes determining a variety of specific proteins, from an outside source. Such a mechanism was not considered until it was demonstrated in strains of *Shigella flexneri* in Japan in 1959 (review by Watanabe[2]). The immediate source of the acquired genes is another bacterial cell and the vector a bacterial plasmid, but the ultimate origin of the resistance genes is still unknown (see papers by Saunders, pp. 54–59 and Cundliffe, pp. 61–67). This evolutionary mechanism, acting in the natural environment, may account for apparently conflicting results between workers studying resistant bacteria selected from pure cultures in the laboratory and those studying clinical isolates; an early example was with sulphonamide-resistant pneumococci.[3,4]

The Japanese workers described the transfer from one bacterium to another of a resistance (R) factor (now referred to as an R plasmid) that conferred resistance simultaneously to four unrelated drugs, chloramphenicol, tetracycline, streptomycin and sulphonamides. The biochemical basis for these resistances are described in this volume by Shaw (pp. 36–41), Chopra (pp. 11–17), Phillips & Shannon (pp. 28–35) and Smith & Amyes (pp. 42–46) but when they were first shown to be transmissible, none of the mechanisms was known. It was known, though, that the penicillin resistance that had become so common in *Staphylococcus aureus* by the late 1950s[5] was mediated by the production of β-lactamase. This did not fit either the mutational or the adaptive theories since exposure of pure cultures of *S. aureus* to penicillin did not yield β-lactamase-producing variants. That β-lactamase production was determined by an extraneous genetic element, or plasmid, was suggested by Novick[6] and has been amply confirmed not only in staphylococci (Lacey, this volume, pp. 77–83) but in many bacterial genera (Medeiros, ibid, pp. 18–27).

Subsequently, many other specific resistances have been found, in an increasingly wide variety of genera, to be plasmid-determined and transmissible by one means or another between bacteria. The biochemical basis of plasmid-determined resistance is very varied, as described in this issue. Some of the resistances are inducible, again by various mechanisms, others are expressed constitutively.

The resistance genes themselves are acquired as new DNA by their plasmid vectors; they are frequently found in transposons, sequences that include genes determining their own replication as they proceed from one DNA molecule to another (Saunders, this volume, pp. 54–60). Thus antibiotic resistance spreads at three levels: carried on transposons between plasmids, plasmids between bacteria, and bacteria between people or animals.

Antibiotic resistance can also result from mutation in genes of the bacterial chromosome. Clinically, this is particularly important in mycobacterial infections (Mitchison, this volume, pp. 84–90) and there are indications that resistance to β-lactam drugs, including the newer cephalosporins not hydrolysed by known β-lactamases, results from mutations (in this volume see Reynolds pp. 3–10, Chopra pp. 11–17 and Medeiros pp. 18–27).

Some of the following papers deal with resistance to particular drugs or determined by particular mechanisms, others deal with resistance in particular bacterial genera or environments. There is, therefore, some overlap but I think this is no disadvantage as the same facts are considered from different view-points. There is no paper devoted specifically to anaerobes. Many of the plasmid-determined resistances discussed, e.g. to tetracycline or chloramphenicol, have been found in anaerobes, as described in the relevant papers. Metronidazole is at present the most important drug in the treatment of anaerobic infections. Anaerobes resistant to metronidazole are fortunately rare; not enough is currently known about such resistance to justify the inclusion of a chapter on the subject.[7]

Advances in knowledge of how bacteria become resistant to antibiotics have not, unfortunately, shown the way towards prevention. The emergence of resistant mutants may be prevented by the use of combined therapy with two or more unrelated drugs (Mitchison, this volume, pp. 84–90). No paper in this volume describes methods for interrupting the spread of resistance genes in or between bacteria. Curing bacteria of R plasmids can sometimes be achieved by chemical or physical means but, for it to have any clinical application, it would be necessary for all cells in a bacterial population to be cured on exposure to some non-toxic compound: such efficiency of curing is not seen even in the controlled environment of laboratory experiments. No means are known for preventing the spread of transposons. The dissemination of resistance genes at the molecular level, therefore, cannot be actively interrupted, though limitation on antibiotic usage at least reduces the selective pressure that encourages the spread of resistance at all levels (Lambert, this volume, pp. 102–106). Methods for preventing the spread of resistant bacteria between people or animals are those that have long been recognized, though not always adequately applied, in the control of bacterial infection.

One outcome of studies on R plasmids and resistance genes is their use in the cloning of foreign DNA. Cloning techiques are being applied rewardingly in many branches of biological science as well as commercially for the production by bacteria of valuable peptides such as mammalian hormones.

Understanding the mechanisms of resistance is of direct importance in the development of new antibacterial drugs. In the early years of the antibiotic era, new drugs were discovered by the empirical testing of great numbers of microbial specimens and organic chemicals. Now synthetic and semisynthetic compounds can be made expressly to overcome some, at least, of the resistance mechanisms of bacteria decribed in this volume. Papers by Sykes (pp. 96–101) and Lambert (pp. 102–106) describe the respective ways in which the pharmaceutical industry and the clinician are overcoming problems posed by the evolutionary miracles achieved by bacteria.

REFERENCES

1 Davies R, Gale EF, eds. Adaptation in Micro-organisms 1953. 3rd symposium of the Society for General Microbiology Cambridge: Cambridge University Press
2 Watanabe T. Infective heredity of multiple drug resistance in bacteria. Bact Rev 1963; 27: 87–115
3 Mirick GS. Enzymatic identification of p-amino benzoic acid (PAB) in cultures of Pneumococcus and its relation to sulphonamide-fastness. J Clin Invest 1942; 21: 628
4 Tillett WS, Cambier MJ, Harris WH. Sulfonamide-fast pneumococci: a clinical report of two cases of pneumonia together with experimental studies on the effectiveness of penicillin and tyrothricin against sulfonamide-resistant strains. J Clin Invest 1943; 22: 249–255
5 Barber M. Drug-resistance of staphylococci with special reference to penicillinase production. Mechanisms of Development of Drug-Resistance in Micro-organisms 1957. CIBA Foundation Symposium, London: Churchill
6 Novick RP. Analysis by transduction of mutations affecting penicillinase formation in *Staphylococcus aureus*. J Gen Microbiol 1963; 33: 121–136
7 Tabaqchali S, Pantosti A, Oldfield S. Pyruvate dehydrogenase activity and metronidazole susceptibility in *Bacteroides fragilis*. J Antimicrob Chemother 1983; 11: 393–400

British Medical Bulletin (1984) Vol. 40, No. 1, pp. 3–10

RESISTANCE OF THE ANTIBIOTIC TARGET SITE

PETER E REYNOLDS MA PhD

Department of Biochemistry
University of Cambridge

1   Penicillin-binding proteins—target of β-lactam antibiotics
2   DNA gyrase—a target of inhibitors of replication
3   RNA polymerase—a target of inhibitors of transcription
4   The ribosome—the target of inhibitors of translation
      a Ribosomal proteins
      b Ribosomal RNA
5   Summary
     References

The precise geometry of the site of binding of an antibiotic to its primary target in cells is not known with certainty even when the interaction is covalent. Such information must await detailed crystallographic analysis at high resolution. In those instances where the antibiotic binds covalently to the active site of an enzyme, it might be imagined that a mutation which affects the binding of the inhibitor (thus resulting in resistance) would also affect the binding of the ordinary substrate. However, other groups in the target are almost certainly involved in the initial, non-covalent, binding either to substrate or inhibitor prior to the subsequent covalent bond formation. Since these secondary sites may be different for inhibitor and substrate, it may be possible for a mutation to resistance to occur without drastic effects on the kinetics of interaction of the altered enzyme and substrate. It would, of course, be virtually impossible for a mutation to occur at the position of the amino acid in the active site involved in covalent bond formation without severe, deleterious effects on the kinetics of the normal reaction. It is most unlikely that such mutations will be found. With targets which interact with antibiotics non-covalently, leading to impairment of function, this problem does not arise. Numerous mutations leading to resistance might be possible without impairing the normal function of the target. The examples cited in this paper illustrate the variety of targets in which alterations have been determined and, in some instances, mapped with precision, but in which the function of the target has not been seriously impaired.

1   Penicillin-Binding Proteins—The Target of β-Lactam Antibiotics

Until the development of β-lactamase-resistant β-lactam antibiotics in recent years, particularly the third generation cephalosporins that are effective in low concentrations against most bacteria in vitro and in vivo, the main defence mechanism against the penicillins and cephalosporins was provided by β-lactamases which destroyed this class of antibiotics before they could reach the primary target. Now that this resistance problem in both gram-positive and gram-negative bacteria has been overcome to some extent, two other mechanisms of resistance to β-lactams have become apparent. One of these mechanisms is restricted to gram-negative bacteria: it results in a decrease in the permeability of the outer membrane through changes in or loss of one or more of the porin proteins[1,2] and is discussed further elsewhere in this issue (pp. 11–17). The second mechanism involves mutation of the primary targets themselves, the penicillin-binding proteins (PBPs) and is detailed below.

Proteins which bind β-lactam antibiotics covalently are located predominantly, if not exclusively, in the cytoplasmic membrane of all bacteria which possess the peptidoglycan polymer in their cell walls.[3] These proteins are believed to catalyse reactions in the terminal stages of peptidoglycan biosynthesis, including the attachment of growing glycan chains (nascent peptidoglycan) to the existing cell wall by transpeptidation, the removal of D-alanine from pentapeptide chains in the glycan (D,D-carboxypeptidase activity) and the splitting of existing peptide cross-bridges during remodelling (endopeptidase activity). Some of the membrane-bound PBPs have been solubilized, purified, partially characterized and shown to possess the enzymic activities referred to above.[4,5] In the few instances in which the interaction of the substrate or inhibitor with the active site has been investigated, the residue to which the antibiotic (or substrate) binds covalently, in ester linkage, has been identified as the amino acid serine. Mutations to β-lactam resistance are therefore unlikely to occur at this position but other amino acids in the enzymes are important in the initial, non-covalent, binding of substrate and/or inhibitor or in stabilizing the inhibitor-enzyme covalent complex, as indicated by kinetic studies[6] and, recently, by X-ray crystallography.[7] Consequently, changes in some of these amino acids could lead to resistance without abolishing enzyme activity.

The different PBPs (as many as 7–10 altogether, though not all are apparently essential) of gram-negative bacteria have different functions in peptidoglycan biosynthesis. PBPs 1a and 1b, the products of different genes, are involved in cell elongation; PBP 2 in the maintenance of cell shape and PBP 3 in septation.[2] Since β-lactam antibiotics vary in their affinities for the different PBPs, resistant mutants are likely to be found particularly to a β-lactam with a high affinity for one of the PBPs and low affinities for the remainder. Mecillinam is such a β-lactam; it binds almost exclusively to PBP 2 of gram-negative bacteria over a wide range of concentrations. Growth of sensitive, rod-shaped organisms in the presence of mecillinam leads to the production of almost spherical forms. Laboratory mutants of *E. coli* resistant to mecillinam have been obtained in which the affinity of PBP 2 for the antibiotic was greatly reduced.[9] Cross-resistance was demonstrated to all β-lactams which bind selectively to PBP 2. Similarly, mutations which affect the affinity of PBP 3 for β-lactam antibiotics which bind selectively to this protein (many cephalosporins) lead to low-level resistance. High-level-resistant mutants have not been obtained, since those cephalosporins which bind to PBP 3 at low concentrations also bind at slightly higher concentrations to other PBPs which are important in cell growth and it is unlikely that multiple mutations will arise sufficiently rapidly to prevent cell death.[10]

A further change in affinity of a single PBP obtained under laboratory conditions by stepwise selection of benzylpenicillin resistant mutants is provided by *Clostridium perfringens*. This organism contains 6 PBPs but the only PBP to show an alteration in affinity for benzylpenicillin in a sequence of ten increasingly resistant mutants that were isolated was PBP 1.[11] The concentration of benzylpenicillin required to half-saturate PBP 1 (measured in intact cells) increased from 0.85 to 7.6 μg ml^{-1}, while the sensitivity of the cells had decreased from 0.06 to 3.0 μg ml^{-1}.

There was no alteration in the actual amount of any of the PBPs. This is a very clear example of how a change in the affinity of a sensitive PBP which is a lethal target of β-lactams can result in the appearance of a resistant strain.

It is relatively easy to induce resistance to β-lactams in *Bacillus* species by growing organisms in increasing concentrations of a β-lactam that is not hydrolysed by gram-positive β-lactamases. A cloxacillin-resistant mutant of *Bacillus subtilis* was shown to have a PBP 2 with much lower affinity for cloxacillin,[12] whereas resistance in *B. megaterium* was achieved by an alteration in the relative amounts of PBPs 1 and 3, but with no obvious alteration in affinity of either PBP. In this particular instance, there was a reduced amount of PBP 1 (shown previously to be an important and indispensible target of β-lactams) and a vastly increased amount of PBP 3, suggesting that PBP 3 with its lower affinity for cloxacillin might be taking over the functions of PBP 1, thus enabling the bacteria to grow at a higher concentration of cloxacillin.[13] The ability of a particular PBP to take over the functions of another was first recognized in *E. coli*. It had been postulated that PBP 1b was the primary transpeptidase in cell elongation but mutants lacking detectable PBP 1b were able to survive. Such mutants were more sensitive than the wild type to cephalosporins that had a high affinity for PBP 1a (as well as for PBP 3) and it is therefore considered that PBP 1a can function in place of PBP 1b in 1b negative mutants. The double mutant, PBP 1a^{ts}, PBP 1b$^-$, grows only at the permissive temperature and lyses at the restrictive temperature.[14]

An analogous situation to that in *B. megaterium* exists in *Streptococcus faecium*: resistant strains isolated both in the laboratory and in the clinic apparently have no change in the actual affinities to benzylpenicillin of what had been considered to be the important PBPs. Further investigation revealed that PBP 5 bound penicillin with very slow kinetics in both sensitive and resistant strains and that resistant strains contained very much more of this protein than sensitive strains.[15] It was postulated that, in resistant strains, this protein could take over the functions of other essential PBPs which were completely saturated with β-lactam antibiotic at concentrations which still permitted growth. It appears that a substantial increase in the amount of a protein which is never saturated with antibiotic (on account of the kinetics of interaction of protein with antibiotic) is sufficient to account for resistance in this organism.

Alterations in the affinities of PBPs have also been detected in clinically resistant strains of *Neisseria gonorrhoeae, Streptococcus pneumoniae* and *Staphylococcus aureus*.

N. gonorrhoeae is an organism that, for many years, could be treated effectively with relatively low concentrations of benzylpenicillin. The reasons for successful treatment were threefold: good penetration, lack of β-lactamases and high affinity of the three membrane-bound PBPs for the β-lactam. In recent years, strains have been isolated which are increasingly resistant (the minimum inhibitory concentration (MIC) has changed from 0.007 μg ml^{-1} to 0.5–8 μg ml^{-1}). Such organisms can still be eliminated with β-lactams, but if further increases in resistance occur then other groups of effective antibiotics will have to be used. Examination of one of the most resistant isolates (designated CDC 77) revealed that PBPs 1 and 2 had reduced affinity for benzylpenicillin compared with a sensitive strain whereas the affinity of PBP 3 was unaltered.[16] DNA isolated from the resistant strain (MIC 2 μg ml^{-1}) was used to produce transformants of the sensitive strain FA 19 (MIC 0.007 μg ml^{-1}). The first stage transformants were approximately ten times more resistant than the parent FA 19 and this low level of resistance resulted from a

change in affinity of PBP 2. This transformed strain was further transformed with DNA from CDC 77, resulting in a further twofold increase in resistance (MIC 0.12 μg ml^{-1}). A third transformation, using the same DNA, produced a strain with an MIC of 0.5 μg ml^{-1}. The PBPs of these last two strains were identical in relation to the affinities for penicillin of their PBPs as those of the first transformant—i.e. the affinity of PBP 2 for benzylpenicillin had not been altered further while that of PBP 1 was identical to that of the sensitive strain.[16] Presumably the increase in MIC from 0.06 to 0.5 μg ml^{-1} had resulted from alteration in the outer membrane proteins with consequent decrease in the rate of penetration of the β-lactam. Although no further increases in resistance have yet been reported using the technique of transformation with DNA from CDC 77, it seems likely that any further change in resistance will result from an altered PBP 1. In sensitive strains, PBP 2 has a higher affinity than PBP 1 for benzylpenicillin so the obvious first step in the acquisition of resistance, assuming that PBPs 1 and 2 are killing targets, is to produce an altered PBP 2 with an affinity for penicillin equal to or lower than that of PBP 1. This might then be followed by further mutation resulting in an alteration in affinity of PBP 1. If mutations occur which alternately decrease the affinities of PBPs 1 and 2 without drastic effects on peptidoglycan synthesis then the MIC will increase in line with such alterations until the organism is so insensitive that it can no longer be treated in the clinical environment.[10]

Analysis of intrinsically resistant strains of *S. pneumoniae* has revealed the complexity of alterations in PBPs that may result in resistance. Since β-lactamases have never been reported in this gram-positive organism, and as the cell wall offers no permeability barrier to β-lactams, mutations resulting in resistance are likely to affect PBPs. Analysis of various resistant strains isolated from a hospital in Oklahoma indicated changes in the β-lactam affinity and the biochemical nature of the PBPs, particularly of groups 1 and 2.[17] These observations were confirmed in studies of the more resistant South African pneumococci in which multiple changes of the PBPs had obviously occurred when compared with a penicillin-sensitive laboratory strain.[18] Five types of changes in binding proteins were detected, ranging from a change in affinity of PBPs 1a and 2a to a complete loss of some PBPs and the appearance of others. This suggests that high-level resistance to β-lactams involves a number of sequential biochemical alterations and confirmation was obtained by transforming a sensitive laboratory strain with DNA isolated from one of the South African strains. A series of transformants was obtained with MICs ranging from 0.012 to 0.8 μg ml^{-1}: examination of the PBPs of these transformants again revealed the same type of alterations that were obvious in the clinical strains.[18] The shift was predictable: the low-level transformants had the typically sensitive pattern while the high-level transformants had the pattern of the resistant strain used as donor of the DNA. This gradual change to increasing resistance rather than a sudden jump, paralleled by small changes in PBPs, is similar to the predicted changes that may be encountered with *N. gonorrhoeae*, but is more complex.

Clinical isolates of *S. aureus* resistant to penicillins such as methicillin which are relatively resistant to staphylococcal β-lactamase have been studied in several laboratories. In many instances, the affinities of the PBPs of the resistant strains have been compared with those of an isogenic strain or a typical laboratory sensitive strain. Interestingly, a variety of different situations have been reported, ranging from an affinity change in a single PBP, or changes in the affinities of all the high-molecular-weight PBPs, to changes in the amount as well as affinity of the

PBP apparently determining resistance. One of the important PBPs for continued growth of *S. aureus* appears to be PBP 3. In one resistant mutant (MR-1) isolated in Yugoslavia, the affinity of PBP 3 for β-lactam antibiotics was reduced approximately 1000-fold with virtually no changes in the other PBPs.[19] The resistant organism itself has a MIC for β-lactam antibiotics approximately 1000-fold higher than sensitive strains so it follows that the organism can apparently survive in the presence of β-lactams with only PBP 3 functioning in peptidoglycan synthesis.

It is probable however that, in *S. aureus*, PBP 3 is not the only PBP of importance. Investigation of a cephradine-resistant mutant indicated that PBP 3 either was missing altogether or had a greatly reduced affinity for benzylpenicillin such that it was not labelled under the experimental conditions.[20] This change was accompanied by an increase in the amount of PBP 2, together with the appearance of a satellite band designated PBP 2′.

These changes are similar to those reported earlier in a strain originally isolated as being methicillin-resistant. This strain differs from MR-1 referred to above in that cell populations are heterogeneous with respect to the level of resistance expressed, although all cells retain the ability to express resistance. The degree of resistance is affected substantially by the environmental conditions: cells grown at 30°C in the presence of 5% NaCl are highly resistant whereas cells grown at 37°C in the absence of 5% NaCl are virtually as sensitive as an ordinary laboratory strain. Examination of the PBPs of the resistant strain and of the isogenic sensitive strain, grown under conditions favouring resistance, revealed that the affinity of PBP 3 for a range of penicillins and cephalosporins was greatly decreased in the former; i.e., it required a much higher concentration of the β-lactam before this PBP was half or fully saturated.[21] In addition to this change in affinity, a very substantial increase in amount of the protein was apparent (possibly as much as tenfold) so that the protein represented between 2 and 5% of the total membrane protein.[21] More careful investigation of the PBPs on gels giving higher resolution revealed further differences. Firstly, what originally appeared to be an altered PBP 3 was really a different protein with a molecular weight intermediate between that of PBP 2 and PBP 3. The vast increase in the amount of the protein obscured this difference in the original gels. Secondly, the original PBP 3 appeared to be absent when the cells were cultured under conditions favouring resistance but was present when cells were grown at 37°C in the absence of salt. The virtual absence of PBP 2′ at the higher temperature suggests it may be thermolabile. Thirdly, the covalent complex of PBP 2′ and benzylpenicillin was much more labile (half-life 2–3 min at 30°C) than those of PBP 2 or 3 of the sensitive strain (half-lives 30–40 min and 2 h respectively). Fourthly, the affinity of this new PBP is approximately 1000-fold lower than that of either PBP 2 or 3 in the sensitive strain—the protein is only just detectable on a fluorogram as a PBP at a concentration of benzylpenicillin of 10μg ml^{-1} and is not fully saturated until a concentration of 60–75μg ml^{-1} is used (D F J Brown and P E Reynolds, unpublished observations).

Any one of the three alterations, namely decrease in affinity, increase in amount or increased rate of breakdown of the protein-inhibitor complex could, in itself, lead to an increase in resistance. The fact that all three have occurred suggests gradual changes in the gene and in the control of its expression during the onset of resistance.

As yet it is unclear whether PBP 2′ is derived from PBP 2 or 3 or neither. Since PBP 3 is apparently not expressed under growth conditions favouring the expression of resistance, whereas PBP 2 is unchanged in amount or sensitivity, it might be considered to be an altered PBP 3, though its higher molecular weight militates against this theory. The fact that the sensitivity of a transpeptidation assay that is almost certainly catalysed by PBP 2 is altered in line with the different affinities of PBP 2 in the sensitive strain and PBP 2′ in the resistant strain provides support for PBP 2′ being an altered PBP 2. However, if this is so, it is unclear why the original PBP 2 remains unchanged in amount or sensitivity while PBP 3 is not expressed.[22] Partial proteolysis and peptide mapping is necessary to establish the relationship of PBP 2′ to PBPs 2 and 3 of the sensitive strain. It seems likely from these results and from other evidence that PBPs 2 and 3 of *S. aureus* can substitute for each other, at least when one of them is absent or non-functional.

These three sets of results in which changes in the MIC to β-lactam antibiotics are paralleled by changes in the affinities of PBPs are at variance with the results of studies with a methicillin-resistant strain isolated from a New York hospital. In this strain it was shown that the affinities for benzylpenicillin of PBPs 1, 2 and 3 were substantially reduced compared with a sensitive strain. When the pH value of the growth medium was reduced from 7.0 to 5.2 a large drop in phenotypic resistance resulted (3000-fold) while the affinities of the PBPs apparently remained unchanged.[23] There was a distinct lack of correlation at pH 5.2 of the sensitivity of the strain and the very low affinity of PBPs 1, 2 and 3 for benzylpenicillin. No satisfactory explanation of these findings has yet been provided.

When benzylpenicillin and other 'early' penicillins were first introduced in the treatment of clinical infections, the vast majority of strains of *Staphylococcus aureus* were very sensitive. With continued and extensive use of the antibiotic, resistant strains arose, most of which produced β-lactamase to destroy the antibiotic. With the introduction of methicillin and other semi-synthetic penicillins that were β-lactamase-resistant, most of the staphylococci isolated from hospital cases, although β-lactamase producers, were still sensitive to these newer compounds. Once the obstacle of β-lactamase has been largely overcome, it was almost inevitable that, sooner or later, strains would arise where resistance was determined by an altered affinity of PBPs important in the biosynthesis of peptidoglycan. This has now proved to be the case with *S. aureus*, *S. pneumoniae* and *N. gonorrhoeae* and presumably will be found to an increasing extent in strains isolated from hospital environments in which β-lactamase-resistant β-lactams are being used, as well as in laboratory strains trained to grow in increasing concentrations of β-lactam antibiotics. A summary of the alterations in PBPs resulting from mutation to resistance is given in Table I.

2 DNA Gyrase—A Target of Inhibitors of Replication

One of the enzymes involved in bacterial DNA replication is DNA gyrase: it introduces negative supercoils (the sense of supercoiling found intracellularly) into closed circular duplex DNA, a process involving the breakage and rejoining of both strands of DNA so that one intact double strand can pass completely through another broken double strand. This is immediately followed by repair of the broken double strand. The supercoiled product has a higher free energy than the starting DNA and ATP hydrolysis is required to drive the reaction.[24] The activities of this enzyme are sensitive to two groups of antibiotics, (a) coumermycin and novobiocin and (b) oxolinic acid and nalidixic acid.[25] When DNA gyrase was isolated from mutants of *Escherichia coli* resistant to either of the two groups of antibiotics it was also found to be drug-resistant. Furthermore, drug resistance

TABLE I. Summary of changes in penicillin-binding proteins resulting in resistance

Organism	Source	Basis of isolation	Alteration resulting in resistance	Reference
E. coli	Laboratory	Resistant to mecillinam	Lower affinity of PBP 2	9
C. perfringens	Laboratory	Resistant to benzylpenicillin	Lower affinity of PBP 1	11
B. subtilis	Laboratory	Resistant to cloxacillin	Lower affinity of PBP 2: loss of PBP 1	12
B. megaterium	Laboratory	Resistant to cloxacillin	Reduction in amount of PBP 1; Increase in amount of the less sensitive PBP 3	13
S. faecium	Laboratory and hospital	Resistant to benzylpenicillin	Increase in amount of the relatively insensitive PBP 5 which binds penicillin with slow kinetics	15
N. gonorrhoeae	Hospital	Resistant to benzylpenicillin	Lower affinity of PBPs 1 and 2	16
S. pneumoniae	Hospital	Resistant to benzylpenicillin	Complex changes: typical alterations involve lower affinity of PBP 1a and 2a, loss of some PBPs and appearance of new ones	17, 18
S. aureus	Hospital	Resistant to methicillin	Lower affinity of PBP 3	19
	Hospital	Resistant to cephradine	Loss of PBP 3; appearance of PBP 2′	20
	Hospital	Resistant to methicillin (degree of resistance dependent on growth conditions)	Increase in amount of PBP 2′ Low affinity of PBP 2′, PBP 2′-β-lactam complex very labile, PBP 3 not expressed	21, 22
	Hospital	Resistant to methicillin	Lower affintiy of PBP's 1, 2 and 3	23

of both the bacteria and of the enzyme was co-transduced by phage P1 suggesting that DNA gyrase is the actual target enzyme.

DNA gyrase from *E. coli*, *Micrococcus luteus* or *B. subtilis* contains two copies of each of two subunits A and B so the holoenzyme is a tetramer A_2B_2. Although neither subunit alone has any of the activities of DNA gyrase,[26] it can be presumed on the basis of antibiotic selectivity that the B subunit catalyses the hydrolysis of ATP (inhibited by coumermycin and novobiocin[27]) and that the A subunit of the holoenzyme catalyses the breakage/rejoining reaction (sensitive to oxolinic and nalidixic acids[28,29]). The inhibition by coumermycin is competitive with respect to ATP binding and, by using an ATP analogue, it has been demonstrated directly that novobiocin prevents the binding of o-ATP to the gyrase B protein.[30] Resistant mutants designated *cou* have been obtained, the mutation mapping at 48′ on the *E. coli* chromosome in the same position as the structural gene for the gyrase B protein. An additional activity of DNA gyrase is that it catalyses the relaxation of negatively supercoiled DNA when ATP is absent: this process is inhibited by oxolinic acid at a concentration comparable to that which blocks supercoiling, whereas novobiocin and coumermycin are without effect.[28,29] Since mutations giving resistance to nalidixic and oxolinic acids map at 82′ on the *E. coli* chromosome in the same position as the gene coding for the gyrase A protein, there is strong circumstantial evidence that the gyrase A subunit catalyses the breakage/rejoining step of the overall reaction. Neither the A nor B subunits of DNA gyrase from sensitive or resistant cells have been sequenced: consequently, the number of different positions at which amino acid substitutions can be tolerated and which result in resistance is unknown.

These results suggest that changes in the target, whether the A or B subunit of DNA gyrase, can lead to resistance to two different groups of antibiotics without drastically affecting the functioning of the protein.

3 RNA Polymerase—A Target of Inhibitors of Transcription

Bacterial RNA polymerases, unlike their mammalian counterparts, are inhibited at low concentrations by ansamycins, a class of antibiotics containing streptovaricins and rifamycins of which the compound rifampicin is the best known example. The RNA polymerase from *E. coli* contains four polypeptide chains (2α, β and β') in the core enzyme and, in addition, associates with another subunit, the σ factor which confers specificity for recognition of the correct promotor site for initiation of transcription on the DNA template. Rifampicin binds strongly and stoichiometrically to the

E. coli purified enzyme in a ratio of one molecule per enzyme monomer. This apparently happens in vivo as well as in vitro: the difference in amount of labelled rifampicin bound to sensitive and resistant strains reflects the estimated number of RNA polymerase molecules present per cell (as many as 1500 molecules).[31]

Investigation of rifampicin-resistant mutants has established that the antibiotic does not bind to the enzyme from resistant cells and, in one instance, the only obvious change was in the electrophoretic mobility of the β subunit.[32] Hybrid molecules of active enzyme can be reconstituted from the individual polymerase subunits obtained from resistant and sensitive strains: the resistance of the reconstituted enzymes to rifampicin is dependent only on the source of the β subunit.[33] This is the case whether the hybrid enzyme molecules are from *E. coli* or are mixtures of subunits obtained from *E. coli* and *Micrococcus luteus* in which the β subunit is smaller than the corresponding polypeptide in *E. coli*.[34] Although rifampicin binds to the purified RNA polymerase enzyme it does not bind to the β subunit alone[33] (or to any of the others): presumably the isolated subunits do not possess the correct conformation for binding to occur (evident also with streptomycin and the isolated S12 protein of *E. coli* ribosomes). The simplest complex which binds rifampicin contains two α subunits and one β,[35] and so corresponds to the core enzyme lacking the β' subunit: it lacks enzymic activity but presumably has the required conformation of the β subunit to permit binding of the antibiotic.

It has been suggested that at least four contact points are involved in the binding of rifampicin: consequently, insensitivity to the antibiotic could be achieved either by mutation at any of these points (a relatively infrequent occurrence) or by alterations in non-contact points which affect the conformation of the β subunit in such a way that binding of the antibiotic is reduced or abolished without affecting enzymic activity too drastically. In view of the frequency with which resistant mutants arise, it is apparent that the interaction of the antibiotic with the β subunit is extremely sensitive to conformational changes.

Rifampicin and streptovaricin both interfere with the RNA polymerase reaction by inhibiting the initiation process: if added after polymerization has been initiated, they have no effect.[36] This distinguishes their action from that of streptolydigin which inhibits the polymerization reaction directly.[37] As with rifampicin, resistance to streptolydigin is a property of the β subunit which has been demonstrated by the properties of hybrid RNA polymerase molecules constructed from subunits isolated from resistant and sensitive strains.[38] The difference in nature of the two resistance mutations was established by several criteria: (a) the two mutations mapped close together (as would be expected since resistance is a property of the β subunit in both instances: presumably the mutation occurs in the structural gene for the β subunit) but not in the identical position;[39] (b) the two markers could be separated by recombination,[40] and (c) the RNA polymerase from a rifampicin-resistant mutant was still sensitive to streptolydigin.[37] This is further evidence that the binding sites of the two antibiotics are different, a fact borne out by the very much weaker and easily reversible interaction of streptolydigin with the enzyme compared with that of rifampicin.[37]

4 The Ribosome—The Target of Inhibitors of Translation

Protein synthesis occurs on polyribosomes, individual ribosomes linked together by messenger RNA which directs the order in which the amino acids are inserted into the polypeptide chain by the ribosome. The ribosome is a complex structure consisting of two subunits, each containing RNA and protein. In prokaryotic cells, the smaller subunit (30S) contains 21 different proteins and 16S RNA, while the large subunit (50S) contains 32 proteins and two pieces of RNA (23S and 5S). The primary structures of all 53 proteins and three different RNAs from *E. coli* are now known,[41] and models for the secondary structure of the ribosomal RNAs have been published. Studies of the secondary and tertiary structure of ribosomal proteins are progressing but the results of such investigations may prove to be of limited value in terms of the identification of antibiotic-binding sites and of discovering the basis of resistance in mutants, since the conformation of individual proteins is likely to be modified, perhaps substantially, by their interaction with other proteins and/or with ribosomal RNA. Investigation of the conformation of proteins in the *intact* ribosomes of sensitive and resistant strains should reveal the differences in three-dimensional shape of ribosomal proteins which result in resistance. Although large numbers of antibiotics inhibit protein synthesis, alterations in the target proteins or RNA of resistant strains that have been reported are relatively few. Furthermore, although amino acid changes in certain ribosomal proteins render the ribosome resistant to a particular antibiotic, there is a conspicuous lack of evidence that the antibiotic actually binds to the unchanged protein in the wild type organism: binding may simply be determined by the presence of the wild type protein. Changes in or loss of ribosomal proteins that result in resistance have been demonstrated for streptomycin, other aminoglycosides such as gentamicin and neomycin, the amino-cyclitol spectinomycin, erythromycin and thiostrepton (Table II). Alterations in RNA, particularly in the degree of methylation, have been shown to determine resistance to kasugamycin, erythromycin and to thiostrepton in the producing organism (Table II). Furthermore, resistance to viomycin is dependent on changes either in the 16S or 23S RNA, the nature of the changes being unknown at present.

a *Ribosomal Proteins*

The mutation to resistance involving a ribosomal protein to be studied earliest was the *strA* mutation which resulted in streptomycin resistance. The sensitivity to streptomycin of hybrid ribosomes using ribosomal subunits from streptomycin resistant and sensitive cells established that the 30S subunit was the determinant of resistance.[42] Subsequently, total reconstitution studies using purified ribosomal proteins and ribosomal RNAs established that protein S 12 (formerly designated P 10), the product of the *rpsL* gene, determined whether strains were streptomycin-sensitive, -resistant or even -dependent.[43] Genetic studies had shown that

the mutation to streptomycin resistance mapped at one of two positions in the *strA* gene; subsequently, biochemical analysis of tryptic peptides derived from the S 12 protein isolated from nine different mutants of *E. coli* indicated that the mutation, to high levels of resistance, involved changes at position 42 (replacement of lys with thr, arg or aspNH$_2$) or at position 87 (replacement of lys with arg).[44] Protein S 12 *determines* the response of 70S ribosomes to streptomycin but does not itself bind the antibiotic—other ribosomal proteins of the small subunit (e.g. S 3, S 5) appear to be involved in this process[45] but, at present, no reports have appeared of mutations in these proteins resulting in resistance to streptomycin.

It is possible to reconstitute partially-active 30S subunits lacking protein S 12 and these defective particles were only weakly active in forming natural initiation complexes: they retained, however, almost full activity in the synthesis of polyphenylalanine directed by poly U, and this process was not sensitive to streptomycin which normally induces misreading under conditions in which protein S 12 is present.

The data for the basis of spectinomycin resistance are as clear-cut as for streptomycin. One-step, high-level, resistant mutants (*spcA* mutants) have been obtained in which the defect has been traced to the 30S subunit[46] and it is interesting that these strains do not demonstrate cross-resistance with streptomycin. Hybrid 30S particles, reconstituted with mixtures of components from *spcA* and wild-type strains, established that spectinomycin resistance was determined by the S 5 protein.[47] The protein isolated from 10 different mutants possessed amino acid substitutions clustered at positions 19–21.[48] With both streptomycin and spectinomycin it is clear that single-step, minor changes in amino acid composition of a single protein can render the ribosome highly resistant to the antibiotic.

The experimental observations linking resistance to other aminoglycoside antibiotics with alterations in ribosomal proteins, in which it is suspected that a change in a particular protein is responsible for resistance, lack the definitive experiments using ribosomal subunits reconstituted from components purified from sensitive and resistant strains. Research has been hindered by a failure to isolate single-step mutants with high-level resistance to such antibiotics as neomycin and gentamicin. This failure may result, in turn, from differences in the mode of interaction of these aminoglycosides with ribosomes: whereas streptomycin binds in a 1:1 ratio and the *strA* mutants have a high level of resistance, aminoglycosides possessing a 2-deoxystreptamine residue have multiple interaction sites with the ribosome and mutants with a high level of resistance have not been detected.[49] The following examples, all taken from studies with *E. coli*, indicate the lack of biochemical precision that has been achieved to date.

Resistance to kanamycin has been shown to map at three locations, one of which (*kanA* mutants) may be in the *rpsL* gene coding for protein S 12[50] (i.e. as for streptomycin resistance). Three independently-isolated, gentamicin-resistant strains apparently did not possess a normal L 6 protein. Genetic analysis involving transduction and reversion experiments revealed a clear correlation between gentamicin resistance and an altered L 6 protein.[51] On the other hand, biochemical analysis of the ribosomes with the altered L 6 protein has not elucidated the mechanism by which the ribosomes were resistant, since the mutant ribosomes were still inhibited by gentamicin although misreading was reduced. It is this last phenomenon that appears to be correlated with the altered L 6 protein.[52] The situation with neomycin-resistant mutants is more involved: it has been reported that alterations have been detected in proteins S 17[53] or in S 5 and S

TABLE II. Summary of alterations in ribosomal proteins and RNAs of resistant strains

Antibiotic	Determinant of resistance	Nature of change in mutant	Reference
Streptomycin	Protein S 12 of 30S subunit	Amino acid changes at two possible sites lys-42 and lys-87	43, 44
Spectinomycin	Protein S 5 of 30S subunit	Amino acid changes at positions 19–21	47, 48
Neomycin	Protein S 17 of 30S subunit	Not determined	53
	Proteins S 5 or S 12 of 30S subunit	S 5: replacement of arg by gly or ser S 12: replacement of pro by leu or gluNH$_2$	54
Gentamycin	Protein L 6 of 50S subunit	Not determined: reduction of mis-reading in mutant	51, 52
Erythromycin	Protein L 4	Not determined	55
Thiostrepton	Protein BM-L 11 (*B. megaterium*)	Protein not present in resistant ribosomes	58
	Protein BS-L 11 (*B. subtilis*)		59
Kasugamycin	16S RNA of 30S subunit	Two adjacent adenine residues near 3′ end not methylated	65, 66
Thiostrepton	23S RNA of 50S subunit in the producing organism	Methylation of adenosine-1067 in *E. coli* 23S RNA by enzyme from producing organism	61
Erythromycin	23S RNA of 50S subunit	Dimethylation of two adenine residues	67, 68
Viomycin	16S RNA or 23S RNA	Not determined	64

12.[54] The position and nature of the amino acid substitutions in the latter have been determined but definitive evidence linking these alterations with the determination of resistance is lacking.

The other inhibitor of protein synthesis for which changes in a ribosomal protein possibly resulting in resistance have been reported is the translocation inhibitor erythromycin. Erythromycin-resistant strains of *E. coli* have been shown to contain alterations in protein L 4 or L 22.[55] The evidence linking an altered protein L 22 with resistance is not strong since one recombinant strain still altered in L 22 was sensitive to erythromycin. Genetic analysis of the other mutant indicated that alteration of protein L 4 co-transduced with resistance and that it was probably the cause of resistance in *eryA* mutants;[55] this gene maps between *strA* and *spcA* on the *E. coli* chromosome and may be identical with the structural gene for protein L 4. Total reconstitution studies with 50S ribosomal subunits could be used to establish whether L 4 determines resistance.

The majority of erythromycin-resistant strains are resistant to the antibiotic by virtue of alterations in the 23S RNA (see section 4b and particularly pp. 47–53).

The mechanism of resistance to thiostrepton has been studied in gram-positive bacteria since *E. coli* is insensitive to the antibiotic, though ribosomes used to investigate the action of the drug in vitro are sensitive. Thiostrepton binds weakly to 23S RNA, but has high affinity for the complex of 23S rRNA and protein L 11;[56] binding is maintained following digestion of the complex with T$_1$ ribonuclease in which approximately 50 residues in the 23S RNA are protected by the presence of protein L 11.[57]

Resistance to the antibiotic results from loss of a single ribosomal protein (BM-L 11 from *B. megaterium*[58] or BS-L 11 from *B. subtilis*[59]). These proteins are serologically homologous with protein L 11 of *E. coli* and the ribosomes from resistant strains which are totally devoid of this protein have an impaired ability to hydrolyse GTP in the presence of elongation factor EF-G.[60] This activity is restored by adding either protein BM-L 11 or L 11 to the defective ribosomes. Furthermore, in *B. subtilis*, revertants to thiostrepton sensitivity have been obtained which possess the BS-L 11 protein missing from the resistant mutants. It is interesting that the 50 base fragment protected against nuclease digestion by protein L 11 contains the adenosine residue that is methylated in the thiostrepton producing organism[61] which renders the ribosomes totally resistant to thiostrepton. However, since ribosomes of *B. megaterium* lacking protein BM-L 11 still bind thiostrepton weakly with similar affinity to isolated 23S RNA, it appears likely that the loss of protein BM-L 11 (and presumably also BS-L 11) results from alterations in the protein rather than in the 23S rRNA.

The antibiotic fusidic acid sequesters factor EF-G and GDP on the ribosome following a single round of GTP hydrolysis: it thus stabilizes what is normally an unstable ternary complex and leads to inhibition of protein synthesis. The drug does not interact primarily with ribosomes and no mutants with fusidic-acid-resistant ribosomes have been reported. Strains resistant to fusidic acid have been described and these contain an altered form of factor EF-G;[62] the factor from the resistant mutant was not sequestered by fusidic acid on ribosomes as evidenced by a lack of inhibition by the antibiotic of uncoupled hydrolysis of GTP catalysed by the factor from resistant mutants.

b *Ribosomal RNA*

Alterations in ribosomal RNA have been shown to be responsible for resistance to kasugamycin, thiostrepton (in the producing organism), erythromycin and viomycin. In the first three instances, the biochemical basis of resistance has been well characterized, but with viomycin, it has proved difficult to elucidate as the drug almost certainly has two binding sites on the ribosome, one to each subunit. Viomycin-resistant strains of *Mycobacteria*, the wild-type strains of which are extremely sensitive to viomycin, possess mutations which affect either the 50S *or* the 30S ribosomal subunit.[63] Total reconstitution studies of both ribosomal subunits using rRNA and proteins from resistant and sensitive strains indicated that the defect lies in some unspecified property of the respective rRNAs: i.e., the strain with resistant 50S subunits has altered 23S RNA whereas the strain with resistant 30S subunits has altered 16S rRNA.[64]

Kasugamycin is an atypical aminoglycoside antibiotic which specifically inhibits polypeptide chain initiation in bacterial systems: strains resistant to it are not cross-resistant to other aminoglycosides. Several different mutations to resistance have been recognized but the *ksgA* mutation results in an altered target in that the 30S subunits of these mutants possess altered 16S RNA.[65] This was demonstrated by total reconstitution studies, and further analysis of the 16S RNA from resistant and sensitive strains showed that the dimethylation of two residues of adenine close to the 3′ terminal end of 16S RNA in wild-type strains did not occur in strains containing the mutation. Extracts of wild-type strains contain a methylase enzyme which catalyses the introduction of four methyl groups into core particles of *ksgA* strains. If these methylated core particles are used in reconstitution studies, the resultant ribosomes prove to be sensitive to kasugamycin.[66] The two adjacent adenine residues are close to the 'Shine and Delgano' sequence of bases believed to be involved in mRNA recognition and it is probably this 3′ end of 16S RNA which base-pairs with 23S RNA when the ribosomal subunits associate.

The basis of resistance in the thiostrepton-producing organism *Streptomyces azureus* is discussed in detail elsewhere in this Bulletin (pp. 61–67): ribosomes are rendered insensitive to thiostrepton by the methylation of a specific adenosine residue. The enzyme involved methylates the pentose moiety of adenosine-1607 in 23S RNA of *E. coli*[61] which is in the 50 base nucleotide fragment protected by protein L 11 against digestion with T_1 ribonuclease.

Resistance to erythromycin (and to other macrolides, to lincomycin and to streptogramin B) can be induced in certain strains of *Staphylococcus aureus* and streptococci. The alteration occurs in the structure of 23S RNA and involves the dimethylation of two molecules of adenine.[67] Dimethyladenine has also been detected in the 23S RNA of the producing organism,[68] whose ribosomes are resistant to erythromycin. (For a full account, see pp. 47–53.)

It is apparent from these examples that resistance to specific antibiotics results either from under- or over-methylation of specific residues in the 16S or 23S rRNA. Binding of antibiotics to targets is dependent on a precise, three-dimensional shape and on certain specific residues in the ribosomal proteins or RNA. If these conditions are not satisfied, the ribosome may still be functional without being sensitive to the particular antibiotic.

5 Summary

Throughout this paper, the examples cited indicate that precise geometrical arrangements are more vital in the interaction of an antibiotic with its target protein than in the interaction of a substrate with its enzyme. If it were not so, organisms resistant to an antibiotic by virtue of a change in the target would not be isolated. Thus, correct conformation of the β subunit is absolutely vital for the interaction of rifampicin with RNA polymerase. Detailed biochemical investigations of the nature of the changes in the resistant organisms should ultimately enable all contact points involved in binding of an antibiotic to its target to be elucidated. When such information is available and stored in computers, it might prove possible to design more powerful inhibitors which fit more tightly into the sites normally occupied by the natural substrate. Would it perhaps be going too far to speculate that the first successful drug designed in this way might be in medical use by the end of the millenium?

REFERENCES

1 Harder KJ, Nikaido H, Matsuhashi M. Mutants of *Escherichia coli* that are resistant to certain beta-lactam compounds lack the *omp F* porin. Antimicrob Agents Chemother 1981; 20: 549–552

2 Zimmermann W. Penetration of β-lactam antibiotics into their target enzymes in *Pseudomonas aeruginosa*: comparison of a highly sensitive mutant with its parent strain. Antimicrob Agents Chemother 1980; 18: 94–100

3 Blumberg PM, Strominger JL. Interaction of penicillin with the bacterial cell: penicillin-binding proteins and penicillin-sensitive enzymes. Bacteriol Rev 1974; 38: 291–335

4 Gale EF, Cundliffe E, Reynolds PE, Richmond MH, Waring MJ. Inhibitors of bacterial and fungal cell wall synthesis. In: Gale EF *et al*. The molecular basis of antibiotic action. 2nd edn. London: Wiley, 1981; 49–174

5 Matsuhashi M, Nakagawa J, Tomioka S, Ishino F, Tamaki S. Mechanism of peptidoglycan synthesis by penicillin-binding proteins in bacteria and effects of antibiotics. In: Mitsuhashi S, ed. Drug resistance in bacteria. Genetics, biochemistry and molecular biology. Tokyo: Japan Scientific Societies Press, 1982: 297–310

6 Ghuysen J-M, Frère J-M, Leyh-Bouille M, Perkins HR, Nieto M. The active centres in penicillin-sensitive enzymes. Philos Trans R Soc Lond [Biol] 1980; B 289: 285–301

7a Dideberg O, Charlier P, Dive G, Joris B, Frère JM, Ghuysen JM. Structure of a Zn^{2+}-containing D-alanyl-D-alanine-cleaving carboxy-peptidase at 2.5 Å resolution. Nature 1982; 299: 469–470

7b Kelly JA, Moews PC, Knox JR, Frère J-M, Ghuysen J-M. Penicillin target enzyme and the antibiotic binding site. Science 1982; 218: 479–481

8 Spratt BG. Distinct penicillin binding proteins involved in the division, elongation and shape of *Escherichia coli* K12. Proc Natl Acad Sci USA 1975; 72: 2999–3003

9 Spratt BG. *Escherichia coli* resistance to β-lactam antibiotics through a decrease in the affinity of a target for lethality. Nature 1978; 274: 713–715

10 Spratt BG. Penicillin-binding proteins and the future of β-lactam antibiotics. J Gen Microbiol 1983; 129: 1247–1260

11 Williamson R. Benzylpenicillin-resistant mutants of *Clostridium perfringens*. In: Hakenbeck R, Holtje J-V, Labischinski H, eds. The target of penicillin. Berlin: W de Gruyter, 1983; 487–492

12 Buchanan CE, Strominger JL. Altered penicillin-binding components in penicillin-resistant mutants of *Bacillus subtilis*. Proc Natl Acad Sci USA 1976; 73: 1816–1820

13 Giles AF, Reynolds PE. *Bacillus megaterium* resistance to cloxacillin accompanied by a compensatory change in penicillin binding proteins. Nature 1979; 280: 167–168

14 Suzuki H, Nishimura Y, Hirota Y. On the process of cellular division in *Escherichia coli*: a series of mutants of *E. coli* altered in the penicillin-binding proteins. Proc Natl Acad Sci USA 1978; 75: 664–668

15 Fontana R, Canepari P, Satta G. The role of a protein that binds penicillin with slow kinetics in physiology and response to penicillin of *Streptococcus faecium* ATCC 9790. In: Hakenbeck R, Holtje J-V, Labischinski H, eds. The target of penicillin. Berlin: W de Gruyter, 1983, 531–536

16 Dougherty TJ, Koller AE, Tomasz A. Penicillin-binding proteins of penicillin-susceptible and intrinsically resistant *Neisseria gonorrhoeae*. Antimicrob Agents Chemother 1980; 18: 730–737

17 Hakenbeck R, Tarpay M, Tomasz A. Multiple changes of penicillin-binding proteins in penicillin-resistant clinical isolates of *Streptococcus pneumoniae*. Antimicrob Agents Chemother 1980; 17: 364–371

18 Zighelboim S, Tomasz A. Penicillin-binding proteins of multiply antibiotic-resistant South African strains of *Streptococcus pneumoniae*. Antimicrob Agents Chemother 1980; 17: 434–442

19 Hayes MV, Curtis NAC, Wyke AW, Ward JB. Decreased affinity of a penicillin-binding protein for β-lactam antibiotics in a clinical isolate of *Staphylococcus aureus* resistant to methicillin. FEMS Microbiol Lett 1981; 10: 119–122

20 Georgopapadakou NH, Smith SA, Bonner DP. Penicillin-binding proteins in a *Staphylococcus aureus* strain resistant to specific β-lactam antibiotics. Antimicrob Agents Chemother 1982; 22: 172–175

21 Brown DFJ, Reynolds PE. Intrinsic resistance to β-lactam antibiotics in *Staphylococcus aureus*. FEBS Lett 1980; 122: 275–278

22 Brown DFJ, Reynolds PE. Transpeptidation in *Staphylococcus aureus* with intrinsic resistance to beta-lactam antibiotics. In: Hakenbeck R, Holtje J-V, Labischinski H, eds. The target of penicillin. Berlin: W de Gruyter, 1983; 537–542

23 Hartman B, Tomasz A. Altered penicillin-binding proteins in methicillin-resistant strains of *Staphylococcus aureus*. Antimicrob Agents Chemother 1981; 19: 726–735

24 Gellert M. DNA topoisomerases. Annu Rev Biochem 1981; 50: 879–910

25 Cozzarelli NR. The mechanism of action of inhibitors of DNA synthesis. Annu Rev Biochem 1977; 46: 641–668

26 Higgins NP, Peebles CL, Sugino A, Cozzarelli NR. Purification of subunits of *Escherichia coli* DNA gyrase and reconstitution of enzymatic activity. Proc Natl Acad Sci USA 1978; 75: 1773–1777

27 Gellert M, O'Dea MH, Itoh T, Tomizawa J-I. Novobiocin and coumermycin inhibit DNA supercoiling catalyzed by DNA gyrase. Proc Natl Acad Sci USA 1976; 73: 4474–4478

28 Sugino A, Peebles CL, Kreuzer KN, Cozzarelli NR. Mechanism of action of nalidixic acid: purification of *Escherichia coli nalA* gene product and its relationship to DNA gyrase and a novel nicking-closing enzyme. Proc Natl Acad Sci USA 1977; 74: 4767–4771

29 Gellert M, Mizuuchi K, O'Dea MH, Itoh T, Tomizawa J. Nalidixic acid resistance: a second genetic character involved in DNA gyrase activity. Proc Natl Acad Sci USA 1977; 74: 4772–4776

30 Mizuuchi K, O'Dea MH, Gellert M. DNA gyrase: subunit structure

and ATPase activity of the purified enzyme. Proc Natl Acad Sci USA 1978; 75: 5960–5963

31 White RJ, Lancini G. Uptake and binding of [³H]rifampicin by *Escherichia coli* and *Staphylococcus aureus*. Biochim Biophys Acta 1971; 240: 429–434

32 Rabussay D, Zillig, W. A rifampicin resistant RNA-polymerase from *E. coli* altered in the β-subunit. FEBS Lett 1969; 5: 104–106

33 Lill UI, Hartmann GR. On the binding of rifampicin to the DNA-directed RNA polymerase from *Escherichia coli*. Eur J Biochem 1973; 38: 336–345

34 Lill UI, Behrendt EM, Hartmann GR. Hybridization *in vitro* of subunits of the DNA-dependent RNA polymerase from *Escherichia coli* and *Micrococcus luteus*. Eur J Biochem 1975; 52: 411–420

35 Stetter KO, Zillig W. Transcription in Lactobacillaceae: DNA-dependent RNA polymerase from *Lactobacillus curvatus*. Eur J Biochem 1974; 48: 527–540

36 Sippel A, Hartmann GR. Mode of action of rifamycin on the RNA polymerase reaction. Biochim Biophys Acta 1968; 157: 218–219

37 Cassani G, Burgess RR, Goodman HM, Gold L. Inhibition of RNA polymerase by streptolydigin. Nature (New Biol) 1971; 230: 197–200

38 Heil A, Zillig W. Reconstitution of bacterial DNA-dependent RNA-polymerase from isolated subunits as a tool for the elucidation of the role of the subunits in transcription. FEBS Lett 1970; 11: 165–168

39 Schleif R. Isolation and characterization of a streptolydigin-resistant RNA polymerase. Nature 1969; 223: 1068–1069

40 Sokolova EV, Ovadis MI, Gorlenko Zh M, Khesin RB. Localizaiton of streptolydigin-resistant mutation in *E. coli* chromosome and effect of streptolydigin on T2 phage development in *stl-r* and *stl-s* strains of *E. coli*. Biochim Biophys Res Commun 1970; 41: 870–876

41 Wittmann HG. Components of bacterial ribosomes. Annu Rev Biochem 1982; 51: 155–183

42 Davies JE. Studies on the ribosomes of streptomycin-sensitive and resistant strains of *Escherichia coli*. Proc Natl Acad Sci USA 1964; 51: 659–664

43 Ozaki M, Mizushima S, Nomura M. Identification and functional characterization of the protein controlled by the streptomycin-resistant locus in *E. coli*. Nature 1969; 222: 333–339

44 Funatsu G, Wittmann HG. Ribosomal proteins: XXXIII Location of amino-acid replacements in protein S12 isolated from *Escherichia coli* mutants resistant to streptomycin. J Mol Biol 1972; 68: 547–550

45 Schreiner G, Nierhaus KH. Protein involved in the binding of dihydrostreptomycin to ribosomes of *Escherichia coli*. J Mol Biol 1973; 81: 71–82

46 Anderson P, Davies J, Davis BD. Effect of spectinomycin on polypeptide synthesis in extracts of *Escherichia coli*. J Mol Biol 1967; 29: 203–215

47 Bollen A, Davies J, Ozaki M, Mizushima S. Ribosomal protein conferring sensitivity to the antibiotic spectinomycin in *Escherichia coli*. Science 1969; 165: 85–86

48 Wittmann-Liebold B, Greuer B. The primary structure of protein S5 from the small subunit of the *Escherichia coli* ribosome. FEBS Lett 1978; 95: 91–98

49 Ahmad MH, Rechenmacher A, Böck A. Interaction between aminoglycoside uptake and ribosomal resistance mutations. Antimicrob Agents Chemother 1980; 18: 798–806

50 Thorbjarnardottir SH, Magnusdòttir RA, Eggertsson G, Kagan SA, Andrésson OS. Mutations determining generalized resistance to aminoglycoside antibiotics in *Escherichia coli*. Mol Gen Genet 1978; 161: 89–98

51 Buckel P, Buchberger A, Böck A, Wittmann HG. Alteration of ribosomal protein L6 in mutants of *Escherichia coli* resistant to gentamicin. Mol Gen Genet 1977; 158: 47–54

52 Kühberger R, Piepersberg W, Petzet A, Buckel A, Böck A. Alteration of ribosomal protein L6 in gentamicin-resistant strains of *Escherichia coli*. Effects on fidelity of protein synthesis. Biochemistry 1979; 18: 187–193

53 Cannon M, Cabezón T, Bollen A. Mapping of neamine resistance: identification of two genetic loci, *nea* A and *nea* B. Mol Gen Genet 1974; 130: 321–326

54 De Wilde M, Cabezón T, Villarroel R, Herzog A, Bollen A. Cooperative control of translational fidelity by ribosomal proteins in *Escherichia coli*. Mol Gen Genet 1975; 142: 19–33

55 Wittmann HG, Stöffler G, Appiron D *et al*. Biochemical and genetic studies on two different types of erythromycin resistant mutants of *Escherichia coli* with altered ribosomal proteins. Mol Gen Genet 1973; 127: 175–189

56 Thompson J, Cundliffe E, Stark M. Binding of thiostrepton to a complex of 23-S rRNA with ribosomal protein L 11. Eur J Biochem 1979; 98: 261–265

57 Schmidt FJ, Thompson J, Lee K, Dijk J, Cundliffe E. The binding site for ribosomal protein L 11 within 23 S ribosomal RNA of *Escherichia coli*. J Biol Chem 1981; 256: 12301–12305

58 Cundliffe E, Dixon P, Srerk M *et al*. Ribosomes in thiostrepton-resistant mutants of *Bacillus megaterium* lacking a single 50S subunit protein. J Mol Biol 1979; 132: 235–252

59 Wienen B, Ehrlich R, Stöffler-Meilicke M, *et al*. Ribosomal protein alterations in thiostrepton- and micrococcin-resistant mutants of *Bacillus subtilis*. J Biol Chem 1979; 254: 8031–8041

60 Stark MJR, Cundliffe E, Dijk J, Stöffler G. Functional homology between *E. coli* ribosomal protein L11 and *B. megaterium* protein BM-L11. Mol Gen Genet 1980; 180: 11–15

61 Thompson J, Schmidt F, Cundliffe E. Site of action of a ribosomal RNA methylase conferring resistance to thiostrepton. J Biol Chem 1982; 257: 7915–7917

62 Kinoshita T, Kawano G, Tanaka N. Association of fusidic acid sensitivity with G factor in a protein-synthesizing system. Biochem Biophys Res Commun 1968; 33: 769–773

63 Yamada T, Masuda K, Shoji K, Hori M. Analysis of ribosomes from viomycin-sensitive and -resistant strains of *Mycobacterium smegmatis*. J Bacteriol 1972; 112: 1–6

64 Yamada T, Mizugichi Y, Nierhaus KH, Wittmann HG. Resistance to viomycin conferred by RNA of either ribosomal subunit. Nature 1978; 275: 460–461

65 Helser TL, Davies JE, Dahlberg JE. Change in methylation of 16S ribosomal RNA associated with mutation to kasugamycin resistance in *Escherichia coli*. Nature (New Biol) 1971; 233: 12–14

66 Helser TL, Davies JE, Dahlberg JE. Mechanism of kasugamycin resistance in *Escherichia coli*. Nature (New Biol) 1972; 235: 6–9

67 Lai CJ, Weisblum B. Altered methylation of ribosomal RNA in an erythromycin-resistant strain of *Staphylococcus aureus*. Proc Natl Acad Sci USA 1971; 68: 856–860

68 Graham MY, Weisblum B. 23S Ribosomal ribonucleic acid of macrolide-producing Streptomycetes contains methylated adenine. J Bacteriol 1979; 137: 1464–1467

British Medical Bulletin (1984) Vol. 40, No. 1, pp. 11-17

ANTIBIOTIC RESISTANCE RESULTING FROM DECREASED DRUG ACCUMULATION

IAN CHOPRA MA PhD

Department of Microbiology
University of Bristol

1   Intrinsic resistance
  a Gram-negative outer membranes
  b Capsules
2   Acquired resistance
  a Plasmid-mediated tetracycline resistance
  b Chromosomal mutations
3   Conclusion
  References

Studies on the nature of antibiotic resistance in bacteria reveal that several biochemical mechanisms may be responsible for resistance. These include:

  (a) alterations of the target site in the cell that eliminate or decrease the binding of drug;
  (b) antibiotic inactivation;
  (c) decreased drug accumulation.

Other contributions to this Bulletin have considered resistance mechanisms in categories a and b and the purpose of this paper is to discuss resistance resulting from category c, i.e., decreased drug accumulation.

Two broad categories of resistance must be considered: intrinsic resistance (or intrinsic insusceptibility) and acquired resistance. The term 'intrinsic' is used to imply that inherent features of the cell are responsible for preventing antibiotic access to the cell interior, and to distinguish this situation from acquired resistance which occurs when resistant strains emerge from previously sensitive bacterial populations usually after exposure to antibiotics. Acquired resistance involving decreased antibiotic accumulation can itself arise either by acquisition of plasmids or by chromosomal mutations.[1] This paper is divided into two main sections to permit separate discussion of intrinsic and acquired resistance. Within the last decade a number of reviews relevant to this paper have been published.[1-15] These papers will provide an extensive guide to the earlier literature on the topic of decreased antibiotic accumulation in bacteria.

1   Intrinsic Resistance

a *Gram-Negative Outer Membranes*

Many antibiotics that are highly toxic for gram-positive bacteria are lethal to gram-negative bacteria only at high concentrations.[2,7] This is widely attributed to exclusion of antibiotics from their sites of action by the outer layers of the gram-negative cell envelope. Nevertheless, detailed studies of the phenomenon have been restricted almost exclusively to *Escherichia coli*, *Salmonella typhimurium*, *Proteus* species and *Pseudomonas aeruginosa*.[2-5,13,15-17] Even within this group of organisms there is considerable variation in the levels of resistance to particular compounds that are again

attributable to differences in antibiotic accumulation. For example the organisms listed above are all resistant to hydrophobic antibiotics such as fusidic acid and rifamycins,[18] but vary in their resistance to hydrophilic drugs with *Ps. aeruginosa* notably resistant to many of these compounds as well.[18,19] The nature of these exclusion mechanisms is beginning to be understood and the following discussion is divided into two sections to consider (i) the almost universal resistance of gram-negative rods to hydrophobic antibiotics, and (ii) the basis by which *Ps. aeruginosa* in particular also displays resistance to a considerable number of hydrophilic antibiotics.

i *Exclusion of Hydrophobic Antibiotics*

The intrinsic resistance of the majority of gram-negative rods to hydrophobic antibiotics is attributable to low drug diffusion rates across the outer membrane.[15,16] Nikaido & Nakae[15] have proposed an attractive model to explain this phenomenon based upon the apparent organization of macromolecules in the outer membrane. Exclusion is attributed to the absence of phospholipid from the outer leaflet of the outer membrane so that membrane regions into which hydrophobic antibiotics could dissolve are not exposed to the environment. Several lines of evidence support this model,[15] but the hypothesis rests partially upon analysis of outer membrane composition in bacteria with complete lipopolysaccharide (LPS) core regions and deep rough LPS mutants. However, there are considerable discrepancies in values for the gross composition of outer membranes from such strains that render equivocal the hypothesis that phospholipid is normally absent from the outer regions of the cell.[20] It seems therefore that certain aspects of the model developed by Nikaido and Nakae may require re-evaluation.

ii *Exclusion of hydrophilic antibiotics by the Pseudomonas aeruginosa outer membrane*

Although the *Ps. aeruginosa* outer membrane has long been suspected of exhibiting low permeability to hydrophilic molecules, direct evidence for this was lacking until a recent report appeared.[17] Many gram-negative bacteria contain outer-membrane proteins, termed porins, which form transmembrane water-filled pores and allow diffusion of hydrophilic molecules below a certain size.[13,15] For *E. coli*, the channel diameter is sufficient to allow the passage of molecules up to about 600 daltons.[13,15] Although porins are also present in *Ps. aeruginosa*,[17] the permeability of the *Pseudomonas* outer membrane to hydrophilic antibiotics and other solutes is markedly reduced compared with *E. coli* (Table I). One explanation for the difference between the two organisms could be the presence in *Ps. aeruginosa* of porins with a smaller channel diameter than in *E. coli*. In fact the opposite is true because porins from *Ps. aeruginosa* form wider channels than those

TABLE I. Comparison of outer membrane permeability to hydrophilic solutes and antibiotics in *Escherichia coli* and *Pseudomonas aeruginosa*

Data from reference 17

Compound	Permeability coefficient (nm/s)*	
	E. coli	*Ps. aeruginosa*
Glucose-6-phosphate	202	0.3 – 1.20
p-Nitrophenyl-phosphate	243	1.57– 3.68
Cephaloridine	500	9.7 –11.7
Cephacetrile	800	5.3 – 9.7

* See references 15 and 17 for definition of this coefficient.

from *E. coli*.[21,22] The intrinsic impermeability of the *Ps. aeruginosa* outer membrane to low-molecular-weight hydrophilic antibiotics has therefore been attributed to special properties of porins in this organism.[17] The features which distinguish the *Ps. aeruginosa* and *E. coli* porins have yet to be determined, but research in this area promises important and exciting developments in the near future.

b *Capsules*

Capsules surround many clinically important micro-organisms that include *Klebsiella* species, *E. coli*, *Streptococcus pneumoniae*, *Neisseria meningitidis* and *Haemophilus influenzae*. Several workers have speculated that capsules comprise an intrinsic barrier to antibiotic penetration,[23] but recent evaluation of the problem suggests that capsules do not contribute to intrinsic antibiotic resistance. This conclusion is based upon a mathematical model which allows estimation of the penetration times of antibiotics through static capsular layers.[23]

2 Acquired Resistance

a *Plasmid-Mediated Tetracycline Resistance*

Early investigations into the molecular basis of plasmid-determined antibiotic resistance led to the conclusion that resistance to a large variety of different compounds resulted primarily from decreased drug accumulation. For instance, in 1963, Watanabe[24] stated that 'multiple drug resistance must be ascribed to reduced permeability of cells to the drugs'. Subsequent studies have proved this statement to be incorrect and resistance to the tetracyclines, fusidic acid[25] and chloramphenicol[26,27] provide the only examples of specific plasmid-determined resistance mechanisms resulting from decreased drug accumulation. The nature of plasmid-mediated reduced fusidic acid and chloramphenicol accumulation is not understood and will not be considered further in this paper. The remainder of this section is therefore devoted to consideration of tetracycline resistance which provides the only well-documented example of a plasmid-determined resistance mechanism resulting from decreased drug accumulation.

i *Resistance Determinants*

Although plasmids which confer resistance to tetracyclines have been found in virtually all bacterial species (Table II), detailed molecular studies on the nature of resistance have been confined to determinants from the Enterobacteriaceae and bacilli (Table III).

DNA–DNA hybridization studies permitted Mendez *et al*.[28] to classify the tetracycline resistance determinants found in the Enterobacteriaceae into four groups, Tet A–D. The resistance determinant in the *Bacillus* plasmid pAB124 was not studied by Mendez *et al*. but is not homologous in hybridization studies with any of the TetA–TetD determinants (S J Eccles & I Chopra, in preparation).

ii *Membrane-located Resistance Proteins*

Although the determinants may encode several products (see section vi) the TetA,B,C and pAB124 determinants each specify a membrane-located protein which promotes energy-dependent efflux of tetracycline (Table III). Proof that these proteins are involved in efflux is provided by tetracycline accumulation studies with derivatives in which the respective structural genes have been deleted or mutated,[38,39] and by the observation that the content of wild-type TetB protein in the membrane correlates with the ability of cells to prevent tetracycline accumulation.[14] Synthesis of the proteins is inducible and involves classical genetic regulatory systems, i.e., there is a regulatory gene specifying a repressor which negatively regulates synthesis of the membrane-located resistance proteins. Figure 1 shows transcriptional maps of the TetA and TetB determinants to illustrate the arrangement of regulatory and structural genes.

iii *Properties of the Resistance Proteins*

The nucleotide sequences of the genes encoding the membrane proteins in the TetA–C determinants have recently become available,[36,37] (S J Waters & J Grinsted, in preparation). These data permit a number of interesting predictions concerning the proteins themselves and also allow comparison between proteins encoded by the different determinants.

TABLE II. Natural bacterial isolates that contain tetracycline resistance plasmids
From Chopra *et al*.[14]

Achromobacter liquefaciens	*Klebsiella pneumoniae*	*Shigella dysenteriae*
Enterobacter cloacae	*Pseudomonas aeruginosa*	*Sh. flexneri*
Bacillus cereus	*Proteus mirabilis*	*Sh. sonnei*
B. stearothermophilus	*Pr. morganii*	*Staphylococcus aureus*
Bacteroides fragilis	*Pr. rettgeri*	*Streptococcus agalactiae*
Campylobacter fetus sub. sp. *jejuni*	*Providencia* sp.	*Strep. faecalis*
Escherichia coli	*Salmonella panama*	*Strep. faecalis* sub. sp. *zymogenes*
Haemophilus influenzae	*Salm. paratyphi* B	*Vibrio cholerae*
	Salm. typhi	
	Salm. typhimurium	

TABLE III. Membrane proteins encoded by different tetracycline resistance determinants that are involved in active efflux of tetracyclines

Determinant*	Prototype plasmid	Properties of the proteins				Tetracyclines extruded§							References
		Molecular weight (k) from		Amino acid residues	Polarity†	Tc	OTc	CTc	DCTc	DDHMTc	Doxy	Min	
		gel electrophoresis	DNA sequences										
TetA	RP1	34	42	399	27	+	+	+					31–35, S J Waters & J Grinsted (in preparation)
TetB	R100	36	43	401	31	+	+	+	+	+	+	+	32–36
TetC	pSC101‡	34	37	338	36	+	+	+	+	+			32–34, 37
	pAB124‡	32				+	+						S J Eccles & I Chopra (in preparation)

* Classification according to the scheme of Mendez *et al*.[28]
† Calculated according to reference 30
‡ pAB124 originated in a thermophilic Bacillus (see reference 29)
§ Abbreviations: Tc = tetracycline, OTc = oxytetracycline, CTc = chlortetracycline, DCTc = demethylchlortetracycline, DDHMTc = 6-demethyl-6-deoxy-5-hydroxy-6-methylenetetracycline, Doxy = doxycycline, Min = minocycline

FIG. 1. Transcriptional maps of the TetA (i) and TetB (ii) determinants

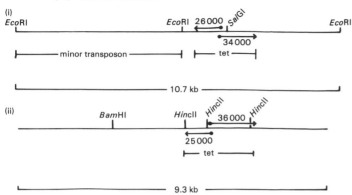

The TetA determinant shown here resides within transposon Tn*1721*, but does not necessarily occur in transposable elements.[8,28] The TetB determinant is invariably located within transposon Tn*10*.[8,28] Arrows above and below the restriction endonuclease sites indicate genes encoding proteins involved in tetracycline resistance or its control. Genes transcribed from left to right encode the membrane-located resistance proteins which in this figure are assigned molecular weights on the basis of their electrophoretic mobilities (see Table III). The genes transcribed from right to left are regulatory genes specifying repressor proteins of apparent molecular weights 26 000 and 25 000. In each determinant the promoters (●) regulating transcription of repressor and resistance proteins overlap.

Abbreviations: tet: tetracycline resistance determinant; kb: kilobase
Maps drawn from data in references 31, 40, 41

The molecular weights of the TetA–C proteins predicted from the DNA sequence are all greater than the apparent molecular weights observed by separation on polyacrylamide gels (Table III). This discrepancy might be explained in two ways: either the resistance proteins are synthesized as molecules which are reduced in length on insertion into the membrane, or the electrophoretic mobility of the proteins is anomalous. The second explanation is more likely because several membrane proteins have been reported to migrate in gels with a higher mobility than would be expected from their known molecular weights (e.g. see reference 42). The variable migration of the TetB membrane protein in different electrophoresis systems[8] also lends support to the idea that the electrophoretic mobility of the resistance proteins is anomalous.

Some cytoplasmic membrane proteins are synthesized as pre-proteins, i.e., with hydrophobic N terminal leader sequences of about 20 amino acids.[43] Leader sequences are required for insertion and translocation of these proteins within the envelope but the pre-proteins are subsequently processed to remove the leader sequences and generate the mature product. The nucleotide sequences at the beginning of the Tet-A, -B and -C structural genes do not predict involvement of leader sequences for membrane insertion of the resistance proteins. Furthermore, the TetB protein has the same electrophoretic mobility whether isolated from minicells or synthesized in vitro,[44] again suggesting that this protein is not processed in vivo.

The predicted amino acid composition of the membrane-located resistance proteins (Fig. 2) permits characterization of their polarities (Table III) and relatedness (Fig. 2, Table IV). Consideration of the polarity values for a number of proteins indicates that soluble proteins have values >47, whereas for membrane proteins the figure is usually <47.[30] Since the resistance proteins have values between 27 and 36 (Table III) one predicts that they are membrane-located, a notion clearly consistent with the reported cellular locations of these proteins.

FIG. 2. Predicted amino acid sequences of membrane proteins coded by Tet-A, -B and -C determinants

```
                                                                       50
MKPNIPLIVI  LSTVALDAVG  IGLIMPVLPG  LLRDLVHSND  VTAHYGILLA
  MNSSTKIA  LVITLLDAMG  IGLIMPVLPT  LLREFIASED  IANHFGVLLA
                                                                      100
LYALVQFACA  PVLGALSDRF  GRRPILLVSL  AGATVDYAIM  ATAPFLWVLY
LYALMQVIFA  PWLGKMSDRF  GRRPVLLLSL  IGASLDYLLL  AFSSALWMLY
        MR  TRSRSTVRPL  WPPPSPARFA  TWSHYRLRDH  GDHTRPVDPL
                                                                      150
IGRIVAGITG  ATGAVAGAYI  ADITDGDERA  RHFGFMSACF  GFGMVAGPVL
LGRLLSGITG  ATGAVAASVI  ADTTSASQRV  KWFGWLGASF  GLGLIAGPII
RRTHRGRHHR  RHRCGCWRLY  RRHHRWGRSG  SPLRAHERLF  RRGYGGRPVA
                                                                      200
GGLMGGFSPH  APFFAAAALN  GLNFLTGCFL  LPESHKGERR  PLRREALNPL
GGFAGEISPH  SPFFIAALLN  IVTFLVVMFW  FRETKNTRDN  TDTEVGVETQ
GGLLGAISLH  APFLAAAVLN  GLNLLLGCFL  MQESHKGERR  PMPLRAFNPV
                                                                      250
SFVRWARGMT  VVAALMAVFF  IMQLVGQVPA  ALWVIFGEDR  FHWDATTIGI
SNSVYITLFK  TMPILLIIYF  SAQLIGQIPA  TVWVLFTENR  FGWNSMMVGF
SSFRWARGMT  IVAALMTVFF  SAQLIGQIPA  ALWVIFGEDR  FRWSATMIGL
                                                                      300
SLAAFGILHS  LAQAMITGPV  AARLGERRAL  MLGMIADGTG  YILLAFATRG
SLAGLGLLHS  VFQAFVAGRI  ATKWGEKTAV  LLEFIADSSA  FAFLAFISEG
SLAVFGILHA  LAQAFVTGPA  TKRFGEKQAI  IAGMAADALG  YVLLAFATRG
                                                                      350
WMAFPIMVLL  ASGGIGMPAL  QAMLSRQVDE  ERQGQLQGSL  AALTSLTSIV
WLDFPVLILL  AGGGIALPAL  QGVMSIQTKS  HEQGALQGSL  VSLTNATGVI
WMAFPIMILL  ASGGIGMPAL  QAMLSRQVDD  DHQGQLQGSL  AALTSLTSIT
                                                                      400
GPLLFTAIYA  ASITTWNGWA  WIAGAALYLL  CLPALRRGLW  SGAGQRADRterm
GPLLFTVIYN  HSLPIWDGWI  WIIGLAFYCI  IILLSITFML  TPQAQGSKQE
GPLIVTAIYA  ASASTWNGLA  WIVGAALYLV  CLPALRRGAW  SRATSTterm
TSAterm
```

The amino acid sequences of membrane-located resistance proteins coded by TetA (upper), TetB (middle) and TetC (lower) are shown, aligned for maximum homology. The proteins are believed to correspond to those shown in Table I and the protein sequences are given by the one-letter amino acid code.[45] Amino acid sequences are those reported by S J Waters & J Grinsted (in preparation) (TetA), Hillen & Schollmeier[36] (TetB), and Sutcliffe[37] (TetC). Bold type indicates common residues.
Abbreviation: term: termination of polypeptide

TABLE IV. Homology between the membrane-located resistance proteins encoded by the Tet-A, -B and -C determinants

Proteins compared	Identical amino acid residues (%)
TetA/TetB	45
TetA/TetC	52
TetB/TetC	25

Since hybridization experiments revealed that the Tet-A, -B and -C determinants are distinct owing to lack of DNA homology,[28] one would also predict that the amino acid sequences of the resistance proteins will differ. Nevertheless, since these proteins are able in common to promote tetracycline efflux, conserved amino acid sequences may exist. Alignment of the Tet-A, -B and -C membrane protein sequences to produce maximum homology (Fig. 2) indicates that the proteins, as anticipated, are dissimilar. Calculation of common amino acid residues (Table IV) shows the Tet-A and -C products to be most closely related, having 52% of their residues in common. Despite differences between the proteins, several amino acid sequences are common to each, particularly in some localized regions of each protein (Fig. 2). Some or all of these conserved regions are therefore likely to be involved in promoting tetracycline efflux. The ability of TetA–C determinants to confer resistance to different tetracycline analogues has been known for some time[28,34] and this is apparently reflected by differences in the capacity of the membrane resistance proteins to promote efflux of the analogues (Table III). Differences in the ability to extrude tetracycline analogues is presumably related to differences in amino acid sequence within the proteins, but at present it is difficult to predict which polypeptide regions are involved in recognition of different tetracyclines.

iv *Mode of Action of Resistance Proteins*

The mechanism by which the plasmid-encoded membrane proteins confer resistance has emerged gradually during the last decade. Initially decreased accumulation was explained solely by reduced antibiotic influx, with no apparent evidence for efflux.[46] This led to a theory suggesting that membrane-located resistance proteins chelate cations involved in tetracycline transport.[47,48] Thus the resistance proteins are assumed to lower the free metal ion concentration in the membrane and prevent entry of tetracycline. However, such theories are no longer tenable and there is now little doubt that the membrane-located resistance proteins promote energy-dependent tetracycline efflux.[32,33,35,49]

Since tetracycline uptake into sensitive bacteria involves active transport,[7,8,10,13,50] do the resistance proteins interact directly with the transport sites to reverse the influx system of the host cell? This possibility has been eliminated by use of membrane vesicles which show that the active efflux systems in resistant bacteria differ from the active influx system in sensitive cells. Thus, the systems differ with respect to kinetic constants, pH, and magnesium requirements (Table V). We can conclude from these data that the plasmid-encoded membrane resistance proteins represent saturable carriers promoting efflux of tetracyclines. The nature of energy coupling to efflux has not been explored in detail, but it appears to be driven by the proton-motive force.[33]

v *Gene Copy Number and Decreased Tetracycline Accumulation*

Gene amplification (i.e., an increase in number) of plasmid-located antibiotic resistance determinants frequently leads to increased levels of antibiotic resistance, e.g. to ampicillin, chloramphenicol and streptomycin.[51] In most cases increased resistance results from elevated levels of soluble enzymes, but in the case of tetracycline resistance the anticipated increase in efflux upon increasing the gene copy number is not realized. As discussed below, this implies that the number of functional binding sites within the membrane that can accommodate the plasmid-specified proteins is limited.

Weibauer *et al.*[52] studied tetracycline gene amplification in *E. coli* using the TetA determinant in transposon Tn*1721*. The transposable element consists of a 'minor transposon' encoding functions required for transposition and a separate tetracycline resistance determinant (Fig. 1). The latter is flanked by two direct repeats which provide sequence homology for amplification of tetracycline resistance genes.[31,52] Multiple tandem repeats of the resistance determinant were generated to study the relationship

between gene dosage and reduced tetracycline accumulation, but increased efflux of the antibiotic was not observed with increasing number of resistance genes in the range of 1–36 copies per chromosome.[52] Although these data imply a limited number of membrane sites at which the resistance proteins can integrate, increased osmotic lability of cells was observed upon increasing the gene copy number.[52] This probably indicates that an excess of resistance protein is accumulating in the cell envelope leading to instability. Therefore, although the ability of the cytoplasmic membrane to accommodate the TetA determined resistance protein may not be limited *per se*, the number of functional sites from which tetracycline efflux can be promoted is probably saturable at the level of one determinant per chromosome.

Studies on gene dosage effects with the TetB determinant have also been conducted, but this has involved cloning the determinant into plasmid vectors having different numbers of copies per chromosome.[53,54] The effect of increasing the number of TetB determinants per cell is more complex than the situation which occurs with TetA. In the case of TetB, increased copy numbers lead to decreased expression of resistance associated with reduced expression of the efflux system.[53] The molecular basis of this response is poorly understood but may represent a regulatory mechanism to prevent overproduction of the membrane-located resistance protein.[54] The reason that TetA and TetB show different responses with respect to gene dosage seems to be related to the ability of TetB determinants to encode minocycline resistance.[53] Possibly the region of the TetB determined membrane protein that causes minocycline efflux can also participate in a regulatory process to limit further transcription or translation of its own product.

Although some progress has been made towards an understanding of the relationship between gene copy number and expression of membrane-located resistance proteins, this has depended on the use of a fluorescence assay to determine tetracycline accumulation. Recently, various limitations concerning the use of this assay have been reported.[55] Therefore it might be desirable to repeat the studies on gene dosage response using an alternative method to study drug accumulation (e.g. using radiolabelled tetracycline).

vi *Are the Membrane-located Resistance Proteins the Only Products Responsible for Resistance?*

Several investigators have commented that the observed decrease in tetracycline accumulation seems insufficient to explain the levels of tetracycline resistance encoded by plasmids.[10,29,33,56] Although the determinant in pSC101 (TetC) apparently specifies four proteins involved in resistance,[8,38] the other determinants appear to encode only a single product (other than repressor proteins) i.e., the membrane-located resistance proteins described above. Recently, genetic complementation data[39,57] have suggested that two resistance proteins are produced by the TetB determinant, but these results could nevertheless be explained by intragenic complementation between mis-sense mutations in different domains of a single polypeptide. Furthermore, nucleic acid sequencing has revealed only one open-reading frame in the TetB determinant, potentially encoding the 44K polypeptide.[36] The apparent discrepancy between resistance levels mediated by plasmids and the decreased tetracycline accumulation they cause may be explained by the involvement of *tet* gene repressors in resistance, i.e., by binding tetracycline, the repressors may actually contribute to resistance themselves.[58]

In previous publications we reported that tetracycline resistance determinants express up to three phenotypic mechanisms of

TABLE V. Properties of tetracycline influx and efflux systems in membrane vesicles from *Pseudomonas putida*[49] and *Escherichia coli*[33,50]

System	Kinetic constants		Optima for influx/efflux	
	K_m (μM)	V_{max} (nmol/min/ mg protein)	pH	[Mg^{2+}] (mM)
P. putida influx	2500	50	ne	ne
E. coli influx	nd	nd	6.9	1
P. putida, TetA-mediated efflux	2.0–3.5	0.15	ne	ne
E. coli, TetB-mediated efflux	6	0.1–1.0	7.7	3–10

Abbreviations: nd: not determinable; ne: not estimated

resistance.[14,56] In the light of new findings described in this paper we can now suggest that mechanism 1 is mediated by repressors[58] and mechanism 2 entails antibiotic efflux promoted by the membrane-located proteins (Table III). Mechanism 3 (coded by the TetB determinant) was previously thought to involve ribosomal alterations.[8,44,56] This, however, is not the case (S W Shales & I Chopra, unpublished work) and the phenotype, like that conferred by mechanism 2, results from minocycline efflux promoted by the membrane-located resistance protein.[35] The inability of TetA and TetC determinants to express minocycline resistance probably results from failure of the respective resistance proteins to promote efflux of the antibiotic (Table III).

b *Chromosomal Mutations*

Many antibiotics utilize envelope components for their passage through this region.[13] This may involve passive diffusion, e.g. through protein porins in gram-negative outer membranes, or active carrier-mediated transport across the cytoplasmic membrane. The utilization of cellular components for antibiotic transport predicts that mutations in their respective chromosomal genes will lead to decreased drug accumulation. The mutations could include lesions in carrier proteins, porins or membrane products involved in the coupling of energy to drug transport. Such changes do indeed occur as mutations in envelope components have been reported which affect the accumulation of aminoglycosides,[6,11–13,59,60] β-lactams,[13,61,62] chloramphenicol,[13] cycloserine,[13] fosfomycin,[13] peptide antibiotics[13] and tetracycline.[13,35,63] Mutations of this type can also act in synergy with other resistance mechanisms, e.g. in conjunction with antibiotic-inactivating enzymes.[64]

3 Conclusion

The impact of antibiotic resistance on chemotherapy is considered in detail elsewhere in this Bulletin (pp. 102–106), but it is nevertheless worthwhile at this point to summarize the extent to which decreased antibiotic accumulation compromises treatment of disease. Intrinsic resistance involving antibiotic exclusion has clearly complicated the therapy of certain infections, notably those caused by *Ps. aeruginosa*,[19,65] but the development of broad-spectrum β lactams has largely overcome these problems.[65,66] The high prevalance of plasmid-determined tetracycline resistance has undoubtedly reduced the value of tetracycline for human and veterinary medicine.[8] Selection pressure with tetracycline in vitro may cause multiplication of resistance gene copies in those plasmids containing amplifiable DNA sequences (e.g. Tn*1721*) (also, see reference 8). Although such amplification may raise resistance levels due to elevated repressor levels,[52] increased quantities of resistance proteins in the membrane may cause physiological problems for the cell (e.g. membrane destabilization: see section 2a,v). Thus even though bacteria harbouring amplifiable tetracycline determinants may possess the capacity to undergo an increase in resistance, in some clinical conditions it may be disadvantageous for them to do so. Failure to amplify tetracycline resistance determinants and thereby maximize resistance levels may not lead to elimination of infecting micro-organisms because tetracyclines are bacteriostatic.[67] The majority of the chromosomal mutants described in section 2 have been isolated under laboratory conditions; it is notoriously difficult to assess whether similar mutations arise during therapy (e.g. see reference 19). Nevertheless, recent studies on *N. gonorrhoeae* provide at least one example where chromosomal mutants have arisen in nature which exhibit decreased antibiotic accumulation.[68]

Finally, an unusual and yet potentially disturbing type of resistance which results in decreased drug accumulation has recently emerged. This involves plasmid-determined suppression of porin synthesis in *E. coli* and is therefore a form of acquired resistance, but differing somewhat from those examples described in section 2. This effect has only been described so far for plasmids of the N incompatibility group[69] and R124, an F-like plasmid of incompatibility group FIV.[70] Nevertheless, it illustrates that, in addition to encoding specific resistance mechanisms, some plasmids have evolved a system to control the level of porins in the outer membrane and thereby confer resistance to those antimicrobial agents that utilize porins to cross the membrane.

Acknowledgements

I thank Dr T G B Howe for helpful comments on the manuscript. Financial support for my work mentioned in the text came from the Medical Research Council.

Addendum

Following completion of this article, a correction was made to the pBR322 (TetC) DNA sequence reported by Sutcliffe.[37] An additional CG base pair has now been inserted at position 526 which lies within the tetracycline resistance region.[71,72] This change adjusts the published sequence to allow an open reading frame from nucleotides 86–1273 (new number) coding for a hypothetical protein of 396 amino acids and molecular weight 41.5 K.[72]

References

1 Davies J, Smith D I. Plasmid-determined resistance to antimicrobial agents. Annu Rev Microbiol 1978; 32: 469–518
2 Franklin T J. Antibiotic transport in bacteria. CRC Crit Rev Microbiol 1973; 2: 253–272
3 Costerton, J W, Cheng K-J. The role of the bacterial cell envelope in antibiotic resistance. J Antimicrob Chemother 1975; 1: 363–377
4 Eagon R G, Stinnett J D, Gilleland H E Jr. Ultrastructure of *Pseudomonas aeruginosa* as related to resistance. In: Brown M R W, ed. Resistance of *Pseudomonas aeruginosa*. London: John Wiley & Sons, 1975; 109–143
5 Brown M R W. The role of the cell envelope in resistance. In: Brown M R W, ed. Resistance of *Pseudomonas aeruginosa*. London: John Wiley & Sons, 1975; 71–107
6 Bryan L E. Resistance to antimicrobial agents: the general nature of the problem and the basis of resistance. In: Doggett R G, ed. *Pseudomonas aeruginosa*. Clinical manifestations of infection and current therapy. New York: Academic Press, 1979; 219–270
7 Chopra I, Howe T G B. Bacterial resistance to the tetracyclines. Microbiol Rev 1978; 42: 707–724
8 Chopra I, Howe T G B, Linton A H, Linton K B, Richmond M H, Speller D C E. The tetracyclines: prospects at the beginning of the 1980s. J Antimicrob Chemother 1981; 8: 5–21
9 Koch A L. Evolution of antibiotic resistance gene function. Microbiol Rev 1981; 45: 355–378
10 Levy S B. The tetracyclines: microbial sensitivity and resistance. In: Gialdroni Grassi G, Sabath L D, eds. New trends in antibiotics: research and therapy. Amsterdam: Elsevier/North-Holland Biomedical Press, 1981; 27–44
11 Hancock R E W. Aminoglycoside uptake and mode of action—with special reference to streptomycin and gentamicin. I. Antagonists and mutants. J Antimicrob Chemother 1981; 8: 249–276
12 Hancock R E W. Aminoglycoside uptake and mode of action with special reference to streptomycin and gentamicin. II. Effects of aminoglycosides on cells. J Antimicrob Chemother 1981; 8: 429–445
13 Chopra I, Ball P R. Transport of antibiotics into bacteria. Adv Microb Physiol 1982; 23: 183–240
14 Chopra I, Ball P R, Shales S W. Methods of studying plasmid-determined resistance to tetracyclines. In: Russell, A. D, Quesnel L B,

eds. Technical series of the Society for Applied Bacteriology vol. 18. London: Academic Press, 1983; 223–244

15 Nikaido H, Nakae T. The outer membrane of Gram-negative bacteria. Adv Microb Physiol 1979; 20: 163–250

16 Nikaido H. Outer membrane of *Salmonella typhimurium.* Transmembrane diffusion of some hydrophobic substances. Biochim Biophys Acta 1976; 433: 118–132

17 Yoshimura F, Nikaido H. Permeability of *Pseudomonas aeruginosa* outer membrane to hydrophilic solutes. J Bacteriol 1982; 152: 636–642.

18 Garrod L P, Lambert H P, O'Grady F. Antibiotic and Chemotherapy. 5th ed. Edinburgh: Churchill Livingstone, 1981

19 Lowbury E J L, Jones R J. Treatment and prophylaxis for *Pseudomonas* infections. In: Brown, M R W, ed. Resistance of *Pseudomonas aeruginosa.* London: John Wiley & Sons, 1975; 237–269

20 Shales S W, Chopra I. Outer membrane composition in *Escherichia coli* and the poor activity of hydrophobic antibiotics against enteric bactreria. J Antimicrob Chemother 1982; 9: 325–327

21 Hancock R E W, Nikaido H. Outer membranes of gram-negative bacteria. XIX. Isolation from *Pseudomonas aeruginosa* PAO1 and use in reconstitution and definition of the permeability barrier. J Bacteriol 1978; 136: 381–390

22 Hancock R E W, Decad G M, Nikaido H. Identification of the protein producing transmembrane diffusion pores in the outer membrane of *Pseudomonas aeruginosa* PAO1. Biochim Biophys Acta 1979; 554: 323–331

23 Slack M P E, Nichols W W. Antibiotic penetration through bacterial capsules and exopolysaccharides. J Antimicrob Chemother 1982; 10: 368–372

24 Watanabe T. Infective heredity of multiple drug resistance in bacteria. Bacteriol Rev 1963; 27: 87–115

25 Chopra I. Mechanisms of resistance to fusidic acid in *Staphylococcus aureus.* J Gen Microbiol 1976; 96: 229–238

26 Gaffney D F, Cundliffe E, Foster T J. Chloramphenicol resistance that does not involve chloramphenicol acetyltransferase encoded by plasmids from gram-negative bacteria. J Gen Microbiol 1981; 125: 113–121

27 Dorman C J, Foster T J. Nonenzymatic chloramphenicol resistance determinants specified by plasmids R26 and R55-1 in *Escherichia coli* K-12 do not confer high-level resistance to fluorinated analogs. Antimicrob Agents Chemother 1982; 22: 912–914

28 Mendez B, Tachibana C, Levy S B. Heterogeneity of tetracycline resistance determinants. Plasmid 1980; 3: 99–108

29 Eccles S, Docherty A, Chopra I, Shales S W, Ball P. Tetracycline resistance genes from *Bacillus* plasmid pAB124 confer decreased accumulation of the antibiotic in *Bacillus subtilis* but not in *Escherichia coli.* J Bacteriol 1981; 145: 1417–1420

30 Capaldi R A, Vanderkooi G. The low polarity of many membrane proteins. Proc Natl Acad Sci USA 1972; 69: 930–932

31 Altenbuchner J, Schmid K, Schmitt R. Tn*1721*-encoded tetracycline resistance: mapping of structural and regulatory genes mediating resistance. J Bacteriol 1983; 153: 116–123

32 Ball P R, Shales S W, Chopra I. Plasmid-mediated tetracycline resistance in *Escherichia coli* involves increased efflux of the antibiotic. Biochem Biophys Res Commun 1980; 93: 74–81

33 McMurry, L, Petrucci R E, Levy S B. Active efflux of tetracycline encoded by four genetically different tetracycline resistance determinants in *Escherichia coli.* Proc Natl Acad Sci USA 1980; 77: 3974–3977

34 Chopra I, Shales S W, Ball P. Tetracycline resistance determinants from groups A to D vary in their ability to confer decreased accumulation of tetracycline derivatives by *Escherichia coli.* J gen Microbiol 1982; 128: 689–692

35 McMurry L M, Cullinane, J C, Levy S B. Transport of the lipophilic analog minocycline differs from that of tetracycline in susceptible and resistant *Escherichia coli* strains. Antimicrob Agents Chemother 1982; 22: 791–799

36 Hillen W, Schollmeier K. Nucleotide sequence of the Tn10 encoded tetracycline resistance gene. Nucleic Acids Res 1983; 11: 525–539

37 Sutcliffe J G. Complete nucleotide sequence of the *Escherichia coli* plasmid pBR322. Cold Spr Harb Symp Quant Biol 1978; 43: 77–90

38 Tait R C, Boyer H W. On the nature of tetracycline resistance controlled by the plasmid pSC101. Cell 1978; 13: 73–81

39 Coleman D C, Chopra I, Shales S W, Howe T G B, Foster T J. Analysis of tetracycline resistance encoded by transposon Tn*10*: deletion mapping of tetracycline sensitive point mutations and identification of two structural genes. J Bacteriol 1983; 153: 921–929

40 Jorgensen R A, Reznikoff W S. Organization of structural and regulatory genes that mediate tetracycline resistance in transposon Tn*10.* J Bacteriol 1979; 138: 705–714

41 Wray L V Jr, Jorgensen R A, Reznikoff W S. Identification of the tetracycline resistance promoter and repressor in transposon Tn*10.* J. Bacteriol 1981; 147: 297–304

42 Noel D, Nikaido K, Ames G F-L. A single amino acid substitution in a histidine-transport protein drastically alters its mobility in sodium dodecyl sulfate-polyacrylamide gel electrophoresis. Biochemistry 1979; 18: 4159–4165

43 Pratt J M, Holland I B, Spratt B G. Precursor forms of penicillin-binding proteins 5 and 6 of the *E. coli* cytoplasmic membrane. Nature 1981; 293: 307–309

44 Yang H-L, Zubay G, Levy S B. Synthesis of an R plasmid protein associated with tetracycline resistance is negatively regulated. Proc Natl Acad Sci USA 1976; 73: 1509–1512

45 IUPAC-IUB Commission on Biochemical Nomenclature. A one-letter notation for amino acid sequences. Tentative rules. Biochem J 1969; 113: 1–4

46 Young T W, Hubball S J. R-factor-mediated resistance to tetracycline in *Escherichia coli* K12. An R-factor with a mutation to temperature-sensitive tetracycline resistance. Biochem Biophys Res Commun 1976; 70: 117–124

47 Bochner B R, Huang H-C, Schieven G L, Ames B N. Positive selection for loss of tetracycline resistance. J Bacteriol 1980; 143: 926–933

48 Herrin G L Jr, Russell D R, Bennett G N. A stable derivative of pBR322 conferring increased tetracycline resistance and increased sensitivity to fusaric acid. Plasmid 1982; 7: 290–293

49 Hedstrom R C, Crider B P, Eagon R G. Comparison of kinetics of active tetracycline uptake and active tetracycline efflux in sensitive and plasmid RP4-containing *Pseudomonas putida.* J Bacteriol 1982; 152: 255–259

50 McMurry L M, Cullinane J C, Petrucci R E Jr, Levy S B. Active uptake of tetracycline by membrane vesicles from susceptible *Escherichia coli.* Antimicrob Agents Chemother 1981; 20: 307–313

51 Uhlin B E, Nordström K. R plasmid gene dosage effects in *Escherichia coli* K-12: copy mutants of the R plasmid R1*drd*-19. Plasmid 1977; 1: 1–7

52 Weibauer K, Schraml S, Shales S W, Schmitt R. Tetracycline resistance transposon Tn*1721*: *recA*-dependent gene amplification and expression of tetracycline resistance. J Bacteriol 1981; 147: 851–859

53 Chopra I, Shales S W, Ward J M, Wallace L J. Reduced expresion of Tn*10*-mediated tetracycline resistance in *Escherichia coli* containing more than one copy of the transposon. J Gen Microbiol 1981; 126: 45–54

54 Coleman D C, Foster T J. Analysis of the reduction in expression of tetracycline resistance determined by transposon Tn*10* in the multicopy state. MGG 1981; 182: 171–177

55 Smith M C M, Chopra I. Limitations of a fluorescence assay for studies on tetracycline transport into *Escherichia coli.* Antimicrob Agents Chemother 1983; 23: 175–178

56 Shales S W, Chopra I, Ball P R. Evidence for more than one mechanism of plasmid-determined tetracycline resistance in *Escherichia coli.* J Gen Microbiol 1980; 121: 221–229

57 Curiale M S, Levy S B. Two complementation groups mediate tetracycline resistance determined by Tn*10.* J Bacteriol 1982; 151: 209–215

58 Beck C F, Mutzel R, Barbé J, Müller W. A multifunctional gene (*tetR*) controls Tn*10*-encoded tetracycline resistance. J Bacteriol 1982; 150: 633–642

59 Ahmad M H, Rechenmacher A, Böck A. Interaction between aminoglycoside uptake and ribosomal resistance mutations. Antimicrob Agents Chemother 1980; 18: 798–806

60 Miller M H, Edberg S C, Mandel L J, Behar C F, Steigbigel N H. Gentamicin uptake in wild-type and aminoglycoside-resistant small-colony mutants of *Staphylococcus aureus.* Antimicrob Agents Chemother 1980; 18: 722–729

61 Sawai T, Hiruma R, Kawana N, Kaneko M, Taniyasu F, Inami A. Outer membrane permeation of β-lactam antibiotics in *Escherichia coli, Proteus mirabilis,* and *Enterobacter cloacae.* Antimicrob Agents Chemother 1982; 22: 585–592

62 Jaffe A, Chabbert Y A, Semonin O. Role of porin proteins OmpF and OmpC in the permeation of β-lactams. Antimicrob Agents Chemother 1982; 22: 942–948

63 Williams G, Smith I. Chromosomal mutations causing resistance to tetracycline in *Bacillus subtilis. MGG* 1979; 177: 23–29

64 Lundbäck A K, Nordström K. Mutations in *Escherichia coli* K-12 decreasing the rate of streptomycin uptake: synergism with R-factor-mediated capacity to inactivate streptomycin. Antimicrob Agents Chemother 1974; 5: 500–507

65 Young L S. Recent advances in the therapy of *Pseudomonas aeruginosa* infection. In: Doggett R G, ed. *Pseudomonas aeruginosa.* Clinical

manifestations of infection and current therapy. New York: Academic Press, 1979; 311–338

66 Gillett A P. Antibiotics against pseudomonas. J Antimicrob Chemother 1982; 9 (Suppl B): 41–48

67 Franklin T J, Snow G A. Biochemistry of Antimicrobial Action. 3rd ed. London: Chapman & Hall, 1981

68 Morse S A, Lysko P G, McFarland L *et al.* Gonococcal strains from homosexual men have outer membranes with reduced permeability to hydrophobic molecules. Infect Immun 1982; 37: 432–438

69 Iyer R, Darby V, Holland I B. Alterations in the outer membrane proteins of *Escherichia coli* B/r associated with the presence of the R plasmid rRM98. FEBS Lett 1978; 85: 127–132

70 Rossouw F T, Rowbury R J. Effects of the resistance plasmid R124 on the level of the OmpF outer membrane protein and on the response of *Escherichia coli* to environmental agents. J Appl Bacteriol 1984; In press

71 Livneh Z. Directed mutagenesis method for analysis of mutagen specificity: application to ultra-violet induced mutagenesis. Proc Natl Acad Sci USA 1983; 80: 237–241

72 Peden K W C. Revised sequence of the tetracycline-resistance gene of pBR322. Gene; 22: 277–280

British Medical Bulletin (1984) Vol. 40, No. 1, pp. 18–27

β-LACTAMASES

ANTONE A MEDEIROS MD

Department of Medicine
The Miriam Hospital
Brown University
Providence, RI

1   Classification of β-lactamases
2   β-lactamases determined by plasmids or transposons
     a   Novel β-lactamases
     b   Transposons determining β-lactamases
     c   Distribution in clinical isolates
3   β-lactamases determined by chromosomal genes
4   Contribution of β-lactamases to β-lactam antibiotic resistance
5   Conclusions
      References

β-lactamases hydrolyse the amide bond in the β-lactam ring of penicillins and cephalosporins, producing acidic derivatives which have no antibacterial properties. They are the major determinants of the resistance to β-lactam antibiotics of most bacterial pathogens. Their variety, their distribution among clinical isolates worldwide and the ways in which they mediate resistance in these isolates will be the principal focus of this review.

Fleming was first to note in 1929 that certain groups of bacteria, such as the 'coli-typhoid' group were not inhibited by penicillin.[1] Abraham & Chain[2] in 1940, pursued this observation by crushing a suspension of *Escherichia coli* with a mill to produce an extract which destroyed the growth-inhibiting properties of penicillin. Heat and papain digestion inactivated the extract leading the investigators to conclude that the active component was an enzyme which they named penicillinase. The enzyme was found also in a penicillin-resistant gram-negative rod contaminating their *Penicillium* cultures but not in a penicillin-sensitive *Staphylococcus aureus*. However, since a penicillin-sensitive culture of *Micrococcus lysodeikticus* also contained penicillinase, the authors concluded that the presence or absence of the enzyme was not the sole factor determining sensitivity or resistance to penicillin. They postulated, also, that because various species of bacteria contain penicillinase, it 'may have a function in their metabolism'.

Four years later, Kirby[3] in comparing penicillin-resistant vs. penicillin-susceptible clinical isolates, of staphylococci, found that acetone–ether extracts of the former, but not the latter, contained penicillinase. From then until the 1960s, most attention focused on staphylococcal penicillinase as the prevalence of penicillin-resistant staphylococci rapidly reached epidemic proportions in hospitals, where penicillin was used widely, and spread then gradually into the community. The advent around 1960 of the semi-synthetic penicillins, methicillin and ampicillin, and the cephalosporins, cephaloridine and cephalothin, shifted the focus of attention on to the β-lactamases of gram-negative bacilli. There were several reasons for this: (a) methicillin and the cephalosporins resisted hydrolysis by staphylococcal β-lactamase, making them effective therapeutic agents against penicillinase-producing sta-

phylococci; (b) as treatment of patients infected with penicillin-resistant staphylococci became more effective, spread within institutions decreased; (c) concomitantly, the prevalence within hospitals of infections due to gram-negative bacilli increased as usage of ampicillin, a broad-spectrum penicillin, widened; (d) these gram-negative bacilli were found to produce a great variety of β-lactamases capable of destroying the newer penicillins and cephalosporins[4] and (e) the more prevalent types of these β-lactamases were discovered to be determined by genetic elements, plasmids[5] and transposons,[6] capable of widespread—almost promiscuous—transfer to other genera. These discoveries accelerated interest in the β-lactamases of gram-negative bacilli and the search for β-lactam antibiotics resistant to these β-lactamases became a major thrust of the pharmaceutical industry. Consequently, several entirely new classes of clinically useful β-lactam antibiotics[7] have come into use and, not unexpectedly, new β-lactamases and other mechanisms of resisting these β-lactams have emerged.

1   Classification of β-Lactamases

Among the gram-positive bacteria, staphylococci are the principal pathogens which produce β-lactamase. Four enzyme types, designated A–D, can be identified serologically but are otherwise indistinguishable.[8] Staphylococcal β-lactamase, a protein of mol. wt. 28 800, preferentially hydrolyses the penicillins and is inducible in most strains. Plasmids, which are transferred from cell to cell by phages (transduction), carry the genes which determine most staphylococcal β-lactamases.[9] One strain of *Streptococcus uberis*[10] and two of *Streptococcus fecalis*[10,11] have been found to produce β-lactamase; one of these strains has been shown to be plasmid-determined. The enzymes have not yet been extensively characterized.

The wide variety of β-lactamases, produced by gram-negative bacteria has led to a number of classification schemes. The earliest[12,13] were based primarily on substrate profiles, i.e. the rate of hydrolysis of penicillins vs. cephalosporins, with additional distinction provided by parameters such as enzyme inhibition and reaction to antisera. Richmond & Sykes[14] elaborated on these criteria, dividing the β-lactamases into five classes, and thus provided the first broadly useful frame of reference. Their class I consists of β-lactamases with a high rate of hydrolysis of cephalosporins (cephalosporinases). This large class includes the chromosomally determined β-lactamases of most of the Enterobactericeae and pseudomonas, except for those of *Proteus* and *Klebsiella* which are more active against penicillins and make up classes II and IV respectively. Class III is made up of the plasmid-determined TEM-type β-lactamases and class V, a heterogenous grouping, contains the oxacillin-hydrolysing and carbenicillin-hydrolysing β-lactamases described below.

The heterogeneity within some of these classes and the problems of determining parameters such as enzyme inhibition by para-chloromercuribenzoate (PCMB) using crude enzyme preparations make it difficult to utilize this classification, especially when additional information on properties such as inducibility of enzyme production or location (chromosome or plasmid) of the β-lactamase genes is lacking.

A major advance occurred when Matthew[4] showed that specific β-lactamases could be identified by flat-bed isoelectric focusing (IEF) in polyacrylamide gel. By developing the gel with a chromogenic cephalosporin overlay, this technique made it possible to identify the active proteins using crude cell extracts even when several β-lactamases co-existed within the same bacterial cell. When concentrated cell extracts were used, the method proved to be highly sensitive, revealing the presence of β-lactamases in virtually all gram-negative bacteria studied. The banding patterns seen with IEF permitted virtual fingerprinting of β-lactamases when side-to-side comparisons with reference β-lactamases were run on the same gel. Coupled with data on enzyme kinetics, the IEF banding patterns have made it feasible to survey the β-lactamases present in large numbers of clinical isolates.

The newer methodologies of amino acid and nucleotide sequencing have yielded further insights into the relationships between different classes of β-lactamases. Based on sequencing data and enzymatic analysis, three evolutionarily distinct classes have been defined.[15,16] Class A β-lactamases have a serine residue at their active site, have molecular weights of around 29 000, show significant amino acid sequence homology, and preferentially hydrolyse penicillins. This group includes the TEM-1 β-lactamase widely prevalent in gram-negative bacilli and those of *S. aureus* PC1 and *Bacillus licheniformis* 749/c. Of interest, there is homology between the amino acid sequence around the penicillin binding sites of the D-alanine carboxypeptidases of *Bacillus stearothermophilus* and *Bacillus subtilis* and the sequence around the active site serine of these Class A β-lactamases, supporting the hypothesis that these β-lactamases may be derived from penicillin-binding proteins (PBPs) involved in peptidoglycan synthesis.[17,18] Class B β-lactamase is a metalloenzyme of mol. wt. 23 000 which attacks cephalosporins and is produced only by *Bacillus cereus*.[15] Class C β-lactamases, on the other hand, are the chromosomally determined cephalosporinases of *E. coli* which show extensive sequence homology with *Shigella* species and lesser homology with *Klebsiella*, *Salmonella*, *Serratia*, and *Pseudomonas* species. They are large proteins (mol. wt. 39 000) that also have serine at their active site but share no sequence homology with the Class A β-lactamases.[16,19,20]

2 β-Lactamases Determined by Plasmids and Transposons

Matthew described 11 types of plasmid-determined β-lactamases.[21,22] All are constitutive and in most cases are produced in greater amounts than the chromosomal β-lactamase of their host strains. They fall into three broad classes: (a) the 'broad-spectrum' penicillinases which hydrolyse benzylpenicillin and cephaloridine at similar rates; (b) the oxacillinases which hydrolyse oxacillin rapidly, and (c) the carbenicillinases which destroy carbenicillin. Each of the β-lactamases has a unique isoelectric point and most have a characteristic banding pattern which consists of a single major band and several accessory bands that appear late following the overlay of nitrocefin. In surveys of several hundred β-lactamases of gram-negative bacilli, these banding patterns have proved to be very characteristic of each type when tested under identical conditions. Figure 1 shows the banding patterns of four of these β-lactamases in polyacrylamide gel and, also, in a newly utilized matrix of highly purified agarose.[23] Both methods produce similar banding patterns, although differences are observed with the HMS-1 and PSE-1 enzymes. The HMS-1 enzyme produces two dense bands in agarose as opposed to a single faint band in polyacrylamide, and the PSE-1 β-lactamase focuses slightly below the TEM-1 in agarose, in contrast to polyacrylamide. The ease of preparation of agarose, lack of toxic hazard, and shorter focusing time make it an attractive medium for characterizing β-lactamases further.

Table I summarizes the properties of the 11 plasmid-determined β-lactamases. TEM-1, SHV-1, and HMS-1 have similar substrate profiles with nearly equal activity against benzylpenicillin and cephaloridine. Cloxacillin inhibits all four enzymes while pCMB inhibits only HMS-1 and SHV-1 (variably). OXA-1, OXA-2, and OXA-3 hydrolyse oxacillin rapidly, as the name implies, and are inhibited by NaCl. On the other hand, the PSE enzymes have a high relative activity against carbenicillin and one, PSE-2, resembles the OXA-hydrolysing enzymes in having a high relative activity against oxacillin as well. The reported molecular weights of these enzymes range between 12 000 and 32 000 except for OXA-2 and OXA-3 which are known to be dimers with molecular weights of 44 600 and 41 200 respectively. Not shown on Table I is the fact that three of these β-lactamases (OXA-1, PSE-1, PSE-2) hydrolyse cefotaxime at a significant rate and two (PSE-2, PSE-3) are active against latamoxef.[24]

Sykes *et al.*[25] and Paul *et al.*[26] have demonstrated immunological

FIG. 1. A comparison of β-lactamase banding patterns obtained using 0.8 mm thick agarose and 2.0 mm thick polyacrylamide as the isoelectric focusing medium

From Vecoli *et al.*[23]

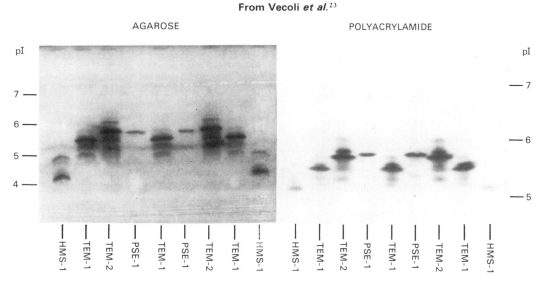

TABLE I. Properties of plasmid-determined β-lactamases
(Adapted from reference 21)

	Relative rate of hydrolysis							Inhibited by			Mol. Wt.	pI	Transposon mediated
	Amp	Carb	Oxa	Meth	Clox	Cer	Cet	Clox	pCMB	NaCl			
Penicillinases— 'broad spectrum'													
TEM-1	106	10	5	0	0	76	20	+	−	−	22000	5.4	+
TEM-2	107	10	5	0	0	74	20	+	−	−	23500	5.6	+
SHV-1	212	8	0	<2	<2	56	8	+	+/−	−	17000	7.6	+
HMS-1	253	14	<2	<2	<2	183	3	+	+	−	21000	5.2	
Oxacillinases													
OXA-1	382	30	197	332	190	30	15	−	+/−	+	23300	7.4	+
OXA-2	179	15	646	23	200	37	25	−	−	+	44600	7.45, 7.7	
OXA-3	178	10	336	29	350	44	10	−	−	+	41200	7.1	
Carbenicillinases													
PSE-1	90	97	<2	<2	<2	18	<2	−	+		26500	5.7	+
PSE-2	267	121	317	803	371	32	<2		+		12400	6.1	
PSE-3	101	253			3	10			−		12000	6.9	
PSE-4	88	150	8	16	<2	40	4	−	−		32000	5.3	+

Abbreviations: Amp: Ampicillin; Carb: Carbenicillin; Oxa: Oxacillin; Clox: Cloxacillin; Cer: Cephaloridine; Cet: Cephalothin

TABLE II. Nomenclature of plasmid-determined β-lactamases

Matthew	Mitsuhashi	Pitton	Labia & Philippon	Richmond & Sykes
TEM-1 ('Temoniera', a patient's name)	Type 1a	TEM-1, type 1		IIIa
TEM-2	Type 1b			IIIa
SHV-1 (Sulphydryl variable)		TEM-1, type 2		IV
HMS-1 (Hedges, Matthew, & Smith)				
OXA-1 (Oxacillin-hydrolysing)	Type II			Va
OXA-2	Type III			Vb
OXA-3				V
PSE-1 (Pseudomonas-specific)	Type IV		CARB-2	V
PSE-2				V
PSE-3			CARB-4	V
PSE-4			CARB-1	V

The nomenclature of these β-lactamases has been a source of considerable confusion. Several investigators have applied different terms to the same enzymes, as shown in Table II. A particular problem arises when β-lactamases are labelled as host-specific, such as with the PSE β-lactamases. The gene determining PSE-1 was initially thought to be on a plasmid restricted to pseudomonas but was later found in clinical isolates of *E. coli*, salmonella,[29] *Serratia liquefaciens* (D. Livermore, personal communication) and *Proteus mirabilis*.[30]

a *Novel β-Lactamases*

More recent surveys of the types of β-lactamase produced by clinical isolates have revealed several novel β-lactamases determined by plasmids and one encoded by an unusual transposon (Table III). Three have a TEM-like substrate profile, five are OXA-type enzymes, one is a PSE-like carbenicillinase and another preferentially hydrolyses cephalosporins. It is likely that more β-lactamases will be discovered. Their characteristics will be of great clinical interest in relation to the range of β-lactam antibiotics available for therapeutic use.

The first of the novel TEM-like enzymes was discovered in a survey of several hundred clinical isolates of *E. coli* resistant to ampicillin.[31] *E. coli* 7604, one of 70 Brazilian strains studied, produced two β-lactamases, i.e. TEM-1 and an enzyme with a substrate profile and molecular weight similar to TEM-1 but with a different pI. The strain carried two plasmids, each of which determined a different β-lactamase along with resistance to other antibiotics.

cross-reactivity between members of these enzyme classes. Antisera to TEM-1 cross-reacts with TEM-2 (as would be expected since they differ in only a single amino acid).[27,28] Anti-TEM-1 also partially inactivates SHV-1 but does not inactivate HMS-1, or the OXA and PSE β-lactamases. Similarly, antisera to OXA-1 does not cross-react with OXA-2 or OXA-3. Antisera to PSE-1 and PSE-4 cross-react but do not inactivate the PSE-2 or PSE-3 β-lactamases. Antiserum to PSE-2, however, does not react with any of the other plasmid-determined β-lactamases.

TABLE III. New β-lactamases determined by plasmids or transposons

Name	Original host	Origin	Plasmid	Transposon	β-lactamase substrate profile	Mol. wt.	pI
	E. coli 7604	Brazil	pMG204b		TEM-like	19800	5.55
ROB-1	*H. influenzae* Rob	Baltimore	R$_{Rob}$		TEM-like		8.1
LCR-1	*P. aeruginosa* 2293E[33]	London	pMG76		TEM-like	44000	6.5 (5.85)*
OXA-4	*E. coli* 7529	Brazil	pMG203	+	OXA-like	23000	7.5
OXA-5	*P. aeruginosa* 76072601	London	pMG54	+	OXA-like	27000	7.62
OXA-6	*P. aeruginosa* Ming	Chicago	pMG329	+	OXA-like	40000	7.8
OXA-7	*E. coli* 7181	Brazil	pMG202		OXA-like	25000	7.65
	B. fragilis[35]	Japan			OXA-like	41500	6.9
AER-1	*A. hydrophila* VL 7711	India	—	Tn798	CARB-like	22000	5.9
CEP-2	*Achromobacter*[36,37] MULB 906	Quebec	pLQ3		Unique (cephalosporinase)	36200	8.1

* The pI value in parenthesis was obtained in our laboratory under experimental conditions different from those of Simpson[33]

The second was found in *Haemophilus influenzae* ROB, a type B strain isolated from a child with meningitis who failed to respond to ampicillin therapy.[32] Although the strain was resistant to ampicillin (minimum inhibitory concentration = 80 µg/ml), the nitrocefin test for β-lactamase was negative. The strain produced a β-lactamase, designated ROB-1, which resembled TEM-1 but hydrolysed carbenicillin at a slightly higher rate and cephaloridine at a lower rate relative to penicillin. The nitrocefin test was positive only with a very dense suspension of *H. influenzae* ROB. Plasmid DNA from *H. influenzae* ROB transformed *E. coli* C600 to ampicillin resistance with synthesis of the ROB enzyme. Sonic extracts of both the wild isolate and an *E. coli* transformant showed an unusual pattern on IEF, i.e. in addition to an enzyme band of pI 8.1, much activity remained at the anodic loading site on the gel, suggesting that enzyme was either an unusually large molecule or membrane-bound. In a survey of 50 ampicillin-resistant isolates of *H. influenzae* from USA, we have found one additional strain producing the ROB-1 enzyme (AA Medeiros, L Rubin, unpublished work).

A third TEM-like β-lactamase encoded by a P group plasmid was identified by Simpson in a carbenicillin-resistant burn isolate of *Pseudomonas aeruginosa*.[33] The β-lactamase had a somewhat higher activity against methicillin than TEM-1 but was otherwise similar in substrate profile. IEF showed a single band nearly equidistant between those of PSE-1 and PSE-2, clearly different from the TEM-1 banding pattern. Interestingly, a carbenicillin-sensitive pseudomonas isolate from the same patient shared a common small plasmid and identical chromosomal β-lactamases, indicating probable acquisition of the resistance plasmid.

Two of the four novel OXA-like β-lactamases were found among the Brazilian *E. coli* isolates, and the remainder in *P. aeruginosa*.[34] Determinants for OXA-4 and OXA-7 are carried out on plasmids which also mediate resistance to streptomycin, sulphonamide and mercury. They have banding patterns on IEF and pIs distinct from other OXA-like enzymes. The OXA-4 enzyme resembles OXA-1 in profile and molecular weight, whereas OXA-6 resembles the OXA-2 and OXA-3 enzymes in having high activity against oxacillin and a high molecular weight. OXA-7 also has high activity against oxacillin but is smaller in molecular weight. OXA-5 has an unusual substrate profile showing slightly higher activity against cloxacillin than oxacillin or methicillin. Of special interest, all four of these novel OXA-type β-lactamases are active against cefotaxime and two (OXA-4 and OXA-5) have low, but measurable, rates of hydrolysis of latamoxef by the pH stat method.

Sato *et al*.[35] reported a novel OXA-like β-lactamase of pI 6.9 and molecular weight 41 500 in a clinical isolate of *Bacteroides fragilis* GN11499. It hydrolysed ampicillin more rapidly than cloxacillin, an unusual pattern for the OXA-type enzymes. The phenotype was transferable by filter-mating to strains of *B. fragilis* and *B. vulgatus*.

A new carbenicillin-hydrolysing β-lactamase, designated AER-1, was found in a blood isolate of *Aeromonas hydrophila* from India (RW Hedges, AA Medeiros, M Cohenford, unpublished data). The enzyme has a pI of 5.9 and focuses slightly higher than the LCR-1 β-lactamase in polyacrylamide gel. Although no plasmid could be found in the clinical isolate, carbenicillin resistance determined by the AER-1 β-lactamase transferred to *E. coli* K12 along with resistance to streptomycin and sulphonamide when a plasmid (of incompatibility group P) was introduced into the host aeromonas. The β-lactamase genes are carried on an aberrant transposon (Tn798) which apparently fails to insert into any mobilizing plasmid but integrates into the *E. coli* K12 chromosome at a unique site, a property more typical of temperate phages.

Levesque *et al*.[36] discovered a plasmid-determined β-lactamase with a unique substrate profile in *Achromobacter* species. It had a pI of 8.1, a molecular weight of 36 200 daltons and it preferentially hydrolysed the cephalosporins. The substrate profile suggested that the CEP-2 enzyme, as it is now designated,[37] might be related to the chromosomal enzyme of *E. coli* K12. However, a higher relative activity against carbenicillin and resistance to inhibition by cloxacillin distinguish it from the chromosomal β-lactamase of *E. coli* K12. Also, after being transformed by plasmid DNA from the *Achromobacter* strain, *E. coli* RL1 produced two β-lactamases, one of low-level activity with pI of 9.8 and the novel cephalosporinase of pI 8.2. The former existed also in the plasmid-less strain and corresponds to the *ampC*-mediated chromosomal β-lactamase of *E. coli* K12. Thus CEP-2 clearly appears to be different from the *ampC*-determined β-lactamase of *E. coli* K12.

Kontomichalou *et al*.[38] had previously reported transfer from *Proteus mirabilis* to *E. coli* K12 of a plasmid which determined production of a cephalosporinase with identical biochemical properties to the K12 chromosomal β-lactamase.[39] Transfer of resistance to other strains of *E. coli* K12 was accompanied by acquisition of new plasmid DNA which shared homologous sequences with the resident Fsp plasmid of the K12 donor. Unfortunately, loss of enzymatic activity from the *P. mirabilis* donor during storage made it impossible to confirm the origin of the transferred β-lactamase gene.

Two *E. coli* K12 clones which acquired β-lactam resistance following mating with strains of *B. fragilis* and *B. vulgatus* produced large amounts of β-lactamase identical to the *E. coli* chromosomal β-lactamase by IEF. The donors, however, produced only β-lactamases of pI 4.7 and 4.9 characteristic of *Bacteroides* species (J Palomares, E Perea, AA Medeiros, unpublished data). No new plasmid DNA was identified in the *E. coli* strains (G Jacoby, personal communication). It is possible that a mutant which hyperproduces the chromosomal β-lactamase was selected during plating, although this occurs rarely. A more interesting possibility, currently under investigation, is that of a transferable genetic element inserted into the *E. coli* operon causing derepression of genes determining the chromosomal β-lactamase.

Conversely, Hafiz *et al*.[40] found that plasmid-containing strains of *Neisseria gonorrhoea* (including one freeze-dried in 1940) acquired the ability to produce β-lactamase upon losing sulphonamide resistance and postulate that the sulphonamide resistance genes suppressed the expression of β-lactamase plasmids.

Murray *et al*.[11] reported finding a clinical isolate of enterococcus which produced β-lactamase that co-transferred with gentamicin resistance. This is the first report of β-lactamase transfer among streptococci.

b *Transposons Determining β-Lactamases*

An increasing number of these β-lactamases are now known to be encoded by transposons,[6] genetic elements capable of transfer among a wide variety of plasmids and between plasmids and chromosomes. Three of the TEM-like β-lactamases are encoded by transposons. TEM-1 is determined by Tn3,[41] and TEM-2 by Tn1, which shares much homology with Tn3.[42] SHV-1, on the other hand, is encoded by a transposon of 15 kilobase pairs (kb) unrelated to Tn1.[43]

Several of the OXA-like β-lactamases and the CARB-type enzymes also are encoded by transposons, some of which are complex units carrying multiple resistance determinants. A 21 kb transposon, Tn2603, determines the OXA-1 β-lactamase along with resistance to streptomycin, sulphonamide and mercury.[44] PSE-1 and PSE-4 are determined by transposons which also carry resistance determinants to streptomycin and sulphonamides and, variably, to mercury.[29,45] A similar linkage of resistance determinants occurs as well in a 22kb transposon, Tn4, which includes Tn3 within its length.[46] The unusual transposon (Tn 798) discussed above, which encodes the AER-1 β-lactamase, also carries resistance to streptomycin and sulphonamides. Yamamoto et al.[47] have emphasized the frequent occurrence of this linkage of resistance determinants (often in conjunction with chloramphenicol and mercury resistance) in transposons encoding different β-lactamases, and have suggested that they may have evolved from a common ancestral transposon.

Overall, six of the well-established plasmid-determined β-lactamases in gram-negative bacteria and four of the novel β-lactamases are determined by transposons (Tables I and III). There is also evidence that a previously described carbenicillin-hydrolysing enzyme from P. aeruginosa, CARB-3,[48] is encoded by a transposon (G Jacoby, personal communication). In addition, Yamamoto et al.[47] recently reported finding in clinical isolates of E. coli, a new transposon which determines a carbenicillin-hydrolysing β-lactamase as yet uncharacterized.

c Distribution in Clinical Isolates

The existence of β-lactamase genes on plasmids and transposons ensures that β-lactamases confined to one group of bacteria sooner or later appear in other groups. Widespread use of antibiotics fosters selection of the resistant organisms which rise in prevalence locally, then spread worldwide. A prime example of this process occurred with the TEM-1 β-lactamase common in enterobacteria. In 1972 strains of H. influenzae producing TEM-1 were first discovered in USA. Rare at first, they have since reached prevalence levels of 38% in some regions.[49] In 1976, strains of N. gonorrhoea producing the plasmid-determined TEM-1 β-lactamase appeared.[50,51] The incidence of gonorrhoea caused by these strains in USA rose from 328 cases in 1979 to 3424 cases reported in the first nine months of 1982, while similar increases in incidence occurred in other countries.[52] Recently, a β-lactamase producing strain of N. meningitidis carrying a plasmid identical to one found in penicillinase-producing N. gonorrhoea was isolated from mixed culture from a patient in Canada. It is believed that the isolate originated in the genitourinary tract and acquired the plasmid by in-vivo transfer from a strain of penicillinase-producing N. gonorrhoea.[53]

The different plasmid-determined β-lactamases, identified by IEF, exhibit different distributions among bacterial genera.[21,54-57] The largest numbers of different types of β-lactamases were found in P. aeruginosa (11) and E. coli (10), followed by P. mirabilis, Klebsiella species, and Salmonella species with five types each. Evidence of the dissemination of β-lactamase

genes is the finding of OXA-1 (A Phillipon, personal communication) and OXA-2 in P. aeruginosa and PSE-1 in E. coli Salmonella (four species), Serratia liquefaciens, and Shigella sonnei. The E. coli isolates which produced PSE-1 came from Brazil, Hong Kong, Indonesia and Thailand while the salmonella isolates came from the USA. The shigella isolate is particularly interesting in that it was obtained from a patient in Canada who acquired it in Brazil, emphasizing the potential for spread of resistance between countries.

The rarest of the well-established β-lactamases is HMS-1, found once only, in an isolate of P. mirabilis.[22] The commonest is TEM-1 which occurred with an overall frequency of 77% among strains studied by Matthew[21] and is most widely distributed geographically. Surveys of ampicillin-resistant E. coli strains from different countries showed some variation in the distribution of β-lactamases, with TEM-1 always the commonest (Table IV). Thirteen percent of isolates produced chromosomal β-lactamase only. The Brazilian collection was extraordinary in that three novel β-lactamases and PSE-1 were found. It is curious, also, that no Brazilian strains had resistance due to chromosomal β-lactamase, which was also true of the strains from Indonesia and Thailand.

In other species, TEM-1 is not the most prevalent β-lactamase. Marre found that all of 16 strains of ampicillin-resistant P. mirabilis isolated in Germany produced TEM-2 (R Marre, personal communication). Philippon, on the other hand, found the following distribution of β-lactamases in 1400 carbenicillin-resistant pseudomonas isolates in Paris: PSE-1 = 51%; OXA-2 = 30%; OXA-1 = 7%; TEM-1 = 5% (A Philippon, personal communication). The extent to which these distributions represent the continued recirculation of a single strain within a particular geographic region is unknown.

There is evidence also that β-lactamase genes may circulate between animal and human isolates. In a study of 113 human and 146 animal isolates of ampicillin-resistant salmonellae from USA, 81% and 77% of human and animal isolates respectively produced TEM-1, similar to results with E. coli[56] (AA Medeiros, TF O'Brien, unpublished work). However, the second commonest β-lactamase in both human and animal isolates was OXA-2, a rare type in E. coli. Moreover, most of the OXA-2-producing isolates belonged to a relatively rare sterotype, i.e., S. typhimurium, var. copenhagen. This unexpected association in both human and animal isolates suggested that they shared the same resistance determinants. Indeed, endonuclease digests of plasmids from isolates of S. typhimurium, var. copenhagen showed that the plasmids from animal and human isolates from different regions of USA were often identical.[58]

TABLE IV. Types of β-lactamases in clinical isolates of ampicillin-resistant *E. coli* from different regions

Geographic origin	Chromosomal only	TEM-1	SHV-1	OXA-1	OXA-2	PSE-1	Novel	TEM-1 + PSE-1	TEM-1 + OXA-1	TEM-1 + Novel	Total
Brazil	0	71 (72)	6	10 (10)		2	3	2	3	1	98 (10)
Providence	6 (12)	41 (82)		2 (4)	1						50
Paris	3 (14)	16 (76)			2						21
Indonesia	0	9 (82)		1 (9)		1					11
South Africa	16 (34)	23 (49)		5 (11)					3		47
Boston	6 (18)	27 (79)		1 (11)							34
Bangkok	0	27 (93)						1	1		29
England (Simpson et al[57])	18	73 (66)	1	17 (16)					1		110
Germany (R Marre, personal communication)	13 (16)	62 (74)	1	8 (10)							84
Total	62 (13)	349 (72)	8 (2)	44 (9)	3	3	3	3	8 (2)	1	484 (10)

() = percent of total.

TABLE V. The β-lactamases of some epidemic strains of ampicillin-resistant salmonellae*

Strain	Source	Plasmid	Inc group	Resistance markers	β-lactamase type
S. typhimurium	Iran	TP181	F‚me	ACKSSuSpT	OXA-1
S. typhi	Algeria	TP160	F‚me	ACKSSuSp	OXA-1
S. typhimurium	UK	NTP101	F‚me	ACSSuSpT	OXA-1
S. wien	Paris				OXA-1
S. ordonnez	Dakar				SHV-1

* The *S. typhimurium* and *S. typhi* strains were received from John Threlfall and the others from Alain Philippon

TABLE VI. Isolates producing multiple plasmid-determined β-lactamases

β-lactamase type	Species	Origin	Number of isolates
TEM-1 + OXA-1	E. coli	Thailand	1
	E. coli	Brazil	3
	E. coli	S. Africa	3
	P. mirabilis		1
	S. st. paul	USA	1
TEM-1 + OXA-2	E. coli	Paris	1
	P. stuartii	Argentina	1
	S. typhimurium var. copenhagen	USA	1
TEM-1 + OXA-3	K. pneumoniae	Boston	1
TEM-1 + PSE-1	E. coli	Brazil	2
	E. coli	Thailand	1
	S. heidelberg	USA	1
	S. johannisberg	Hong Kong	1
TEM-1 + SHV-1	Morganella morganii[57]	England	1
	K. pneumoniae	Boston	1
TEM-1 + "pMG204b"	E. coli	Brazil	1
OXA-2 + PSE-1	P. aeruginosa	Boston	4
TEM-1 + OXA-2 + PSE-1	P. aeruginosa	Boston	1

The prevalence of different β-lactamases can be expected to vary in time and place when strains become epidemic. Table V underscores this point by showing the different types of β-lactamase produced by strains which caused large-scale epidemics of salmonellosis in Europe, Africa, and the Middle East (AA Medeiros, unpublished work).

Table VI lists isolates known to produce two and, in one instance, three plasmid-determined β-lactamases. In all but one case, TEM-1 was one of the β-lactamases produced. The strain of *P. aeruginosa* which produced OXA-2 plus PSE-1 as well as the single isolate which also produced TEM-1 came from an outbreak of infections in a children's hospital in Boston. Interestingly, a single plasmid, pMG209, carried both the TEM-1 and PSE-1 genes.[29] The high proportion of strains from South America and the Far East which produced two plasmid-mediated β-lactamases and which had novel β-lactamases suggests that the bacterial flora of those regions provides fertile ground for cultivating new resistance mechanisms.

3 β-Lactamases Determined by Chromosomal Genes

Matthew & Harris[10] found that virtually all gram-negative bacteria produce some chromosomally-determined β-lactamase and that the types of β-lactamase produced are often specific for species and sometimes for subspecies.[59,60] The amount of β-lactamase activity is frequently very low, particularly in ampicillin-susceptible isolates, but may increase because of induction or alterations in the number of β-lactamase genes on the chromosome or their regulation.[61,62] These genetic alterations are often accompanied by resistance to β-lactam antibiotics.

Most of the chromosomally-determined β-lactamases preferentially hydrolyse the cephalosporins, including many of the newer β-lactams which are resistant to hydrolysis by the plasmid-determined β-lactamases. Sawai[63] describes two major groups: (1) 'cephalosporinases with broad substrate specificity' which hydrolyse benzylpenicillin, ampicillin, and carbenicillin as well as cephalosporins, and (2) 'typical cephalosporinases' which have little or no activity against these penicillins.

A prototypic enzyme of the first group is the inducible β-lactamase produced by *Proteus vulgaris*. Another important broad-spectrum enzyme is that produced by *Klebsiella pneumoniae* which some classify as a 'penicillinase'. Indole + strains of *Klebsiella* have been described which have activity against cefuroxime and monobactams, i.e. *K. aerogenes* K1[64] and *K. oxytoca*.[65] Gentamicin-resistant strains of the latter species caused an outbreak in a Liverpool hospital.[65] β-lactamase from one of the isolates from that outbreak, *K. oxytoca* 3859, is active against latamoxef and ceftazidime as well as cefuroxime.

β-lactamases of many species comprise the 'typical cephalosporinase' group. They are the constitutive enzymes produced by *Proteus morganii*, *Citrobacter freundii*, *Enterobacter cloacae*, *E. coli*, and *B. fragilis*. Inducible enzymes produced by *Enterobacter aerogenes*, *Enterobacter cloacae*, *Providencia rettgeri*, *Pseudomonas aeruginosa*, *Acinetobacter anitratum* and *Serratia marcescens* also belong to this latter category. As newer β-lactam antibiotics have become available, their interaction with β-lactamases has led to further classification schemes. Thus Mitsuhashi classifies the β-lactamases of *P. cepacia*, *P. vulgaris*, and *B. fragilis* as cefuroximases while Labia divides the β-lactamases into groups based on their affinity for latamoxef and the degree to which they are inactivated by it.[66]

Saino et al.[67] have found a novel β-lactamase in *Pseudomonas maltophilia* GN 12873 which destroys *N*-formimodoyl thienamycin. Thus, it appears likely that no class of β-lactam antibiotic escapes attack by some β-lactamase. Table VII lists β-lactamases, both chromosomally-mediated and plasmid-mediated, which hydrolyse newer β-lactam antibiotics. Strains producing both plasmid- and chromosomally-determined enzymes pose a potentially serious threat.

With one exception, none of these chromosomally-determined β-lactamases are identical in their biochemical properties to the plasmid-determined enzymes. The exception is a chromosomal β-lactamase found in many isolates of *K. pneumoniae*, which is indistinguishable by kinetic analysis and IEF from the SHV-1 β-lactamase. Nugent & Hedges[43] found that *K. pneumoniae* 1529E, carried two copies of the SHV-1 structural gene, one on a plasmid

TABLE VII. Some β-lactamases which hydrolyse the newer β-lactam antibiotics

Antibiotic	β-Lactamase type	
	Chromosomal	Plasmid
Cefuroxime or cefotaxime	P. cepacia GN11164[68]	OXA-1
	P. vulgaris GN 7919[69]	OXA-4
	B. fragilis MULB-1008[70]	OXA-5
	K. oxytoca R30[71]	OXA-6
	K. aerogenes K1[64]	OXA-7
	(indole +)	PSE-1
		PSE-2
Ceftazidime		OXA-1
		OXA-2
Latamoxef	K. oxytoca 3859[65]	OXA-4
		OXA-5
		PSE-2
		PSE-3
Monobactams	K. oxytoca 3859[65]	
	K. aerogenes K-1[72]	
	(indole +)	
Imipenam	P. maltophilia GN12873[67]	

(R1293) and another on a non-transmissible replicon, probably the bacterial chromosome. They suggest that the SHV-1 β-lactamase gene evolved as a chromosomal gene in *Klebsiella* and was later incorporated into a plasmid. As yet no such ancestral chromosomal gene has been found for the much more common TEM-1 β-lactamase nor for any of the other plasmid-determined β-lactamases. Thus the origins of most of the plasmid-determined β-lactamases remain unknown.

4 Contribution of β-Lactamases to β-Lactam Antibiotic Resistance

Several parameters contribute to the level of antibiotic resistance mediated by a particular β-lactamase in a population of bacteria. The efficiency of the β-lactamase in hydrolysing an antibiotic depends both on its rate of hydrolysis (V_{max}), usually expressed as a ratio relative to benzylpenicillin or cephaloridine, and its affinity for the antibiotic (K_m), a value often difficult to obtain with substrates which are weakly hydrolysed. Another variable is the amount of β-lactamase produced by the bacterial cell. Since the amount may vary with phase of cell growth or even conditions of incubation,[62] a single value may be misleading. An example is J53-R997, an *E. coli* K12 strain which produces the plasmid-determined HMS-1 β-lactamase. The strain was highly resistant to ampicillin yet we could find barely detectable levels of β-lactamase activity in sonic extracts of overnight cells. Extracts of cells in log phase, however, unexpectedly yielded values 100 times greater.[73]

Within the bacterial cell, β-lactamases contribute to antibiotic resistance in several ways. The simplest model is that of penicillinase-producing staphylococci in which the bacteria, upon exposure to penicillin, begin to produce β-lactamase which they excrete into the medium. Two events then take place concurrently: (1) penicillin lyses bacteria, and (2) β-lactamase hydrolyses penicillin. If viable bacterial cells remain after the level of penicillin has fallen below the minimal inhibitory concentration, regrowth of bacteria occurs.[74]

The second model shows a similar kinetic effect. It is exemplified by gram-negative bacilli which (a) produce a β-lactamase that remains trapped in the periplasmic space, and which (b) have no barrier to antibiotic penetration. An example is *H. influenza* strains that produce the TEM-1 β-lactamase.[75] In both of these models a marked inoculum effect occurs in which MICs of antibiotic using small inocula (c. 10^2 CFU/ml) may rise a thousandfold using large inocula (c. 10^6 CFU/ml). The low level of resistance of single cells has made it possible for ampicillin to cure some infections caused by β-lactamase-producing strains *H. influenza*, when the inoculum of infecting bacteria was low.[76,77]

The third model is exemplified by resistance to ampicillin of *E. coli* strains which produce the TEM-1 β-lactamase. These bacteria have a barrier to entry of β-lactam molecules (the outer membrane) and they produce a β-lactamase which remains localized to the periplasmic space. In this model, the kinetics are more complicated. The enzymes which are strategically situated between the antibiotic penetration barrier (outer membrane) and the antibiotic targets (PBPs on the cytoplasmic membrane) can sequentially destroy antibiotic molecules as they make their way through the barrier, analogous to a rifleman with abundant ammunition who aims at targets passing through a single entry point. As a consequence, high levels of resistance occur with single bacterial cells, unlike the previous example.[74,78,79]

Variations on this model may occur when the amount of β-lactamase produced increases with exposure to a β-lactam (induction), as occurs in enterobacter and pseudomonas species. High levels of β-lactamase are produced only after a period of exposure to the inducing antibiotic, and so resistance may be expressed late. This sometimes causes a problem for the clinical microbiologist, in that the disk susceptibility test may give falsely susceptible results. An example occurs with disk testing for susceptibility to cefamandole of enterobacter strains, which falsely appear susceptible unless pre-incubated with cefamandole prior to testing. A further problem arises when enterobacter strains are exposed to two β-lactam antibiotics, one of which is a potent inducer (e.g. cefoxitin) of a β-lactamase highly active against the other (e.g. cefamandole). Antagonism between the two antibiotics results.[80]

One of the more puzzling aspects of this antagonism is that, for some antibiotics, the induced enzyme hydrolyses the 'antagonized' antibiotic (e.g. carbenicillin) poorly or not at all. It has been postulated that the β-lactamases protect the cell by binding rather than splitting the antibiotic molecules, acting in a sense as periplasmic sponges which keep the antibiotics from reaching their target sites on the cytoplasmic membrane.[81–83] However, not all antibiotics (e.g. *N*-formimodoyl thienamycin) that bind tightly to the induced enterobacter β-lactamase are antagonized.[84] which suggests that additional mechanisms may be operative.

Wiedemann has objected to this concept of binding as a sole resistance mechanism on the grounds that the amount of enzyme required to block the antibiotic is probably in excess of the amount present in the bacterial cell (B Wiedemann, personal communication). Our own calculations support this objection, if one assumes that one molecule of enzyme binds one molecule of antibiotic. In order for a β-lactamase of 30 000 mol. wt. to block the action of 1 μg/ml of latamoxef on 10^5 bacterial cells/ml, approximately 0.5 ng of pure β-lactamase protein are needed in each cell. The measured amount of total protein per bacterial cell, in our hands, is usually about 2 pg. This order of magnitude difference makes it unlikely that non-hydrolytic binding can fully explain these antagonisms.

An alternative explanation is that the enzyme–substrate complex of β-lactamase and inducing β-lactam blocks certain penicillin binding proteins making them inaccessible to attack by other β-lactams. In support of this hypothesis is the fact that some 'antagonized' antibiotics (e.g. carbenicillin) produce, over a broad concentration range, effects on bacteria (e.g. filament formation in enterobacter) which occur only over a narrow concentration range in the absence of inducer. This suggests that the carbenicillin molecules may have been diverted to other target sites, i.e. those which determine filamentation.[80]

Documented treatment failures due to emergence of resistance during therapy were rare prior to the use of third-generation cephalosporins.[85] There has been, however, a recent increase in such reports, mainly in patients treated with cefamandole, cefoxitin, cefotaxime, latamoxef, ceftazidime and ceftriaxone for infections due to *Enterobacter*, *Serratia*, and *Pseudomonas* species.[86–89] A disturbing feature of some of these reports is that the strains isolated during therapy with one cephalosporin have decreased susceptibility to other third-generation cephalosporins, such as latamoxef, cefamandole, cefotaxime, and cefoperazone.[90] Studies of treatment failures due to emergence of resistance in enterobacter during cefamandole treatment have shown that the resistant strains produce increased amounts of β-lactamase[91] probably due to mutation in the locus regulating β-lactamase expression.[92] Increase in production of chromosomal β-lactamase has been found also in strains of *E. coli* isolated from patients who failed treatment with cephalothin[93] and ampicillin.[94]

Acquired resistance to cephalosporins has been found also in a strain of *Salmonella typhimurium* isolated from a patient during treatment with cephalexin, in which the resistant isolate had acquired a permeability barrier to cephalosporins but showed no increase in β-lactamase production.[95] The resistant mutant produces only one of the two porins, protein channels through which β-lactams enter the bacterial cell, produced by the parent strain. (H Nikaido, personal communication). This provides an example of another type of resistance mechanism acquired during therapy. The potential threat of selecting resistant strains during therapy with the newer β-lactam antibiotics has led some clinicians to recommend combined therapy with aminoglycosides, especially in treating *Enterobacter, Serratia,* and *Pseudomonas* infections.

5 Conclusions

Clinical pathogens worldwide possess a vast armoury of β-lactamases, the genetic determinants for many of which can be transferred from one bacterial cell to another, even across boundaries of species and genera. Consequently, clinical isolates often have the capacity to produce several β-lactamases in response to antibiotic selection pressures. Also, alterations may occur in the genes which regulate the production of these enzymes resulting in hyperproduction of β-lactamase, often in direct response to exposure to the antibiotic. In addition, as Abraham & Chain[2] surmised, the β-lactamases are not the sole factors determining resistance. They are known to interact with permeability barriers, and probably with PBPs in effecting resistance. Little is known yet of the interaction between β-lactamases and the cytoplasmic membrane in clinical isolates. It seems likely, however, that this structure which regulates the secretion of β-lactamase protein into the periplasm[96] will be found to contribute to β-lactam antibiotic resistance as well. All of these elements would seemingly guarantee that clinical pathogens will continue to manifest remarkable virtuosity in counteracting new β-lactam antibiotics.

ACKNOWLEDGEMENTS

I thank George Jacoby, Margaret Matthew and Thomas F. O'Brien for many helpful discussions. This work was supported by The Miriam Hospital Research Trust.

REFERENCES

1 Fleming. A. On antibacterial action of cultures of a penicillium with special reference to their use in isolation of *B. influenzae.* Br J Exp Path 1929; 10: 226–235

2 Abraham EP, Chain E. An enzyme from bacteria able to destroy penicillin. Nature 1940; 146: 837

3 Kirby WMM. Extraction of a highly potent penicillin inactivator from penicillin resistant staphylococci. Science 1944; 99: 452–453

4 Matthew M, Harris AM, Marshall M, Ross GW. The use of analytical isoelectric focusing for detection and identification of β-lactamases. J Gen Microbiol 1975; 88: 169–178

5 Datta N, Knotomichalou P. Penicillinase synthesis controlled by infectious R factors in Enterobacteriaceae. Nature 1965; 208: 239–241

6 Hedges RW, Jacob AE. Transposition of ampicillin resistance from RP4 to other replicons. Mol Gen Genet 1974; 132: 31–40

7 Brown AG. β-lactam nomenclature. J Antimicrob Chemother 1982; 10: 365–368

8 Richmond MH. Wild-type variants of exopenicillinase from *Staphylococcus aureus* Biochem J 1965; 94: 584–593

9 Dyke KGH. β-lactamases of *Staphylococcus aureus.* In: Hamilton-Miller JMT, Smith JT, eds. Beta-lactamases. London: Academic Press, 1979; 291–310

10 Matthew M, Harris AM. Identification of β-lactamases by analytical isoelectric focusing: correlation with bacterial taxonomy. J Gen Microbiol 1976; 94: 55–67

11 Murray BE, Mederskisamoraj, B. Transferrable β-lactamase in a clinical isolate of *Streptococcus faecalis.* In: Program and abstracts of the twenty-second interscience conference on antimicrobial agents and chemotherapy. Miami Beach: American Society for Microbiology, 1982; 714

12 Sawai T, Mitsuhashi S, Yamagishi S. Drug resistance of enterobacteria. 14. Comparison of β-lactamases in gram-negative rod bacteria resistant to alpha-aminobenzylpenicillin. Jpn J Microbiol 1968; 12: 423–434

13 Jack GW, Richmond MH. A comparative study of eight distinct β-lactamases synthesized by gram-negative bacteria. J Gen Microbiol 1970; 61: 43–61

14 Richmond MH, Sykes RB. The β-lactamases of gram-negative bacteria and their possible physiological role. In: Rose AH, Tempest DW, eds. Advances in Microbial Physiology. London and New York: Academic Press, 1973; 9: 31–88

15 Ambler RP. The structure of β-lactamases. Philos Trans R Soc Lond [Biol] 1980; 289: 321–331

16 Bergström S, Olsson O, Normark S. Common evolutionary origin of chromosomal beta-lactamase genes in enterobacteria. J Bacteriol 1982; 150: 528–534

17 Yocum RR, Waxman, DJ, Rasmussen JR, Strominger JL. Mechanism of penicillin action: penicillin and substrate bind covalently to the same active site serine in two bacterial D-alanine carboxypeptidases. Proc Natl Acad Sci USA 1979; 76: 2730–2734

18 Waxman DJ, Amanuma H, Strominger JL. Amino acid sequence homologies between *Escherichia coli* penicillin-binding protein 5 and class A β-lactamases. FEBS Lett 1982; 139: 159–163

19 Jaurin B, Grundström T. *AmpC* cephalosporinase of *Escherichia coli* K-12 has a different evolutionary origin from that of β-lactamases of the penicillinase type. Proc Natl Acad Sci USA 1981; 78: 4897–4901

20 Knott-Hunziker V, Petursson S, Jayatilake GS, Waley SG, Jaurin B, Grundström T. Active sites of β-lactamases. The chromosomal β-lactamases of *Pseudomonas aeruginosa* and *Escherichia coli.* Biochem J 1982; 201: 621–627

21 Matthew M, Plasmid-mediated β-lactamases of gram-negative bacteria: properties and distribution. J Antimicrob Chemother 1979; 5: 349–358

22 Matthew M, Hedges RW, Smith JT. Types of β-lactamase determined by plasmids in gram-negative bacteria. J Bacteriol 1979; 138: 657–662

23 Vecoli C, Prevost FE, Ververis JJ, Medeiros AA. A comparison of polyacrylamide and agarose gel thin-layer isoelectric focusing for the characterization of beta-lactamase. Antimicrob Agents Chemother 1983; 24: 186–189

24 Simpson IN, Plested SJ, Harper PB. Investigation of the β-lactamase stability of ceftazidime and eight other new cephalosposin antibiotics. J Antimicrob Chemother 1982; 9: 357–368

25 Sykes RB, Matthew M. Detection, assay and immunology of beta-lactamases. In: Hamilton-Miller JMT, Smith JT, eds, Beta-lactamases. London: Academic Press, 1979: 17–49

26 Paul G, Philippon A, Barthelemy M, Labia R, Nevot P. Immunological distinction between constitutive beta-lactamases of gram-negative rods with antisera TEM-1 and CARB-3. In: Program and abstracts of the 21st interscience conference on antimicrobial agents and chemotherapy. Chicago: American Society for Microbiology, 1981; 681

27 Sutcliffe JG. Nucleotide sequence of the ampicillin resistance gene of *Escherichia coli* plasmid pBR322. Proc Natl Acad Sci USA 1978; 75: 3737–3741

28 Ambler RP, Scott GK. Partial amino acid sequence of penicillinase coded by *Escherichia coli* plasmid R6K. Proc Natl Acad Sci USA 1978; 75: 3732–3736

29 Medeiros AA, Hedges RW, Jacoby GA. Spread of a "*Pseudomonas*-specific" beta-lactamase to plasmids of enterobacteria. J Bacteriol 1982; 149: 700–707

30 Katsu K, Inoue M, Mitsuhashi S. Plasmid-mediated carbenicillin hydrolyzing beta-lactamases of *Proteus mirabilis.* J Antibiot 1981; 34: 1504–1506

31 Medeiros AA, Ximenez J, Blickstein-Goldworm K, O'Brien TF, Acar, J. β-lactamases of ampicillin-resistant *Escherichia coli* from Brazil, France and the United States. In: Nelson JD, Grassi, C, eds. Current chemotherapy and infectious disease. Washington DC: American Society for Microbiology, 1980; 761–762

32 Rubin LG, Medeiros AA, Yolken RH, Moxon ER. Ampicillin treatment failure of apparently β-lactamase-negative *Haemophilus influenzae* type b meningitis due to novel β-lactamase. Lancet 1981; ii: 1008–1010

33 Simpson IN, Plested SJ, Budin-Jones MJ, Lees J, Hedges RW, Jacoby GA. Characterization of a novel plasmid-mediated beta-lactam resistance in *Pseudomonas aeruginosa.* FEMS Microbiol Lett 1983; 19: 23–27

34 Medeiros AA, Jacoby GA. Five novel plasmid-determined beta-lactamases found in *E. coli* and pseudomonas. In: Program and abstracts of the twenty-second interscience conference in antimicrobial agents and chemotherapy. Miami Beach: American Society for Microbiology, 1982; 191

35 Sato K, Matsuura Y, Inoue M, Mitsuhashi S. Properties of a new penicillinase type produced by *Bacteriodes fragilis*. Antimicrob Agents Chemother 1982; 22: 579–584

36 Levesque R, Roy P, Letarte R, Pechere J-C. A plasmid-mediated cephalosporinase from *Achromobacter* species. J Infect Dis 1982; 145: 753–761

37 Levesque R, Roy PH. Mapping on the plasmid (pLQ3) from Achromobacter and cloning of its cephalosporin gene in *Escherichia coli*. Gene 1982; 18: 69–75

38 Kontomichalou PM, Papachristou EG, Levis G. R-mediated β-lactamases and episomal resistance to the β-lactam drugs in different bacterial hosts. Antimicrob Agents Chemother 1974; 6: 60–72

39 Bobrowski MM, Matthew M, Barth PT *et al*. Plasmid-determined β-lactamase indistinguishable from the chromosomal β-lactamase of *Escherichia coli*. J Bacteriol 1976; 125: 149–157

40 Hafiz S, McEntegart MG, Gooch H. Did *Neisseria gonorrhoeae* acquire the ability to produce β-lactamase in 1976? Lancet 1982; i: 558

41 Heffron FR, Kostriken R, Morita C, Parker R. Tn3—Encodes a site-specific recombination system: Identification of essential sequences, genes, and the actual site of recombination. Cold Spring Harbor Symp Quant Biol 1981; 45: 259–268

42 Rubens, C, Heffron F, Falkow S. Transposition of a plasmid deoxyribonucleic acid sequence that mediates ampicillin resistance: Independence from host *rec* functions and orientation of insertion. J Bacteriol 1976; 128: 425–434

43 Nugent ME, Hedges RW. The nature of the genetic determinant for the SHV-1 beta-lactamase. Mol Gen Genet 1979; 175: 239–243

44 Yamamoto T, Tanaka M, Nohara C, Fukunaga U, Yamagishi S. Transposition of the oxacillin-hydrolyzing penicillinase gene. J Bacteriol 1981; 145: 808–813

45 Katsu K, Inoue M, Mitsuhashi S. Transposition of the carbenicillin-hydrolyzing beta-lactamase gene. J Bacteriol 1982; 150: 483–489

46 Hyde DR, Tu C-PD. Insertion sites and the terminal nucleotide sequences of the Tn4 transposon. Nucleic Acids Res 1982; 10: 3981–3993

47 Yamamoto T, Watanabe M, Matsumoto K, Sawai T. Tn2610, a transposon involved in the spread of the carbenicillin-hydrolyzing β-lactamase gene. Mol Gen Genet 1983; 189: 282–288

48 Labia R, Guionie M, Barthelemy M. Properties of three carbenicillin-hydrolyzing beta-lactamases (CARB) from *Pseudomonas aeruginosa*: identification of a new enzyme. J Antimicrob Chemother 1981; 7: 49–56

49 Thornsberry C, McDougal LK. Ampicillin-resistant *Haemophilus influenzae*. 1. Incidence, mechanism, and detection. Postgrad Med 1982; 71: 133–145

50 Percival A, Rowlands J, Corkhill JE *et al*. Penicillinase-producing gonococci in Liverpool. Lancet 1976; 2: 1379–1382

51 Perine PL, Thornsberry C, Schalla W *et al*. Evidence for two distinct types of penicillinase-producing *Neisseria gonorrhoeae*. Lancet 1977; ii: 993–995

52 Centers for Disease Control. Global distribution of penicillinase-producing *Neisseria gonorrhoeae* (PPNG). Conn Med 1982; 46: 223

53 Dillon JR, Pauzé M, Yeung KH. Spread of penicillinase-producing and transfer plasmids from the gonococcus to *Neisseria meningitidis*. Lancet 1983; 1: 779–781

54 Medeiros AA, Ximenez J, Blickstein-Goldworm K, O'Brien TF, Acar J. β-lactamases of ampicillin-resistant *Escherichia coli* from Brazil, France, and the United States. In: Nelson JD, Grassi C, eds. Current chemotherapy and infectious disease. Washington DC: American Society for Microbiology, 1980; 761–762

55 Jacoby GA, Sutton L, Medeiros AA. Plasmid-determined β-lactamase of *Pseudomonas aeruginosa*. In: Nelson JD, Grassi C, eds. Current chemotherapy and infectious disease. Washington DC: American Society for Microbiology, 1980; 769–771

56 Medeiros AA, Gilleece ES, O'Brien TF. Distribution of plasmid type β-lactamases in ampicillin-resistant salmonellae from humans and animals in the United States. In: Levy SB, Clowes RC, Koenig EL, eds. Molecular biology, pathogenicity, and ecology of bacterial plasmids. New York: Plenum Press, 1981; 634

57 Simpson IN, Harper PB, O'Callaghan CH. Principal β-lactamases responsible for resistance to β-lactam antibiotics in urinary tract infections. Antimicrob Agents Chemother 1980; 17: 929–936

58 O'Brien TF, Hopkins JD, Gilleece ES *et al*. Molecular epidemiology of antibiotic resistance in salmonella from animals and human beings in the United States. N Engl J Med 1982: 307: 1–6

59 Mathew M, Cornelis G, Wauters G. Correlation of serological and biochemical groups of *Yersinia enterocolitica* with the β-lactamases of the strains. J Gen Microbiol 1977: 102: 55–59

60 Marre R, Medeiros AA, Pascule AW. Characterization of the beta-lactamases of six species of *Legionella*. J Bacteriol 1982; 151: 216–221

61 Normark S, Edlund T, Grundström T, Bergstrom S, Wolf-Watz H. *Escherichia coli* K-12 hyperproducing chromosomal β-lactamase by gene repetitions. J Bacteriol 1977; 132: 912–922

62 Jaurin B, Grundstrom T, Edlund T, Normark S. The *E. coli* β-lactamase attenuator mediates growth rate-dependent regulation. Nature 1981; 290: 221–225

63 Sawai T, Kanno M, Tsukamoto K. Characterization of eight β-lactamases of gram-negative bacteria. J Bacteriol 1982; 152: 567–571

64 Richmond MH. The β-lactamase stability of a novel β-lactam antibiotic containing a 7α-methoxyoxacephem nucleus. J Antimicrob Chemother 1980; 6: 445–453

65 Hart CA, Percival A. Resistance to cephalosporins among gentamicin-resistant klebsiellae. J Antimicrob Chemother 1982; 9: 275–286

66 Labia R. Moxalactam: An oxa-β-lactam antibiotic that inactivates β-lactamases. Rev. Infect Dis 1982; 4 (suppl): S529–S535

67 Saino Y, Kobayashi F, Inoue M, Mitsuhashi S. Purification and properties of inducible penicillin β-lactamase isolated from *Pseudomonas maltophilia*. Antimicrob Agents Chemother 1982; 22: 564–570

68 Hirai K, Iyobe S, Inoue M, Mitsuhashi S. Purification and properties of a new β-lactamase from *Pseudomonas cepacia*. Antimicrob Agents Chemother 1980; 17: 355–358

69 Matsubara N, Yotsuji A, Kumano K, Inoue M, Mitsuhashi S. Purification and some properties of a cephalosporinase from *Proteus vulgaris*. Antimicrob Agents Chemother 1981; 19: 185–187

70 Pechère JC, Guay R, Dubois J, Letarte R. Hydrolysis of cefotaxime by a beta-lactamase from *Bacteroides fragilis*. Antimicrob Agents Chemother 1980; 17: 1001–1003

71 Labia R, Kazmierczak A, Guionie M, Masson JM. Some bacterial proteins with affinity for cefotaxime. J Antimicrob Chemother 1980; 6 (suppl A): 19–23

72 Sykes RB, Bonner DP, Bush K, Georgopapadakou NH, Wells JS. Monobactams—monocyclic β-lactam antibiotics produced by bacteria. J Antimicrob Chemother 1981; 8 (suppl E): 1–16

73 Bisson JW, Medeiros AA. Effect of growth phase on production of plasmid-determined β-lactamase by β-lactam resistant bacteria. In: Abstracts of the annual meeting of the American society of microbiology. Dallas: American Society for Microbiology 1981: 11

74 Sykes RB, Matthew M. The β-lactamases of gram-negative bacteria and their role in resistance to β-lactam antibiotics. J Antimicrob Chemother 1976; 2: 115–517

75 Medeiros AA, O'Brien TF. Ampicillin-resistant *Haemophilus influenzae* type B possessing a TEM-type β-lactamase but little permeability barrier to ampicillin. Lancet 1975; 1: 716–718

76 Moxon ER, Medeiros AA, O'Brien TF. Beta-lactamase effect on ampicillin treatment of *Haemophilus influenzae* B bacteremia and meningitis in infant rats. Antimicrob Agents Chemother. 1977; 12: 461–464

77 Murphy D, Todd J. Treatment of ampicillin-resistant *Haemophilus influenzae* in soft tissue infections with high doses of ampicillin. J Pediatr 1979; 94: 983–987

78 Pervival A, Brumfitt W, de Louvois J. The role of penicillinase in determining natural and acquired resistance of gram-negative bacteria to penicillins. J Gen Microbiol 1963; 32: 77–89

79 Medeiros AA, Kent RL, O'Brien TF. Characterization and prevalence of the different mechanisms of resistance to beta-lactam antibiotics in clinical isolates of *Escherichia coli*. Antimicrob Agents Chemother 1974; 6: 691–801

80 Graham WC, Medeiros AA. Antagonism of carbenicillin by cephalosporins in gram-negative bacilli. In: Nelson JD, Grassi C, eds. Current chemotherapy and infectious disease. Washington DC: American Society for Microbiology, 1980; 489–491

81 Sanders C. Novel resistance selected by the new expanded-spectrum cephalosporins: a concern. J Infect Dis 1983; 147: 585–589

82 Labia R, Bequin-Billecoq R, Guionie M. Behaviour of ceftazidime towards β-lactamases. J Antimicrob Chemother 1981; 8 (suppl B): 141–146

83 Yokota T, Azuma E. Biochemical aspects of bacterial resistance to new beta-lactam drugs non-hydrolyzable by beta-lactamases. In: Mitsuhashi A, Rosival L, Krcméry V, eds. Antibiotic resistance: transposition and other mechanisms. Berlin: Springer Verlag, 1980; 333–337

84 Sanders CC, Sanders WE Jr, Goering RV. In vitro antagonism of beta-lactam antibiotics by cefoxitin. Antimicrob Agents Chemother 1982; 21: 968–975

85 Sugarman B, Pesanti E. Treatment failures secondary to in vivo

development of drug resistance by microorganisms. Rev Infect Dis 1980; 2: 153 168

86 Preheim LC, Penn RG, Sanders CC, Goering RV, Giger DK. Emergence of resistance to β-lactam aminoglycoside antibiotics during moxalactam therapy of *Pseudomonas aeruginosa* infections. Antimicrob Agents Chemother 1982; 22: 1037–1041

87 Beckwith DG, Jahre JA. Role of a cefoxitin-inducible β-lactamase in a case of breakthrough bacteremia. J Clin Microbiol 1980; 12: 517–520

88 Sanders CC, Moellering RC Jr, Martin RR *et al.* Resistance to cefamandole: a collaborative study of emerging clinical problems. J Infect Dis 1982; 145: 118–125

89 Then RL, Angehrn P. Trapping of nonhydrolyzable cephalosporins by cephalosporinases in *Enterobacter cloacae* and *Pseudomonas aeruginosa* as a possible resistance mechanism. Antimicrob Agents Chemother 1982; 21: 711–717

90 Murray PR, Granich GG, Krogstad DJ, Niles AC. In vivo selection of resistance to multiple cephalosporins by *Enterobacter cloacae*. J Infect Dis 1983; 147: 590

91 Olson B, Weinstein RA, Nathan C, Kabins SA. Broad spectrum β-lactam resistance in *Enterobacter:* emergence during treatment and mechanisms of resistance. J Antimicrob Chemother 1983; 11; 299–310

92 Gootz TD, Sanders CC, Goering RV. Resistance to cefamondole: Derepression of β-lactamases by cefoxitin and mutation in *Enterobacter cloacae*. J Infect Dis 1982; 146: 34–42

93 Kabins SA, Sweeney HM, Cohen S. Resistance to cephalothin in vivo associated with increased cephalosporinase production. Ann Intern Med 1966; 65: 1271–1277

94 Medeiros AA, Mandel MD. In vivo acquired resistance to β-lactam antibiotics due to hyperproduction of β-lactamase. In: Abstracts of the annual meeting of the American society for microbiology. Los Angeles: American Society for Microbiology, 1979: 6

95 Medeiros AA, O'Brien TF. Acquisition of resistance to different beta-lactam antibiotics without change in isolate beta-lactamase activity. In: Proceedings of the 13th interscience conference on antimicrobial agents and chemotherapy, 1973: 151

96 Daniels CJ, Bole DG, Quay SC, Oxender DL. Role for membrane potential in the secretion of protein into the periplasm of *Escherichia coli*. Proc Natl Acad Sci USA 1981; 78: 5396–5400

British Medical Bulletin (1984) Vol. 40, No. 1, pp. 28–35

AMINOGLYCOSIDE RESISTANCE

IAN PHILLIPS MD FRCP FRCPath
KEVIN SHANNON BSc PhD MRCPath

Department of Microbiology
St Thomas's Hospital Medical School
London

1   Aminoglycoside-modifying enzymes
    a   Phosphotransferases
    b   Adenylyltransferases
    c   Acetyltransferases
    d   How do aminoglycoside-modifying enzymes produce
        resistance?
2   Reduced uptake of aminoglycosides
3   Resistance in clinical isolates
    a   Mechanisms
    b   Prevalence
4   Conclusion
    References

Before considering resistance to aminoglycosides, it is necessary briefly to consider the structure and mode of action of these compounds. The aminoglycosides, most of which strictly speaking should be called aminoglycosidic aminocyclitols, may be divided into two main groups on the basis of whether they contain streptidine or 2-deoxystreptamine, although a few compounds (notably fortimicin) contain neither of these aminocyclitols. Spectinomycin, a pure aminocyclitol, is usually included among the aminoglycosides for convenience.

The only member of the streptidine-containing group that is of any importance in medicine is streptomycin. The larger 2-deoxystreptamine-containing group can itself be divided into two main subgroups depending upon whether the 2-deoxystreptamine is substituted at positions 4 and 5 (neomycin, paromomycin and butirosin) or positions 4 and 6 (kanamycin, amikacin, tobramycin, gentamicin, sissomicin and netilmicin). Gentamicin as used therapeutically consists of a mixture of gentamicins C_1, C_{1a} and C_2 with perhaps a little C_{2b}, neomycin consists predominantly of neomycin B with some neomycin C, and kanamycin consists predominantly of kanamycin A.

The way in which aminoglycosides are taken up into the bacterial cell has been elucidated by the work of Bryan *et al.*[1–4] who have found that uptake occurs in three phases. There is an initial, energy-independent phase which consists of binding to the exterior of the cell. This is followed by energy-dependent phase I, so named because it is abolished by conditions that prevent energy metabolism, in which aminoglycosides are thought to associate with membrane 'transporters' on the basis of their positive electrical charge and be driven across the cytoplasmic membranes by the electrical potential difference, which is negative on the interior of the membrane. Damper & Epstein[5] doubt that transporters are involved and believe that uptake is due solely to the potential difference across the membrane. A second, faster energy-dependent phase II occurs at a later stage than ribosome binding and may be related to the increased membrane potential associated with loss of potassium ions.

The mode of action of streptomycin has been studied more than that of the other compounds though it is assumed that all act in similar ways. The primary target of streptomycin is thought to be the 30S subunit of the bacterial ribosome with the drug acting to inhibit protein synthesis mainly by preventing binding of the ribosome to messenger RNA.[6,7] Hancock[8,9] disputes the view that inhibition of protein synthesis is the main mode of action of aminoglycosides and suggests that direct effects on the cell membrane are important.

Resistance to aminoglycosides can be divided into three categories. Firstly, there is ribosomal resistance, which does not seem to be an important mechanism of resistance to 2-deoxystreptamine aminoglycosides in clinical isolates. Mutations at the *rpsL* locus (formerly known as *strA*) can lead to resistance to high levels of streptomycin in *Escherichia coli* K-12 and clinical isolates with this mechanism of streptomycin resistance have been reported in *Neisseria gonorrhoeae*,[10] enterococci,[11] *Staphylococcus aureus*[12] and *Pseudomonas aeruginosa*[13] and presumably occur in most species of bacteria. Secondly, there are a number of enzymes that modify aminoglycosides and, thirdly, uptake of aminoglycosides can be diminished.

1   Aminoglycoside-Modifying Enzymes

There are three classes of aminoglycoside-modifying enzymes and a number of specific sites at which they can act (Table I). The numbering system used for the aminoglycoside rings and the sites of modification by aminoglycoside-modifying enzymes are shown in Fig. 1. It is now customary to use the abbreviation AAC for acetyltransferases, which acetylate amino groups on the aminoglycoside, AAD for adenylyltransferases and APH for phosphotransferases. Both AAD and APH enzymes modify hydroxyl groups. The term 'nucelotidyltransferase' (ANT) might be preferable for adenylyltransferases since many of the enzymes can use nucleoside triphosphates other than ATP as cofactor.

A number of methods are used to detect and identify these enzymes. We believe the most convenient to be the cellulose phosphate paper binding method.[14,15] This method has proved useful also in the clinical assay of aminoglycosides. However, definitive identification of an aminoglycoside-modifying enzyme requires identification of the structure of its product.

a   *Phosphotransferases*

APH(3″) and APH(6). Both of these enzymes phosphorylate streptomycin but not spectinomycin or the 2-deoxystreptamine aminoglycosides. The degree of resistance conferred is variable, with streptomycin minimum inhibitory concentrations (MICs) of 64 mg/l in some cases but much higher in others. The APH(3″) specified by plasmid JR35 is said to require ATP or GTP as cofactor whereas that synthesized by *P. aeruginosa* H9 can use ATP, GTP, CTP or UTP.[16]

An enzyme that phosphorylated the 6-position of streptomycin was found in *P. aeruginosa* GN 573.[17] It had an isoelectric point of 4.7. Its K_m for streptomycin was 10 μM and for ATP was 83 μM. An APH(6) has also been found in a streptomycin-producing *Streptomyces* strain.[18]

APH(3′). There are at least four types of this enzyme, all of which phosphorylate neomycin and kanamycin: types I–III are distinguished on the basis of phosphorylation of lividomycin and butirosin. The degree of resistance conferred by production of these enzymes is variable with MICs of kanamycin ranging from 16–>4096 mg/l and MICs of neomycin mostly somewhat lower.

TABLE I. Aminoglycoside-modifying enzymes

Enzyme	Modification of									Organisms where found
	Streptomycin	Spectinomycin	Neomycin B and C	Kanamycin A	Amikacin	Tobramycin	Gentamicin C sissomicin	Netilmicin	Apramycin	
APH(3")	+	−	0	0	0	0	0	0	0	Gram-negative and gram-positive organisms
APH(6)	+	0	0	0	0	0	0	0	0	Pseudomonas
APH(3')	0	0	+	+	variable	0	0	0	0	Gram-negative and gram-positive organisms
APH(2")	0	0	0	+	±	+	+	±	0	Gram-positive organisms
AAD(3")(9)	+	+	0	0	0	0	0	0	0	Gram-negative organisms
AAD(6)	+	0	0	0	0	0	0	0	0	Staphylococci
AAD(9)	−	+	0	0	0	0	0	0	0	Staphylococci
AAD(4')(4")	0	0	+	+	+	+	0	0	0	Staphylococci
AAD(2")	0	0	0	+	variable	+	+	±	0	Gram-negative organisms
AAC(3)I	0	0	−	−	−	±	+	±	−	Gram-negative organisms
AAC(3)II	0	0	−	±	−	+	+	+	−	Gram-negative organisms
AAC(3)III	0	0	+	+	−	+	+	±	−	Gram-negative organisms
AAC(3)IV	0	0	+	+	−	+	+	+	+	Gram-negative organisms
AAC(2')	0	0	+	0	0	+	+	+	0	Providencia
AAC(6')I	0	0	+	+	+	+	variable*	+	0	Gram-negative organisms
AAC(6')II	0	0	+	+	+	+	variable*	+	0	Moraxella
AAC(6')III	0	0	+	+	±	+	variable*	+	0	Pseudomonas
AAC(6')IV	0	0	±	+	+	+	variable*	+	0	Gram-positive organisms

Symbols: + modified; − not modified; ± poorly modified; 0 substituent necessary for modification absent

* Gentamicin C_1 0, gentamicins C_{1A} and C_2 and sissomicin +

FIG. 1. Structures of some aminoglycosides and spectinomycin

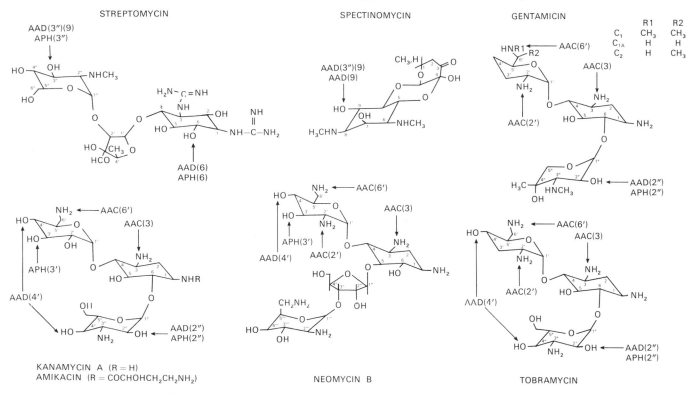

The arrows indicate the sites of attack by aminoglycoside-modifying enzymes

APH(3')I, which phosphorylates lividomycin but not butirosin, was the first to be described.[19] Lividomycin lacks a 3'-hydroxyl group so cannot be modified at this site. Instead it is phosphorylated at the 5" position, which is located near to the 3' position. Not all forms of APH(3')I are identical: Matsuhashi *et al.*[20] found differences in molecular weight and affinities for ATP, kanamycin and lividomycin between enzymes from different sources. A variant, termed APH(3')Ib, from *Haemophilus parainfluenzae* has been described for which kanamycin was a poorer substrate than for the usual form of the enzyme.[21]

APH(3')II phosphorylates butirosin but not lividomycin. In contrast to the situation with APH(3')I, enzymes from different sources seem to have similar properties.[20] APH(3′)II is more stable than APH(3′)I and has been purified to homogeneity: the K_m for ATP is about 24μM and that for neomycin is about 3.9μM.[22] There is no immunological cross-reaction between APH(3′)I and APH(3′)II.[22]

APH(3′)III, found in a strain of *P. aeruginosa*, phosphorylates both lividomycin and butirosin.[23] This enzyme may have been found also in *Providencia stuartii*, though it is possible that the strain produced APH(3′)I plus APH(3′)II.[24]

A superficially similar enzyme is found in neomycin-resistant staphylococci,[25,26] though unlike most other forms of APH(3′) this enzyme, APH(3′)IV, phosphorylates amikacin. Nevertheless, strains that produce this enzyme are mostly said to be sensitive to amikacin though a later report[27] states that for four strains of *S. aureus* producing this enzyme MICs of amikacin were 16–128mg/l. The apparent explanation for amikacin sensitivity is that amikacin has an appreciably higher K_m for the enzyme than do neomycin or kanamycin and, therefore, is phosphorylated more slowly at the low concentrations that are sufficient for inhibition of bacterial growth. APH(3′)IV has been found also in highly neomycin- and kanamycin-resistant strains of *Streptococcus faecalis.*[28]

Amikacin-resistant variants (MICs of amikacin up to 5000mg/l) of strains of *E. coli* that carry plasmids specifying APH(3′)II have been produced in the laboratory. Perlin & Lerner[29] attribute this to broadening of the spectrum of the enzyme. In contrast, Bongaerts & Kaptijn[30] believe that both their own results and those of Perlin & Lerner can be explained by an increase in copy number of the plasmid leading to much enhanced enzymic activity.

APH(5″). APH(3′) enzymes that phosphorylate lividomycin do so at the 5″ position and thus, strictly speaking, should be called APH(3′)(5″). Kida *et al.*[31] reported an enzyme that preferentially phosphorylated the 5″-hydroxyl group of ribostamycin but that also phosphorylated the 3′-hydroxyl. There is also a report of an enzyme that was said to phosphorylate lividomycin, neomycin and paromomycin at the 5″ position.[32] However, further work has shown it to be APH(3′)I.[33] Thus it is not yet certain whether or not there are any enzymes that are specific for the 5″-hydroxyl group.

APH(2″). Gentamicin-resistant staphylococci generally produce two enzymes, AAC(6′) and APH(2″). The phosphotransferase, which phosphorylates gentamicin, tobramycin and kanamycin, but not neomycin or amikacin, has not yet been found without AAC(6′). However, it does not seem that the two activities are dual aspects of a single polypeptide since it has been possible to separate the functions by polyacrylamide gel electrophoresis.[34] The isoelectric point of the phosphotransferase is 5.8 whereas that of the accompanying acetyltransferase is 5.7.[35] MICs of gentamicin and tobramycin for staphylococci that produce APH(2″) plus AAC(6′) can be as low as 4mg/l but are mostly higher and may exceed 128mg/l. Since, as far as we know, no gentamicin-resistant staphylococci produce APH(2″) without AAC(6′), or vice versa, it may be that both enzymes are needed to produce resistance, as with neomycin resistance due to production of APH(3′) + AAC(3) in *Streptomyces fradiae* (see Cundliffe, pp. 61–67). APH(2″) + AAC(6′) occur also in highly aminoglycoside-resistant strains of *S. faecalis.*[36]

b *Adenylyltransferases*

AAD(3″)(9). This enzyme, which confers resistance to streptomycin (MICs 16–>4096mg/l) and spectinomycin, and is usually plasmid-mediated, modifies streptomycin at the 3″ position and spectinomycin at position 9. It can use ATP and dATP but not other nucleoside triphosphates as cofactor.[37] AAD(3″)(9) appears to be confined to gram-negative organisms. An enzyme that adenylylates spectinomycin but not streptomycin has been reported in a spectinomycin-resistant isolate of *S. aureus*: it has not been studied in any detail but is assumed to be AAD(9).[22]

AAD(6). An enzyme that adenylylates streptomycin, at position 6, but not spectinomycin has been reported from a streptomycin-resistant (MIC 400mg/l), spectinomycin-sensitive strain of *S. aureus.*[38]

AAD(2″). This enzyme, specified by a transferable plasmid, was first found in *Klebsiella* by Benveniste & Davies.[39] It confers resistance to gentamicin, tobramycin and kanamycin (MICs mostly 16–128mg/l) but not to neomycin or amikacin. The enzyme can use ATP, GTP, CTP and UTP as cofactor[37] and would, therefore, perhaps be better known as ANT(2″). It has been partially purified: its K_m for ATP is 61μM; K_ms for gentamicin, tobramycin and kanamycin are in the range 0.8 to 2.3μM.[40]

A variant, AAD(2″)II, that adenylylates amikacin has been found in Australia.[41] It is not clear from the original description whether it confers resistance to amikacin though a later report[42] suggests that it does not.

AAD(4′)(4″). This enzyme, which so far has been found only in staphylococci, mostly adenylylates its substrates at the 4′ position though equatorial 4″-hydroxyl groups (as in dibekacin) but not polar 4″-hydroxyl groups (as in gentamicin) can also be modified.[43] Production of AAD(4′)(4″) confers only a small degree of resistance to dibekacin, amikacin and neomycin B (MICs 6.25mg/l) but a greater degree of resistance to kanamycin and tobramycin (MICs 100mg/l).

c *Acetyltransferases*

AAC(3)I. There are a number of distinct enzymes that acetylate aminoglycosides at position 3. The first to be described, AAC(3)I,[44] confers resistance to gentamicin and sissomicin (MICs mostly 8–32mg/l) but not to tobramycin. Nevertheless, tobramycin is acetylated readily in vitro at high substrate concentrations. The apparent explanation for this discrepancy is that its K_m for tobramycin is 2.3μM whereas that for gentamicin C_{1A} is 0.3μM and that the V_{max} for tobramycin is 0.48units/mg while that for gentamicin C_{1A} is 3units/mg. Thus, at low substrate concentrations, tobramycin is acetylated much more slowly than gentamicin. Although, from its activity on 2-deoxystreptamine aminoglycosides, AAC(3)I appears to have a narrow spectrum of activity, it is in fact the only aminoglycoside-modifying enzyme so far known for which fortimicin, which does not contain 2-deoxystreptamine, is a substrate.[45]

The term AAC(3)Ia has been used for a phenotype (resistance to gentamicin and netilmicin but sensitivity to tobramycin) found in *P. aeruginosa.*[27] The enzymological basis of the phenotype is not known.

AAC(3)II. Le Goffic *et al.*[46] described a plasmid that conferred resistance to gentamicin and tobramycin, and a reduction in sensitivity to kanamycin. An acetyltransferase, AAC(3)II, that modified gentamicin, tobramycin and kanamycin was detected. Its isoelectric point was 6.4, compared to 7.4 for AAC(3)I. Organisms that produce AAC(3)II are more resistant to gentamicin (MICs >64mg/l) than those that produce AAC(3)I: MICs of tobramycin and netilmicin are generally about one quarter of those of gentamicin.

AAC(3)III. This enzyme was first described in a strain of *P. aeruginosa.*[47] Despite the ready acetylation of neomycin, the strain that produced this enzyme was fairly sensitive to the drug (MIC 8mg/l) though resistant to gentamicin and tobramycin (MICs >128mg/l).

AAC(3)IV. Davies & O'Connor[48] reported an enzyme that acetylated the veterinary aminoglycoside apramycin in addition to the substrates of AAC(3)III. Kanamycin is not such a good substrate of AAC(3)IV as are gentamicin, tobramycin, neomycin or apramycin and, in our experience, strains that produce this enzyme are sensitive to kanamycin and amikacin (MICs 2–8 mg/l) in the absence of another mechanism to produce resistance to one or both drugs. Only a moderate degree of resistance to neomycin is conferred (MICs 4–16 mg/l) but MICs of gentamicin, tobramycin and netilmicin are in the range 32–128 mg/l.

It is suggested from time to time that various AAC(3) enzymes may be related. However, T J White (quoted in Davies & Smith[22]) found no immunological cross-reaction between AAC(3)I and AAC(3)II, AAC(3)III and AAC(3)IV.

AAC(3)V. These are two reports of enzymes termed AAC(3)V. Gomez-Lus *et al.*[49] provisionally used the term for an enzyme that seems very similar to AAC(3)II. Coombe & George[50] detected an AAC(3) enzyme that acetylated amikacin, though it is implied that the strain of *P. aeruginosa* that was the source of the enzyme was sensitive to this drug. Further information is needed before the status of either of these enzymes can be established.

AAC(2'). An enzyme that acetylated the 2'-amino group of gentamicin, tobramycin and neomycin was first found in an isolate of *Providencia stuartii*.[51] The enzyme does not appear to be plasmid-determined[52] and seems to be associated mostly with Providencia. Davies & Smith[22] state, 'AAC(2') has also been isolated from several clinical isolates of Proteus strains and is found to be plasmid coded in these cases'. However, there is no evidence for AAC(2') production reported in the reference they cite.[53]

An AAC(2') enzyme has been found also in *Streptomyces spectabilis*, the organism that synthesizes spectinomycin.[54] It has been suggested that this enzyme be called AAC(2')I and the one from Providencia be called AAC(2')II.[55]

AAC(6'). The first type of AAC(6') to be described was that coded by the plasmids R5 and NR79.[56] This enzyme has a broad substrate range, including amikacin but excluding gentamicin C_1. In our hands, a strain of *E. coli* that carries plasmid R5 is resistant to kanamycin, amikacin, tobramycin, netilmicin (MICs > 128 mg/l) and neomycin (MIC 32 mg/l) but only moderately resistant to gentamicin (MIC 4 mg/l).

Since this first report, various other forms of AAC(6') have been described. Unfortunately, their nomenclature is confusing with several incompatible schemes having developed.

Mitsuhashi[55] suggested subdivision into types I to IV on the basis of a progressively broadening spectrum. AAC(6')I acetylates kanamycin: in addition AAC(6')II acetylates gentamicins C_{1a} and C_2. AAC(6')III adds amikacin to the substrates of AAC(6')II, and AAC(6')IV acetylates dibekacin plus the substrates of AAC(6')II. Thus, the enzyme coded by plasmids R5 and NR79 is AAC(6')IV. A major limitation of this scheme is that no account is taken of acetylation of neomycin.

A rather different scheme has developed in Europe and North America and is used in this review. The enzyme coded by R5 and NR79 is called AAC(6')I. AAC(6')II is an enzyme from an isolate of Moraxella with a somewhat different substrate profile and an isoelectric point of 7.6 in contrast to 5.4 for AAC(6')I.[57] AAC(6')III is an enzyme with little activity against amikacin that has been found in Pseudomonas.[58–60] Strains of *P. aeruginosa* that produce AAC(6')III are resistant to gentamicin, netilmicin and tobramycin (MICs 16–64 mg/l) but sensitive to amikacin. The enzyme that accompanies APH(2″) in gentamicin-resistant staphylococci has poor activity against neomycin[34,35] and is called AAC(6')IV in this scheme.

Miller *et al.*[27] recognize only two types of AAC(6'). What they call AAC(6')II corresponds to AAC(6')III in this review.

Other acetyltransferases. Dowding[61] reported an *N*-acetyltransferase from a clinical isolate of Acinetobacter that most readily acetylates compounds with a 2'-hydroxyl group (notably kanamycin A, amikacin and gentamicin B). An acetyltransferase that confers resistance to neomycin, paromomycin and apramycin (MICs 32–64 mg/l) has been detected in an isolate of *E. coli* from a pig (R W Hedges & K P Shannon, manuscript in preparation). The product of acetylation of neomycin by this enzyme is distinguishable from the products of AAC(3)IV, AAC(2') and AAC(6') by high performance liquid chromatography (A Lovering, D S Reeves & L O White, personal communication).

d How Do Aminoglycoside-Modifying Enzymes Produce Resistance?

It is not entirely clear how these enzymes produce resistance to aminoglycosides. Davies & Smith[22] argue that modified aminoglycoside blocks further entry of aminoglycosides into the cell. However, since the modified aminoglycoside is ineffective in inhibiting protein synthesis by ribosomes in vitro,[62] and since possession of aminoglycoside-modifying enzymes does not seem to prevent the uptake of aminoglycosides in energy-dependent phase I,[63] some regard this resistance mechanism as one of inactivation.[8,64]

Production of an aminoglycoside-modifying enzyme that modifies a particular aminoglycoside does not always result in resistance to the drug. In some cases, for example AAC(3)I and tobramycin, this is explained by the aminoglycoside having poor affinity for the enzyme. Alternatively, as with 6'-*N*-acetylneomycin,[56] the modified aminoglycoside may retain appreciable antibacterial activity. Conversely, some organisms are resistant to drugs that are not observably modified by the enzymes produced: the most widely reported example of this is the resistance of AAC(6')III producers to gentamicin.[58–60] There is no satisfactory explanation for this phenomenon though a possibility is the production of a second, undetected, enzyme.

Sometimes resistance to an aminoglycoside is not expressed although the gene coding for a modifying enzyme is present: for example, plasmid-mediated resistance to gentamicin in *P. aeruginosa* has been found not to be expressed in *E. coli*;[65] conversely Prince & Neu found that transfer of a gentamicin resistance gene from *P. aeruginosa* to *E. coli* enhanced detection of a modifying enzyme.[66]

2 Reduced Uptake of Aminoglycosides

There are a number of laboratory strains with mutations affecting membrane-energy metabolism, that reduce the potential difference across the membrane, and show reduced uptake of, and resistance to, aminoglycosides.[3,4,8] There are also many aminoglycoside-resistant clinical isolates, of species that are usually aminoglycoside-sensitive, in which aminoglycoside modifying enzymes cannot be detected and in which the mechanism of resistance is assumed to be some sort of 'impermeability'. In most such cases there is no direct evidence that uptake of aminoglycosides is reduced compared to that in sensitive strains, though Price *et al.*[67] observed diminished uptake of radiolabelled amikacin by most such strains. Organisms that exhibit 'impermeability' are cross-resistant to all the aminoglycosides though the levels of resistance are not very high (MICs of gentamicin and tobramycin mostly 4–16 mg/l; MICs of kanamycin and amikacin mostly 16–64 mg/l).

Poor uptake of aminoglycosides seems also to be the cause of the resistance of obligately anaerobic bacteria to aminoglycosides[68] and may account for the relative resistance of streptoccoci to the drugs. Reduction of the potential difference across the membrane and, in consequence, reduced uptake of aminoglycosides may well be the cause of the reduced sensitivity of facultatively anaerobic bacteria under anaerobic conditions.[69]

3 Resistance in Clinical Isolates

a *Mechanisms*

There have been a number of surveys of mechanisms of aminoglycoside resistance in clinical isolates. Most, however, concern the organisms from a single hospital and may be of no relevance to the situation elsewhere. For example, in Sydney, Australia most gentamicin-resistant isolates were found to produce AAC(3)I or AAD(2″)II[42] whereas in Saragossa, Spain none of the isolates adenylylated gentamicin but most produced either AAC(3)V (which we would probably have called AAC(3)II) or AAC(3)I.[70]

Results for organisms from St Thomas' Hospital are shown in Table II. Up to 1977, except for Providencia, resistance was almost entirely due to production of AAC(3)I or a non-enzymic mechanism.[59,71] When the mechanisms of resistance were surveyed again in 1981, a considerable change was noted with the emergence of AAC(3)II and AAD(2″) as frequent mechanisms of gentamicin resistance. It should be noted that since only gentamicin-resistant strains were studied, AAC(6′) producers might well have been missed.

The most comprehensive study of mechanisms of aminoglycoside resistance is that conducted by Bristol Laboratories in USA.[67] Aminoglycoside-resistant enterobacteria generally owed their resistance to production of modifying enzymes, though non-enzymic resistance was common in *E. coli*. Except for Serratia, which mostly produced AAC(6′) with or without another enzyme, AAD(2″) was the enzyme most commonly produced, with AAC(3)I in second place followed by other forms of AAC(3). Among *P. aeruginosa* and other non-fermenters, non-enzymic resistance was the most common. Miller *et al.*[27] came to similar conclusions though they based their identification of resistance mechanisms on sensitivity patterns rather than detection of the enzymes.

In a study of klebsiellae from several countries, Knight[72] found AAD(2″) to be the most common mechanism of gentamicin resistance (23 out of 61 isolates) followed by AAC(3)I (15 isolates) and AAC(3)II (10 isolates). Gentamicin-modifying enzymes were not detected in 12 isolates.

Although many bacteria produce a gentamicin-modifying enzyme plus neomycin/kanamycin phosphotransferase and a streptomycin-modifying enzyme, production of two gentamicin-modifying enzymes has been uncommon in the past except for production of AAC(6′) plus APH(2″) by resistant staphylococci and enterococci and, perhaps, AAC(6′) plus another enzyme by Serratia.[67,71] However, at least in some locations, production of two gentamicin-modifying enzymes appears to be becoming more common. The production of AAD(2″)II plus other enzymes in Sydney[42] has been mentioned already. Most of the seven strains from Central Europe reported by Kettner *et al.* produced more than one gentamicin-modifying enzyme[73] and we detected production of two such enzymes in six of the strains isolated in 1981 (AAC(3)I + AAD(2″)) by isolates of *E. coli* and *Citrobacter freundii*, AAC(2′) + AAC(6′) by an isolate of Providencia, AAC(6′) + AAD(2″) by an isolate of *P. aeruginosa* and AAC(3)I + AAC(6′) by two isolates of Serratia).

b *Prevalence*

Resistance to the older aminoglycosides (streptomycin, neomycin and kanamycin) was more common than that to the newer ones (gentamicin, tobramycin, amikacin and netilmicin) in 1975–78[74] though, since the older ones have been largely superseded by the newer ones and sensitivity to them is rarely tested, it is hard to know if this is still true. Geographical differences in prevalence of resistance have been reported, particularly for gentamicin and tobramycin. Resistance is more common in France and Central Europe[74–76] than in the USA.[76,77] Resistance is also commoner in Klebsiella than in *E. coli*.[74,76] Table III outlines what has happened with regard to gentamicin resistance among gram-negative organisms at our own hospital within the past few years (unfortunately, information is not available for 1978). Gentamicin resistance was uncommon in enterobacteria, apart from Providencia, in 1976. It became more common in Klebsiella in 1977 and in the few strains of Serratia that we isolated in 1978, but has remained rare in *E. coli* and other enterobacteria. There has been no clear trend in the frequency of gentamicin-resistant isolates of *P. aeruginosa* during the period of the study but resistance had become common in Acinetobacter by 1979. Amikacin resistance has remained rare in all organisms throughout the study.

TABLE II. Aminoglycoside-modifying enzymes produced by bacteria isolated at St. Thomas' Hospital in 1974–77 and 1981

Organism	Number of isolates with indicated mechanism of resistance in 1981						
	AAC(3)I	AAC(3)II	AAC(3)IV	AAC(2′)	AAC(6′)	AAD(2″)	Non-Enzymatic
E. coli	1 (1) *	2				5	7 (6)
Proteus spp							
M. morganii							
Citrobacter	7 (9)	2				8	2 (1)
E. cloacae							
Klebsiella	11 (12)	30				24 (1)	1 (4)
Serratia	3				3 (2)	1	
Providencia				26 (25)	1		
Acinetobacter	20				0 (5)		
P. aeruginosa	6 (4)				2 (4)	4 (2)	9 (24)
Pseudomonads	0 (1)				0 (1)		7 (17)
Alkaligenes	1		4				1

* Results for 1974–77 are shown in parentheses
The following gentamicin-resistant organisms isolated in 1981 were not tested for production of aminoglycoside-modifying enzymes: four isolates of Acinetobacter, four isolates of *P. aeruginosa* and two isolates of *E. coli*.

TABLE III. Resistance to aminoglycosides at St. Thomas' Hospital 1976–1981

Organism	1976		1977				1979				1980				1981			
	No. of isolates	% Resistant to Gent	No. of isolates	% Resistant to			No. of isolates	% Resistant to			No. of isolates	% Resistant to			No. of isolates	% Resistant to		
				Gent	Tobra	Amik		Gent	Tobra	Amik		Gent	Tobra	Amik		Gent	Tobra	Amik
E. coli	1980	0.2	2340	0.4	0.4	0.1	2578	0.9	1.0	0.3	2532	0.6	0.5	0.4	2780	0.6	0.6	0.3
Proteus spp.																		
M. morganii																		
Citrobacter }	798	0.5	890	1.1	0.4	0.2	909	3.0	2.2	0.4	987	1.9	1.7	0.4	883	2.2	1.6	0.2
E. cloacae																		
Klebsiella	596	1.3	621	8.0	3.0	0.2	663	11	10	0.3	686	8.7	7.4	0.1	636	9.9	8.1	0.2
Providencia	14	28	29	59	48	3.4	30	63	66	0	36	67	69	0	29	83	83	0
Serratia	10	0	13	0	0	0	27	15	15	0	32	16	13	0	33	12	12	0
P. aeruginosa	473	4	407	6.1	2.9	2.7	406	4.6	1.5	1.9	458	6.1	2.4	1.9	444	5.4	1.8	1.1
Acinetobacter	77	2.6	66	4.5	0	0	113	40	4.4	0	144	36	4.1	4.9	122	20	1.6	2.4

Abbreviations: Gent: gentamicin; Tobra: tobramycin; Amik: Amikacin

4 Conclusion

Ribosomal resistance, especially to streptomycin, is the mechanism of aminoglycoside resistance that has been most intensively studied in academic circles, though it is the least important in clinical practice. Microbiologists and others interested in bacteria of medical importance mostly have studied aminoglycoside-modifying enzymes and pharmaceutical companies have put considerable effort—with success in the cases of amikacin and netilmicin—into the production of compounds that are resistant to these enzymes. Aminoglycoside-modifying enzymes have been found useful in the clinical assay of aminoglycosides. It may well be, as suggested by Davies,[78] that compounds analogous to the β-lactamase inhibitors, clavulanic acid and sulbactam, will be developed in the future as an alternative way of overcoming aminoglycoside-modifying enzymes. The mechanism of aminoglycoside resistance that has been neglected most (except by Canadians) is impaired uptake of the drugs—probably because it is the most difficult to study. It should perhaps be considered the most important resistance mechanism, as it seems to be the one that determines the spectrum of antibacterial activity of the aminoglycosides.

REFERENCES

1 Bryan LE, Van Den Elzen HM. Gentamicin accumulation by sensitive strains of *Escherichia coli* and *Pseudomonas aeruginosa*. J Antibiot 1975; 28: 696–703

2 Bryan LE, Van Den Elzen HM. Streptomycin accumulation in susceptible and resistant strains of *Escherichia coli* and *Pseudomonas aeruginosa*. Antimicrob Agents Chemother 1976; 9: 928–938

3 Bryan LE, Van Den Elzen HM. Effects of membrane-energy mutations and cations on streptomycin and gentamicin accumulation by bacteria: a model for the entry of streptomycin and gentamicin in susceptible and resistant bacteria. Antimicrob Agents Chemother 1977; 12: 163–177

4 Bryan LE, Nicas T, Holloway BW, Crowther C. Aminoglycoside-resistant mutation of *Pseudomonas aeruginosa* defective in cytochrome c_{552} and nitrate reductase. Antimicrob Agents Chemother 1980; 17: 71–79.

5 Damper PD, Epstein W. Role of the membrane potential in bacterial resistance to aminoglycoside antibiotics. Antimicrob Agents Chemother 1981; 20: 803–808

6 Gale ED, Cundliffe E, Reynolds PE, Richmond MH, Waring MJ. The molecular basis of antibiotic action. London: Wiley, 1972; 290–306

7 Moellering RC Jr. Clinical microbiology and the in vitro activity of aminoglycosides. In: Whelton A, Neu HC, eds The aminoglycosides. Microbiology, clinical use and toxicology. New York: Marcel Dekker 1981: 65–95

8 Hancock REW. Aminoglycoside uptake and mode of action—with special reference to streptomycin and gentamicin. I. Antagonists and mutants. J Antimicrob Chemother 1981; 8: 249–276

9 Hancock REW. Aminoglycoside uptake and mode of action—with special reference to streptomycin and gentamicin. II. Effects of aminoglycosides on cells. J Antimicrob Chemotherapy 1981; 8: 429–445

10 Maness MJ, Foster GC, Sparling PF. Ribosomal resistance to streptomycin and spectinomycin in *Neisseria gonorrhoeae*. J Bacteriol 1974; 120: 1293–1299

11 Zimmermann RA, Moellering RC Jr, Weinberg AN. Mechanisms of resistance to antibiotic synergism in enterococci. J Bacteriol 1971; 105: 873–879

12 Lacey RW, Chopra I. Evidence for mutation to streptomycin resistance in clinical strains of *Staphylococcus aureus*. J Gen Microbiol 1972; 73: 175–180

13 Tseng JL, Bryan LE, Van Den Elzen HM. Mechanisms and spectrum of streptomycin resistance in a natural population of *Pseudomonas aeruginosa*. Antimicrob Agents Chemother 1972; 2: 136–141

14 Ozanne B, Benveniste R, Tipper D, Davies J. Aminoglycoside antibiotics: inactivation by phosphorylation in *Escherichia coli* carrying R factors. J Bacteriol 1969; 100: 1144–1146

15 Shannon KP, Phillips I. Detection of aminoglycoside-modifying strains of bacteria. In: Russell AD, Quesnel LB, eds. Antibiotics. Society for applied bacteriology technical series no. 18. London: Academic Press, 1983; 183–198

16 Doi O, Ogura M, Tanaka N, Umezawa H. Inactivation of kanamycin, neomycin and streptomycin by enzymes obtained in cells of *Pseudomonas aeruginosa*. Appl Microbiol 1968; 16: 1276–1281

17 Kida M, Asako T, Yoneda M, Mitsuhashi S. Phosphorylation of dihydrostreptomycin by *Pseudomonas aeruginosa*. In: Mitsuhashi S, Hashimoto H, eds. Microbial drug resistance. Tokyo: University Park Press, 1975; 441–448

18 Walker JB, Skorvaga M. Phosphorylation of streptomycin and dihydrostreptomycin by *Streptomyces*. Enzymatic synthesis of different diphosphoryated derivatives. J Biol Chem 1973; 248: 2435–2440

19 Umezawa H, Okanishi M, Kondo S *et al*. Phosphorylative inactivation of aminoglycosidic antibiotics by *Escherichia coli* carrying R factor. Science 1967; 157: 1559–1561

20 Matsuhashi Y, Yagisawa M, Kondo S, Takeuchi T, Umezawa H. Aminoglycoside 3′-phosphotransferases I and II in *Pseudomonas aeruginosa*. J Antibiot 1975; 28: 442–447

21 Le Goffic F, Moreau N, Siegrist S, Goldstein FW, Acar JC. La résistance plasmidique de *Haemophilus* sp. aux antibiotiques amino-glycosidiques isolement et etudié d'une nouvelle phosphotransferase. Ann Microbiol (Paris) 1977; 128A: 388–391

22 Davies J, Smith DH. Plasmid-determined resistance to antimicrobial agents. Ann Rev Microbiol 1978; 32: 469–518

23 Umezawa Y, Yagisawa M, Sawa T *et al.* Aminoglycoside 3'-phosphotransferase III, a new phosphotransferase resistance mechanism. J Antibiot 1975; 28: 845–853

24 Marengo PB, Chenoweth ME, Overturf GD, Wilkins J. Phosphorylation of kanamycin, lividomycin A and butirosin B by *Providencia stuartii.* Antimicrob Agents Chemother 1974; 6: 821–824

25 Kayser FH, Devaud M, Biber J. Aminoglycoside 3'-phosphotransferase IV: a new type of aminoglycoside phosphorylating enzyme found in staphylococci. Microbios Lett 1976; 3: 63–68

26 Courvalin P, Davies J. Plasmid mediated aminoglycoside phosphotransferase of broad substrate range that phosphorylates amikacin. Antimicrob Agents Chemother 1977; 11: 619–624

27 Miller GH, Sabatelli, Hare RS, Waitz JA. Survey of aminoglycoside resistance patterns. Dev Indust Microbiol 1980; 21: 91–104

28 Courvalin PM, Shaw WV, Jacob AE. Plasmid-mediated mechanisms of resistance to aminoglycoside-aminocyclitol antibiotics in group D streptococci. Antimicrob Agents Chemother 1978; 13: 716–725

29 Perlin MH, Lerner SA. Amikacin resistance associated with a plasmid-borne aminoglycoside phosphotransferase in *Escherichia coli.* Antimicrob Agents Chemother 1979; 16: 598–604

30 Bongaerts GPA, Kaptijn GMP. Aminoglycoside phosphotransferase-II-mediated amikacin resistance in *Escherichia coli. Antimicrob Agents Chemother* 1981; 20: 344–350

31 Kida M, Igarasi S, Okutani T, Asako T, Hiraga K, Mitsuhashi S. Selective phosphorylation of the 5''-hydroxy group of ribostamycin by a new enzyme from *Pseudomonas aeruginosa.* Antimicrob Agents Chemother 1974; 5: 92–94

32 Yamaguchi M, Koshi T, Kobayashi F, Mitsuhashi S. Phosphorylation of lividomycin by *Escherichia coli* carrying an R factor. Antimicrob Agents Chemother 1972; 2: 142–146

33 Umezawa H. Biochemical mechanisms of resistance to aminoglycosidic antibiotics. Adv Carbohydr Chem Biochem 1974; 30: 183–225

34 Dowding JE. Mechanisms of gentamicin resistance in *Staphylococcus aureus.* Antimicrob Agents Chemother 1977; 11: 47–50

35 Le Goffic F, Martel A, Moreau N, Capmau MI, Sossy CJ, Duval J. 2''-O-Phosphorylation of gentamicin components by a *Staphylococcus aureus* strain carrying a plasmid. Antimicrob Agents Chemother 1977; 12: 26–30

36 Courvalin P, Carlier C, Collatz E. Plasmid-mediated resistance to aminocyclitol antibiotics in group D streptococci. J Bacteriol 1980; 143: 541–551

37 Benveniste R, Davies J. Mechanisms of antibiotic resistance in bacteria. Annu Rev Biochem 1973; 42: 471–506

38 Suzuki I, Takahashi N, Shirato S, Kawabe H, Mitsuhashi S. Adenylylation of streptomycin by *Staphylococcus aureus*: a new streptomycin adenylyltransferase. In: Mitsuhashi S, Hashimoto H, eds. Microbioal drug resistance. Tokyo: University Park Press, 1975; 463–473

39 Benveniste R, Davies J. R-Factor mediated gentamicin resistance: a new enzyme which modifies aminoglycoside antibiotics. FEBS Letts 1971; 14:293–296

40 Smith AL, Smith DH. Gentamicin:adenine mononucleotide transferase: partial purification, characterization, and use in the clinical quantitation of gentamicin. J Infect Dis 1974; 129: 391–401

41 Coombe RG, George AM. New plasmid-mediated aminoglycoside adenylyltransferase of broad substrate range that adenylylates amikacin. Antimicrob Agents Chemother 1981; 20: 75–80

42 Groot Obbink DJ, George AM, Coombe RG. Aminoglycoside-modifying enzymes associated with hospital isolates of Gram-negative rods. J Antimicrob Chemother 1983; 11: 525–533

43 Schwotzer U, Kayser FH, Schwotzer W. R-Plasmid mediated aminoglycoside resistance in *Staphylococcus epidermidis*: structure determination of the products of an enzyme nucleotidylating the 4'- and 4''-hydroxyl group of aminoglycoside antibiotics. FEMS Microbiol Lett 1978; 3: 29–33

44 Brzezinska M, Benveniste R, Davies J, Daniels PJL, Weinstein J. Gentamicin resistance in strains of *Pseudomonas aeruginosa* mediated by enzymatic N-acetylation of the deoxystreptamine moiety. Biochemistry 1972; 11: 761–766

45 Sato S, Iida T, Okachi R, Shirahata K, Nara T. Enzymatic acetylation of fortimicin A and seldomycin factor 5 by aminoglycoside 3-acetyltransferase I [AAC(3)I] of *E. coli* KY 8348. J Antibiot 1977; 30: 1025–1027

46 Le Goffic F, Martel A, Witchitz J. 3-N Enzymatic acetylation of gentamicin, tobramycin and kanamycin by *Escherichia coli* carrying an R factor. Antimicrob Agents Chemother 1974; 6: 680–684

47 Biddlecome S, Haas M, Davies J, Miller GH, Rane DF, Daniels PJL. Enzymatic modification of aminoglycoside antibiotics: a new 3-N-acetylating enzyme from a *Pseudomonas aeruginosa* isolate. Antimicrob Agents Chemother 1976; 9: 951–955

48 Davies J, O'Connor S. Enzymatic modification of aminoglycoside antibiotics: 3-N-acetyltransferase with broad specificity that determines resistance to the novel aminoglycoside apramycin. Antimicrob Agents Chemother 1978; 14: 69–72

49 Gomez-Lus R, Rubio-Calvo MC, Larrad L, Navarro M, Lasierra P, Vitoria MA. 3-*N*-Aminoglycoside-acetylating enzymes produced by R-plasmid-carrying bacteria isolated in a general hospital. In: Nelson JD, Grassi C, eds. Current chemotherapy and infectious disease. Proceedings of the 11th international congress of chemotherapy and the 19th interscience conference on antimicrobial agents and chemotherapy. Vol 1. Washington DC: American Society for Microbiology, 1980; 708–710

50 Coombe, RG, George AM. Purification and properties of an aminoglycoside acetyltransferase from *Pseudomonas aeruginosa.* Biochemistry 1982; 21: 871–875

51 Chevereau M, Daniels PJL, Davies J, Le Goffic F. Aminoglycoside resistance in bacteria mediated by gentamicin acetyltransferase II, an enzyme modifying the 2'-amino group of aminoglycoside antibiotics. Biochemistry 1974; 13: 598–603

52 Yamaguchi M, Mitsuhashi S, Kobayashi F, Zenda H. A 2'-N-acetylating enzyme of aminoglycosides. J Antibiot 1974; 27: 507–515

53 Shafi MS, Datta N. Infections caused by *Proteus mirabilis* strains with transferable gentamicin-resistance factors. Lancet 1975; 1: 1355–1357

54 Benveniste R, Davies J. Aminoglycoside antibiotic-inactivating enzymes in actinomceytes similar to those present in clinical isolates of antibiotic-resistant bacteria. Proc Natl Acad Sci USA 1973; 70: 2276–2280

55 Mitsuhashi S. Proposal for a rational nomenclature for phenotype, genotype, and aminoglycoside-aminocyclitol modifying enzymes. In: Mitsuhashi S, ed. Drug action and drug resistance in bacteria. 2. Aminoglycoside antibiotics. Tokyo: University Park Press, 1975; 269–275

56 Benveniste R, Davies J. Enzymatic acetylation of aminoglycoside antibiotics by *Escherichia coli* carrying an R factor. Biochemistry 1971; 10: 1787–1796

57 Le Goffic F, Martel A. La resistance aux aminosides provoquée par une isoenzyme la kanamycine acetyltransferase. Biochimie 1974; 56: 893–897

58 Haas M, Biddlecome S, Davies J, Luce CE, Daniels PJL. Enzymatic modification of aminoglycoside antibiotics: a new 6'-N-acetylating enzyme from a *Pseudomonas aeruginosa* isolate. Antimicrob Agents Chemother 1976; 9: 945–950

59 Phillips I, King BA, Shannon KP. The mechanisms of resistance to aminoglycosides in the genus Pseudomonas. J Antimicrob Chemother 1978; 4: 121–129

60 King BA, Shannon KP, Phillips I. Aminoglycoside 6'-N acetyltransferase production by an isolate of *Pseudomonas maltophilia.* J Antimicrob Chemother 1978; 4: 467–468

61 Dowding JE. A novel aminoglycoside-modifying enzyme from a clinical isolate of Acinetobacter. J Gen Microbiol 1979; 110: 239–241

62 Yamada T, Tipper D, Davies J. Enzymatic inactivation of streptomycin by R-factor resistant *Escherichia coli.* Nature (London) 1968; 219: 288–291

63 Dickie P, Bryan LE, Pickard MA. Effect of enzymatic adenylylation on dihydrostreptomycin accumulation in *Escherichia coli* carrying an R factor: model explaining aminoglycoside resistance by inactivating mechanisms. Antimicrob Agents Chemother 1978; 14: 569–580

64 Shannon KP, Phillips I. Mechanisms of resistance to aminoglycosides in clinical isolates. J Antimicrob Chemother 1982; 9: 91–102

65 Kato T, Sato Y, Iyobe S, Mitsuhashi S. Plasmid-mediated gentamicin resistance of *Pseudomonas aeruginosa* and its lack of expression in *Escherichia coli.* Antimicrob Agents Chemother 1982; 22: 358–363

66 Prince AS, Jacoby GA. Cloning the gentamicin resistance gene from a *Pseudomonas aeruginosa* plasmid in *Escherichia coli* enhances detection of aminoglycoside modification. Antimicrob Agents Chemother 1982; 22: 525–526

67 Price KE, Kresel PA, Farchione LA, Siskin SB, Karpow SA. Epidemiological studies of aminoglycoside resistance in the U.S.A. J Antimicrob Chemother 1981; 8 Suppl A: 89–105

68 Bryan LE, Kowand SK, Van den Elzen HM. Mechanism of aminoglycoside antibiotic resistance in anaerobic bacteria: *Clostridium perfringens* and *Bacteroides fragilis.* Antimicrob Agents Chemother 1979; 15: 7–13

69 Reynolds AV, Hamilton-Miller JMT, Brumfitt W. Diminished effect of gentamicin under anaerobic or hypercapnic conditions. Lancet 1976; 1: 447–449

70 Gomez-Lus R, Rubio-Calvo MC, Navarro M, Vitoria MA, Chocarro MP, Larrad L. Plasmid-determined resistance to aminocylitols in enterobacteria. In: Periti P, Grassi GG, eds. Current chemotherapy and immunotherapy. Proceedings of the 12th international congress of chemotherapy. Washington DC: American Society for Microbiology, 1982: 218–219

71 Shannon KP, Phillips I, King, BA. Aminoglycoside resistance among Enterobacteriaceae and *Acinetobacter* species. J Antimicrob Chemother 178; 4: 131–142

72 Knight S. Plasmids from gentamicin-resistant klebsiellae and other enterobacteria. London: University of London, 1982. PhD Thesis.

73 Kettner M, Navarová J, Rýdl Z, Knothe H, Lebek G, Krcmery V. Occurrence of aminoglycoside-modifying enzymes in resistant strains of enterobacteria and *Pseudomonas aeruginosa* from several countries. J Antimicrob Chemother 1981; 8: 175–181

74 Langmaack H. Prevalence of drug resistance of bacteria (1975–1978): results of an international study. In: Nelson JD, Grassi C eds. Current chemotherapy and infectious disease. Proceedings of the 11th international contress of chemotherapy. Vol 1. Washington DC: American Society for Microbiology, 1980; 716–718

75 Witchitz JL. Epidemiologal aspects of aminoglycoside resistance in France. J Antimicrob Chemother 1981; 8 Suppl A: 71–82

76 O'Brien TF, Acar JF, Medeiros AA, Norton RA, Goldstein F, Kent RL. International comparison of prevalence of resistance to antibiotics. J Am Med Assoc 1978; 239: 1518–1523

77 Young LS, Meyer-Dudnik DV, Hindler J, Martin WJ. Aminoglycosides in the treatment of bacteraemic infections in the immunocompromised host. J Antimicrob Chemother 1981; 8 Suppl A: 121–132

78 Davies JE. Resistance to aminoglycosides; mechanisms and frequency. Rev Infect Dis 1983; 5: S261–267.

British Medical Bulletin (1984) Vol. 40, No. 1, pp. 36–41

BACTERIAL RESISTANCE TO CHLORAMPHENICOL

WILLIAM V SHAW BA MD

Department of Biochemistry
University of Leicester

1   Chemistry and properties of chloramphenicol
2   Chloramphenicol resistance by enzymic acetylation
3   Variants of chloramphenicol acetyltransferase
4   Expression of genes for chloramphenicol acetyltransferase
5   Non-enzymic chloramphenicol resistance
6   Clinical considerations and chemotherapy
    References

Chloramphenicol has played an important role in the drama of antimicrobial therapy over three decades, a role which has become limited in recent years by concern for its potential toxicity and by the emergence of other natural and semi-synthetic antibiotics as reasonable alternatives for most clinical problems. Reasons for the continued use of chloramphenicol are several and include the chemical and biological properties of the antibiotic and the fact that resistance to β-lactams and other alternative antibiotics has become widespread.[1-3] Although microbial resistance to chloramphenicol has been well known since the early years of its clinical use, it is relatively uncommon in a number of life-threatening infections for which chloramphenicol is a first-line antibiotic. In this category are typhoid fever and other invasive salmonella infections, some anaerobic infections, bacterial meningitis (*Haemophilus influenzae* in particular), and rickettsial infections.[1-4] But the grey baby syndrome and the idiosyncratic aplastic anaemia (and pancytopenia) associated with chloramphenicol administration are powerful deterrents to more general use of an otherwise admirable antibiotic. The toxic manifestations attributed to chloramphenicol have been reviewed elsewhere;[4,5] the most serious of them, bone marrow aplasia, is (a) not dose-related and (b) *may* not extend to certain analogues of chloramphenicol which lack the *p*-nitro and *N*-dichloroacetyl substituents of the parent antibiotic.[6,7] The former functional group has received considerable attention as the necessary precursor for production in vivo of the *p*-nitroso compound, proposed as the elusive metabolite suspected to be the cause of the irreversible and often fatal aplastic anaemia, observed with an incidence of 1 in approximately 30 000 courses of therapy.[4]

1   Chemistry and Properties of Chloramphenicol

The structure of chloramphenicol is deceptively simple and also instructive in guiding thinking about its biologic and pharmacologic properties.[8-10] Chloramphenicol is not ionized at any pH attainable in vivo and has amphiphilic properties due to the presence of hydrophobic components (the *p*-nitrophenyl moiety and the *N*-dichloroacetyl substituent) and a hydrophilic dihydroxypropane side chain which confers reasonable solubility in aqueous systems. The stereochemistry of the propanediol side chain at C-1

and C-2 should be noted since only one of the four possible diastereoisomers of chloramphenicol (the D-*threo* isomer) is active as an antibiotic. Its action is to inhibit the peptidyl transferase centre of prokaryotic ribosomes. The preference of the ribosomal 50S subunit for D-*threo* chloramphenicol is mirrored in the specificity of the enzyme responsible for resistance to the antibiotic, chloramphenicol acetyltransferase.[10] The ability of chloramphenicol (and closely related analogues) to traverse the blood–brain barrier readily and to gain access to abscesses and the aqueous and vitreous humours is likely to be due to its being a neutral molecule with relatively high lipid solubility.

2   Chloramphenicol Resistance by Enzymic Acetylation

The relative simplicity of the structure of chloramphenicol prompted the development of economic routes to its chemical synthesis, making it the first totally synthetic antibiotic of pharmaceutical importance. The natural product was characterized after its isolation from a soil bacterium (*Streptomyces venezuelae*); analogous compounds ('corynecins' wherein the *N*-dichloroacetyl substituent is replaced by non-halogenated acyl groups) have been isolated from certain corynebacteria.[11] All micro-organisms known to synthesize chloramphenicol (or its congeners) are prokaryotes with 70S ribosomes (comprised of 50S and 30S sub-units) and it is not known precisely how they synthesize and secrete a potent inhibitor of microbial protein synthesis without evident ill effects. The general problem is addressed by Cundliffe in this Bulletin[12] but, unlike the picture which seems to be emerging for producers of other antibiotics which inhibit ribosome function, the mechanism of resistance or tolerance of *S. venezuelae* to chloramphenicol is not that which is widespread among non-antibiotic-producing bacteria (see below).

Chloramphenicol became available for clinical use in 1948 and was soon accepted as the prototype broad-spectrum antibiotic, active against virtually all gram-positive and many gram-negative bacteria including rickettsia. Clinical isolates resistant to chloramphenicol were recognized within a few years of its introduction, but the earliest reported studies on this resistance (as well as resistance to penicillin and streptomycin) were on its use as a model system for investigating heredity in bacteria.[13] The appearance in 1955 of epidemic strains of shigella, resistant to chloramphenicol and three other unrelated antibiotics, led eventually to the recognition of the phenomenon of plasmid-mediated transmissible antibiotic resistance.[14] The dramatic association of clinically important chloramphenicol resistance with plasmids, in gram-negative bacteria wherein transmissibility was first observed, and also in gram-positive pathogens such as *Staphylococcus aureus* and streptococci, is discussed elsewhere in this Bulletin.

Miyamura was the first to observe (1964) that *Escherichia coli* strains which harboured transmissible elements conferring chloramphenicol resistance were able to inactivate the antibiotic rapidly and completely.[15] He also noted that some clinical isolates of *S. aureus* had this property, an observation made independently and simultaneously by an American group.[16] Within a few years it became clear that chloramphenicol resistance in most clinical isolates was plasmid-borne and due to the presence in resistant bacteria of an enzyme, chloramphenicol acetyltransferase (CAT), which catalyses the acetyl-CoA dependent acetylation of the antibiotic at the C-3 hydroxyl group.[17-19] Enzymic acetylation occurs only at the primary hydroxyl group and not at the secondary C-1 hydroxyl. The latter does, however, play an interesting role in the overall transformation of chloramphenicol to the final inactivation product, 1,3-diacetoxychloramphenicol. The CAT

FIG. 1. The structure of chloramphenicol shown by three conventions

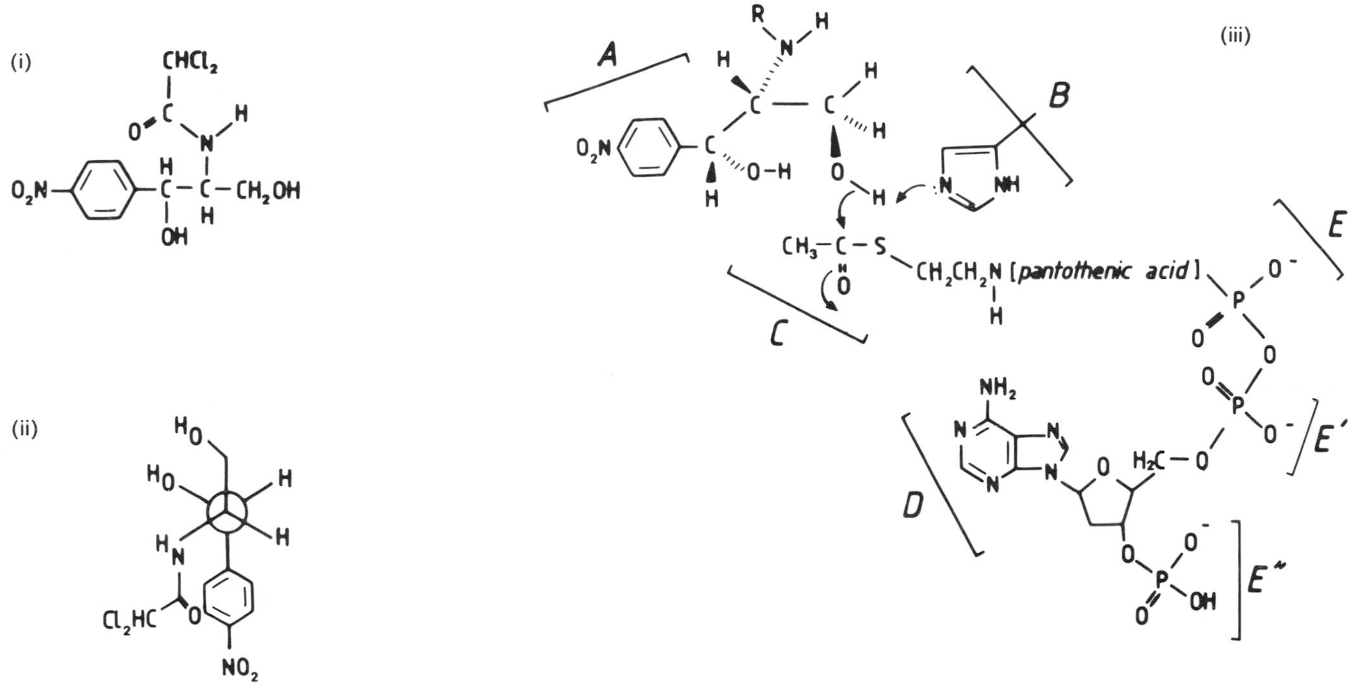

Diagram (i) gives the familiar planar depiction. Structure (ii) is drawn to emphasize rotation along the C_1–C_2 axis and the favoured conformational isomer deduced from spectroscopic and crystallographic studies.[48] The possibility for stabilization of the preferred conformer by hydrogen bond formation between the two hydroxyl groups is clear from structure ii and the depiction of chloramphenicol in diagram (iii). The latter includes the structure of acetyl-CoA and suggests an early step in the mechanism for formation of the tetrahedral intermediate via a general base role for the N-3 atom of the imidazole group (B) believed to play a critical role in catalysis. The collapse of the proposed intermediate to yield 3-acetoxy chloramphenicol and CoA is not shown. Chemical modification and kinetic studies (summarized in reference 10) have implicated an aromatic 'pocket' (A) and an adenine binding site (D) at the active site; further stabilization of the CoA moiety by critically disposed arginine residues at one or more sites (designated E, E', and E") seems likely. A constraint on the size and properties of the acyl group is designated by site C.

R = dichloroacetyl

catalysed acetylation yields 3-acetoxychloramphenicol, which undergoes non-enzymic intramolecular rearrangement to yield 1-acetoxychloramphenicol. The latter undergoes further enzymic modification by addition of a second acetyl group but at a rate at least two orders of magnitude slower than that of the first acetylation. Since the initial product, 3-acetoxychloramphenicol, fails to bind to bacterial ribosomes and lacks antibiotic activity, the subsequent chemical and enzymic events are largely irrelevant to the expression of the resistance phenotype.[10] The overall schema is as follows:

$$\text{CAT}$$
(1) chloramphenicol + acetyl-S-CoA → 3-O-acetyl chloramphenicol + HS-CoA
(2) 3-O-acetyl chloramphenicol ⇌ 1-O-acetyl chloramphenicol
$$\text{CAT}$$
(3) 1-O-acetyl chloramphenicol + acetyl-S-CoA → 1,3-diacetyl chloramphenicol + HS-CoA

Since steps (1) and (3) couple the cleavage of a thio-ester with the synthesis of a conventional oxy-ester, the equilibrium for both acetylation steps lies far to the right. The crucial first enzymic step is therefore essentially irreversible and the inactivated antibiotic is subject to isomerization and a second acetylation if it remains within the bacterial cell.

The kinetic mechanism of chloramphenicol acetylation has been determined for one naturally occurring variant of CAT (reviewed in reference 10). The reaction does not involve a kinetically detectable acetyl–enzyme intermediate but proceeds via the formation of a ternary complex of enzyme, chloramphenicol, and acetyl-CoA. The order of addition of substrates is random and the formation of the ternary complex is not rate-determining so that the apparent Michaelis constant (K_m) for each substrate approximates the experimental dissociation constant (K_d) for the appropriate binary complex. The K_d for chloramphenicol in all instances examined falls in the range of 5–20μM (1.6–6.5μg ml^{-1}), a necessary prerequisite for an efficient resistance mechanism since most bacteria are inhibited by chloramphenicol at comparable concentrations. Whilst natural selection has led to a common and acceptably high affinity for chloramphenicol by CAT variants, there is much evidence for evolutionary divergence in segments or domains of the protein structure which are not intimately concerned with substrate binding.[10]

3 Variants of Chloramphenicol Acetyltransferase

Whereas earlier analyses of the mechanism of chloramphenicol resistance emphasized the enzymology and the consequences of acetylation, more recent studies have concentrated on the extent of variation within the CAT enzyme family of proteins.[10, 20–22] In every instance examined, CAT exists in the native state as a tetramer composed of four identical monomeric polypeptide subunits, each of which contributes to the formation of an active site. The monomeric polypeptide in each CAT consists of approximately 220 amino acids, and the corresponding apparent molecular weight (M_r) of the tetrameric enzyme is of the order of 100000. Early studies suggested that the CAT specified by plasmids in gram-negative bacteria was different from that found in *S. aureus*, but the full extent of heterogeneity has only become apparent with the advent of direct amino acid sequence determinations on CAT variants[23] and, more recently still, the application of rapid methods for DNA sequence analysis to various structural genes for CAT.[24–26] Shown in Table I are partial primary structures for six CAT variants. The type I enzyme is specified by many R plasmids found in enteric bacteria and by the CAT gene of transposable element Tn9. Enzyme types II and III, encoded by other plasmids in gram-negative bacteria, show substantial segments of homology with the type I polypeptide as well as with other variants, but their complete primary structures are not yet known.[10] The plasmid-specified CAT variants of staphylococci (types A–D and that specified by plasmid pC194) are more closely related to one another than is the case within the gram-negative subgroup (types I–III above). The staphylococcal variants are also structurally similar to the recently described CAT of *Bacillus pumilus* which is the product of a chromosomal gene.[27] The most striking homology amongst the CAT structures presently known is the segment centred at residue 193 of the type I polypeptide.

Histidine-193 (and its counterparts in other variants) appears to play a critical role in catalysis, and the conservation of primary structure in this region reflects its likely functional importance and the need for proper folding of this segment of polypeptide. The overall folding pathway for CAT variants seems likely to be a common one in view of (a) the identity of proline residues in a number of positions likely to be within abrupt turns or bends in the tertiary structure and (b) conservation of many hydrophobic residues which are prime candidates for the interior of the CAT monomer (or the interfaces between subunits) wherein constraints on correct chain folding and packing of amino acid side chains are most marked. The evidence bearing on these points has been presented elsewhere.[10] Since a structure based upon X-ray diffraction data is not yet available, further speculation about the relation of structure to function is premature.

One of the central problems arising from study of plasmid-specified resistance mechanisms in general, and CAT in particular, is that of their origin. Strains of *E. coli* or *S. aureus* which lack plasmids (and which have not been the subject of genetic manipulation) are uniformly and characteristically sensitive to chloramphenicol concentrations of the order of 3μM (3μg ml^{-1}). There is abundant evidence in *E. coli* that laboratory selection for chloramphenicol resistance yields strains tolerant to the presence of the antibiotic by virtue of mechanisms which do not involve enzymic acetylation by CAT.[28–29] Pleiotropic mutations involving changes in the permeability of the cell envelope are the rule, but there are no unambiguous examples of (a) the appearance of CAT in clones derived from cells which formerly lacked the enzyme or

TABLE I. Selected properties of chloramphenicol acetyltransferase variants

Enzyme types	Binding to chloramphenicol-substituted agarose*	K_m^{app} (μM) chloramphenicol	K_m^{app} (μM) acetyl-CoA	Relative V_{max} (%)†	DTNB sensitivity	Reaction with antiserum to CAT$_I$	Reaction with antiserum to CAT$_{III}$	Reaction with antiserum to CAT$_C$‡
I	5	12	76	10–20	0	+	–	–
II	4	18	57	5–10	5	–	–	–
III	3	16	80	[100]	1	–	+	–
Proteus mirabilis	5	15	82	~8	3	+	–	–
Haemophilis influenzae	3	n.d.	n.d.	5–10	5	–	–	–
Agrobacterium tumefaciens	3	21	133	<10	2	–	–	–
Flavobacterium sp.§	1	n.d.	n.d.	<5	n.d.	n.d.	n.d.	n.d.
Streptomyces acrimycini§	3	17	143	<5	4	–	–	–
Bacteroides fragilis	2	5	n.d.	n.d.	5	n.d.	n.d.	n.d.
Staphylococcus sp.								
A	3	2.6	57	~4	0	–	–	+
B	3	2.7	56	~2	0	–	–	+
C	3	2.5	61	~2	0	–	–	+
D	3	2.7	46	~3	0	–	–	+
Streptococcus agalactiae	3	9.3	101	<5	1	–	–	+
Streptococcus faecalis	3	n.d.	n.d.	<5	1	–	–	+
Streptococcus pneumoniae	2	10	15	n.d.	1	–	–	(+)
Clostridium perfringens	2	22	85	n.d.	2	–	–	(+)

Enzyme type	Primary structures of polypeptides‖
	1 5 10 15 20 190 195 200 → C-terminus
I (Tn9)	Met Glu Lys Lys Ile Thr Gly Tyr Thr Thr Val Asp Ile Ser Gln Trp His Arg Lys Glu --- Gln Val His His Ala Val Cys Asp Gly Phe His ---
II	Met Asn Phe Thr Arg Ile Asp Len Asn Thr Trp Asn --- not determined ---
III	
C (pC221)¶	Met Asn Tyr Thr Lys Phe Asp Val Lys Asn Trp Val Arg Arg Glu --- Gln Val His His Ala Val Cys Asp Gly Phe His ---
(pC194)	[Met] Thr Phe Asn Ile Ile Lys Leu Glu Asn Trp Asp Arg Lys Glu --- Gln Val His His Ala Val Cys Asp Gly Tyr His ---
B. pumilus	Met Asn Phe Asn Ile Ile Lys Leu Asp Asn Trp Lys Arg Lys Glu --- Gln Val His His Ala Val Ser Val Asp Gly Tyr His ---
	Met Thr Phe Asn Ile Ile Lys Leu Glu Asn Trp Asp Arg Lys Glu --- Gln Val His His Ala Val Cys Asp Gly Tyr His --- ↑

The properties of CAT variants have been summarized from previous reports[10,20–27,52,56] save for those marked (§)
* Graded from 0–5 where 0 = no binding to affinity resin or inhibition by DTNB (5,5′-dithio-bis-2 nitrobenzoate)
† Relative V_{max} estimate of maximum catalytic rate in presence of saturating concentrations of both substratres. The turnover number (k_{cat}) for the Type III enzyme purified from *E. coli* (R387) is 1500 sec^{-1} and is taken as 100
‡ The anti-CAT$_c$ serum neutralized all gram-positive variants but did not give precipitation reaction with *S. pneumoniae* or *C. perfringens*. These results are indicated by (+). All others marked + give both precipitation and neutralization
§ Data from unpublished experiments in the author's laboratory
‖ The amino acid sequences shown have been selected from more extensive compilations published elsewhere[10,22] with the addition of selected segments of the CAT primary structure for *B. pumilus*.[27] The segments shown demonstrate the high degree of homology around the catalytic imidazole group of His-193, less conservation in the amino-terminal region, and the five residue difference between the start of the type I polypeptide and all others
¶ The type C enzyme variant encoded by pC221 has the N-terminal sequence Thr-Phe-Asn- - - whereas the DNA sequences of the genes for CAT from pC194[26] and *B. pumilus*[27] are believed to specify amino-terminal Met via ATG and TTG. Post-translational removal of the amino terminal Met residue occurs with the pC221 specified CAT and may occur with all CAT variants from gram-positive bacteria

(b) resistance to chloramphenicol due to mutations in genes for ribosomal proteins. That is, there is no direct evidence that genes for the many CAT variants now found to be associated with plasmids in gram-negative and gram-positive bacteria of clinical importance have a readily identifiable immediate chromosomal ancestor. Although the extent of homology amongst CAT variants is compatible with the notion of divergent evolution from an ancestral gene, the evidence is incomplete and circumstantial.

The phenomenon of plasmid-mediated antibiotic resistance is best understood in gram-negative bacteria in which plasmid transmissibility is common and genetic exchange is known to occur by both 'legitimate' recombination and mechanisms independent of the usual host *rec* genes. In the case of chloramphenicol resistance, such exchanges have been described for a transposon (Tn9) wherein the gene for a type I enzyme variant is flanked by direct repeat of the IS1 insertion sequence.[24,25] Recent studies have suggested a likely origin for this transposable element, the resistance determinant, (r-det) region of plasmids such as NR1 which is also flanked by direct repeats of IS1.[30-32] The finding of a gene for the type I variant CAT on the chromosome of a gram-negative bacterium, especially in conjunction with a flanking IS1 element, is more likely to be the consequence of transposition than evidence for the evolutionary 'origin' of CAT.

There are several genera or species of bacteria in which genuinely novel CAT variants have been detected and the genes appear to be chromosomal. The three most intriguing examples, *Agrobacterium tumefaciens*, several species of streptomyces, and a flavobacterium, belong to the soil eco-system in which genes for antibiotic synthesis abound. The CAT polypeptides produced in the above cases are different from one another and distinct from those encoded by plasmids in clinically important bacteria.[22] It is curious that *S. venezuelae* which synthesizes chloramphenicol does not contain CAT, and the mechanism by which it is tolerant to its own product remains obscure.[33] DNA sequences of the structural and regulatory regions of genes for CAT from these soil micro-organisms may yield new and important clues about the evolution of the CAT family of proteins and, in a larger sense, the evolution of medically important drug resistance plasmids. Hughes & Datta[34] showed that many bacteria of medical importance isolated prior to the discovery and use of antibiotics possessed plasmids lacking resistance genes. The acquisition of genes for CAT variants by such plasmids from micro-organisms indigenous to soil is plausible and more likely than the independent evolution of specificity for chloramphenicol on the part of diverse acetyltransferase enzymes in diverse bacterial genera.

4 Expression of Genes for Chloramphenicol Acetyltransferase

All known variants of CAT encoded by plasmids in gram-negative bacteria are synthesized constitutively. By contrast, their counterparts in staphylococci,[35] streptococci,[36-37] and *B. pumilus*[38,39] are inducible in the presence of the antibiotic (or one of a number of closely related analogues).

The discovery of an inducible CAT phenotype posed several problems which have yet to be solved. Chloramphenicol is the prototype inhibitor of protein synthesis amongst antibiotics and particularly effective as an experimental tool for inhibiting induced enzyme synthesis. Early experiments in *S. aureus* demonstrated that protein synthesis was necessary for the synthesis of CAT and that the product of the reaction, 3-acetoxychloramphenicol, was not an inducer.[40] The kinetics of induction were observed to be sigmoid and rapid induction occurred only with concentrations of chloramphenicol less than $100\mu M$ ($33\mu g\,ml^{-1}$). The use of 3-deoxy-

chloramphenicol, a 'gratuitous' inducer, showed (a) that a compound which was neither an inhibitor of protein synthesis nor a substrate, could be an effective inducer and (b) that *linear* kinetics of induction were obtained after a short lag (4–6 minutes) interpreted as the time required for specific transcription (mRNA synthesis) and translation (protein synthesis) of the CAT gene. Although the phenomenon of induction of CAT in gram-positive bacteria by chloramphenicol is not in doubt, there are now reasons to question the original proposal for transcriptional control of expression. The DNA sequences are now known for two CAT variants specified by plasmids (pC221 and pC194) in staphylococci[26,41] and for the chromosomal gene in *B. pumilus*. All three are inducible and similar in structure. Where small DNA segments from each (containing only the gene for CAT) are cloned in *E. coli*, the resistance phenotype is still inducible.[27,39,41] A suspicion that CAT itself might be the regulatory protein ('autogenous' regulation of transcription) has faded in the light of new knowledge; the *B. pumilus* structural gene for CAT can be interrupted by the insertion of a foreign gene which is then subject to induction by chloramphenicol in *B. subtilis* even when the CAT polypeptide is no longer synthesized.[39] Although such genetic fusions have not been made for the CAT variants of staphylococcal plasmids, the genes for the latter have striking similarities with their *B. pumilus* counterpart; namely, the presence in the deduced mRNA of an inverted complementary repeat yielding a predicted stem-loop structure immediately 5' to the start of the polypeptide and which incorporates a characteristic sequence (GGAGG) at the base of the stem. The latter is complementary to the 3' end of ribosomal RNA (16S) from gram-positive bacteria and serves as the ribosome-binding site required for efficient translation of the mRNA. It has been suggested that translation of the message occurs only when chloramphenicol (or any congener which induces CAT) is bound to the ribosome and induces it to display an enhanced affinity for the GGAGG sequence, thereby competing effectively with the Watson–Crick base pairing of the stem-loop structure, and allowing CAT synthesis to proceed.[39] Since the CAT gene from *B. pumilus* in the construction under study lacked its natural promoter, it remains to be seen whether the proposed post-transcriptional model for control of CAT expression is the only one operating in the natural host. There are now a number of examples of gene regulation effected by transcriptional (repression) as well as translational (attenuation) mechanisms,[42] and there is no reason, *a priori*, why CAT in gram-positive bacteria need be controlled only by the latter.

Viewed from the therapeutic point of view, the most important difference between the expression of CAT in gram-negative bacteria compared with gram-positive ones is the level of chloramphenicol resistance attained. In most cases of the former, the constitutive synthesis of CAT promotes levels of resistance to chloramphenicol *at least* five-fold higher than are found in gram-positive bacteria. However, where pre-induced by prior exposure to low levels of chloramphenicol, the latter are characteristically resistant to chloramphenicol concentrations in excess of 0.5mM ($162\mu g\,ml^{-1}$), a level of resistance typical of most clinical isolates of *E. coli* harbouring a low-copy-number plasmid specifying the type I variant of CAT. Gene dosage (number of gene copies per cell) necessarily plays an important role in the observed resistance phenotype. Whilst most naturally occurring R plasmids in the enteric bacteria are low-copy-number replicons, the small plasmids carrying chloramphenicol resistance in staphylococci have characteristically high copy numbers (20–40 per chromosome), a factor which, to some degree, must compensate for the special problems inherent in the inducible synthesis of CAT.

5 Non-Enzymic Chloramphenicol Resistance

Most clinical isolates of chloramphenicol-resistant bacteria owe their phenotype to plasmid-borne CAT genes. An exception is *Pseudomonas aeruginosa* which, although occasionally a host for plasmids which specify CAT, is characteristically tolerant to high levels ($> 100 \mu g\,ml^{-1}$) of chloramphenicol by virtue of an exclusion mechanism yet to be defined in detail.[43] Foster and his colleagues have, however, studied one example of a plasmid-encoded, non-enzymic resistance mechanism[44] which is expressed in *E. coli* and can occur in isolation or co-exist with CAT.[45,46] Recent experiments have shown that this inducible mechanism is associated with the synthesis of a 33K polypeptide associated with the cell envelope (TJ Foster; personal communication). Although the effect appears to be one of reduced net influx of chloramphenicol into the cell, the details are not yet clear. Nor is it known how prevalent is the gene for this non-enzymic mechanism. There is circumstantial evidence for such a mechanism in chloramphenicol resistant isolates of *H. influenzae*[47] which lack CAT and which are resistant not only to chloramphenicol but to its 3-fluoro analogues which are not susceptible to inactivation by CAT (see below).

6 Clinical Considerations and Chemotherapy

Unlike the proliferation of useful antibiotics of the β-lactam family, there have been rather few successes in the development of analogues of chloramphenicol with enhanced (or more selective) antimicrobial activity or effectiveness against resistant strains. No compounds significantly more active than the parent have been synthesized and there is, as yet, no convincing animal or in-vitro test system for the toxic effects that have prevented wider use of chloramphenicol. Two synthetic efforts are, however, worthy of mention.

An analogue of chloramphenicol wherein the aromatic nitro group (see Fig. 1) is replaced by CH_3SO_2- has proved to be clinically useful and *may* be free of the potentially lethal haematological toxicity.[4-7] A more recent development was the preparation of the 3-fluoro analogue of chloramphenicol in which the primary hydroxyl target for acetylation is replaced by fluorine.[48] The compound is active against CAT-producing bacteria as is a related analogue which combines 3-fluoro substitution with the presence of CH_3SO_2- as the para substituent of the 1-phenyl moiety.[47,49] Chloramphenicol itself is, however, the therapeutic standby for those few clinical situations for which it remains a first-line antibiotic. Plasmid-bearing and multi-resistant epidemic strains of *Salmonella typhi* containing CAT have been described, but the presence of the resistance phenotype is unusual in isolates from sporadic cases. Resistance to chloramphenicol and the presence of CAT are well documented in *H. influenzae* type b[50-52] but the incidence of chloramphenicol resistance and CAT amongst isolates of *Haemophilus influenzae* and *S. pneumoniae* remains very low in most countries, and the vast majority of clinical isolates of *Bacteroides fragilis* remain sensitive to chloramphenicol. Since chloramphenicol is bactericidal against sensitive strains of *H. influenzae* type b at concentrations which can be achieved in the cerebrospinal fluid,[53-55] it is the drug of choice for the treatment of infection, especially with β-lactamase-producing strains. The usefulness of chloramphenicol in the treatment of *Bacteroides fragilis* remains unchallenged in spite of a report demonstrating resistance and CAT in a clinical isolate.[56] A survey in USA in 1981 revealed uniform sensitivity to chloramphenicol for some 750 isolates collected at nine centres.[57]

A recent therapeutic review of its efficacy in paediatric practice has spoken of the 'renaissance of chloramphenicol'. Although prospects for a return to the wide usage of chloramphenicol seen in the first decade of its clinical life seem remote, there are sound reasons for keeping it firmly in mind for serious infections in which resistance to β-lactam antibiotics is common, the high degree of diffusibility of the antibiotic is a valuable asset, and likelihood of encountering chloramphenicol resistance remains low.

ACKNOWLEDGEMENTS

This work is supported by the Medical Research Council and the Wellcome Trust.

REFERENCES

1 Laferriere CI, Marks MI. Chloramphenicol: properties and clinical use. Pediatr Infect Dis 1982; 1: 257–264
2 Dajani AS, Kauffman RE. The renaissance of chloramphenicol. Pediatr Clin North Am 1981; 28: 195–202
3 Lietman PS. Chloramphenicol and the neonate—1979 view. Clin Perinatol 1979; 6: 151–162
4 Sande MA, Mandell GL. Chloramphenicol. In: Gilman AG, Goodman, LS, Gilman A, eds. Goodman and Gilman's the pharmacological basis of therapeutics. 6th ed. New York: Macmillan, 1980; 1191–1199
5 Yunis AA. Chloramphenicol-induced bone marrow suppression. Semin Hematol 1973; 10: 225–234
6 Keiser G. Co-operative study of patients treated with thiamphenicol. Comparative study of patients treated with chloramphenicol and thiamphenicol. Postgrad Med J 1974; 50 (suppl 5): 143–151
7 Murray T, Downey KM, Yunis AA. Degradation of isolated deoxyribonucleic acid mediated by nitroso-chloramphenicol. Possible role in chloramphenicol-induced aplastic anemia. Biochem Pharmacol 1982; 31: 2291–2296
8 Pongs O. Chloramphenicol. In: Hahn FE, ed. Mechanism of action of antibacterial agents. Berlin: Springer, 1979; 26–42
9 Gale EF, Cundliffe E, Reynolds PE, Richmond MH, Waring MJ. The molecular basis of antibiotic action. 2nd ed. London: Wiley, 1981; 462–468
10 Shaw WV. Chloramphenicol acetyltransferase: enzymology and molecular biology. CRC Crit Rev Biochem 1983; 14: 1–46
11 Nakano H, Tomita F, Suzuki T. Biosynthesis of corynecins by *Corynebacterium hydrocarboclastus*: on the origin of the N-acyl group. Agric Biol Chem 1976; 40: 331–336
12 Cundliffe E. Self defence in antibiotic-producing organisms. Br Med Bull 1984; 40: 61–67
13 Cavalli-Sforza LL. Indirect selection and origin of resistance. In: Wolstenholme GEW, O'Connor CM, eds. Ciba Foundation symposium on drug resistance in micro-organisms. London: Churchill, 1957; 30–46
14 Watanabe T. Infective heredity of multiple drug resistance in bacteria. Bacteriol Rev 1963; 27: 87–115
15 Miyamura S. Inactivation of chloramphenicol by chloramphenicol-resistant bacteria. J Pharm Sci 1964; 53: 604–607
16 Dunsmoor CL, Pim KL, Sherris JC. Observations on the inactivation of chloramphenicol by chloramphenicol-resistant staphylococci. In: Sylvester JC, ed. Antimicrobial agents and chemotherapy—1963. Ann Arbor MI: American Society for Microbiology, 1964; 500–506
17 Okamoto S, Suzuki Y. Chloramphenicol, dihydrostreptomycin, and kanamycin-inactivating enzymes from multiple drug-resistant *Escherichia coli* carrying episome R. Nature 1965; 208: 1301–1303
18 Shaw WV. The enzymatic acetylation of chloramphenicol by extracts of R factor-resistant *Escherichia coli*. J Biol Chem 1967; 242: 687–693
19 Suzuki Y, Okamoto S. The enzymatic acetylation of chloramphenicol by the multiple drug-resistant *Escherichia coli* carrying R factor. J Biol Chem 1967; 242: 4722–4730
20 Gaffney DF, Foster TJ, Shaw WV. Chloramphenicol acetyltransferases determined by R plasmids from Gram-negative bacteria. J Gen Microbiol 1978; 109: 351–358

21 Fitton JE, Shaw WV. Comparison of chloramphenicol acetyltransferase variants in staphylococci. Biochem J 1979; 177: 575–582

22 Zaidenzaig Y, Fitton JE, Packman LC, Shaw WV. Characterization and comparison of chloramphenicol acetyltransferase variants. Eur J Biochem 1979; 100: 609–618

23 Shaw WV, Packman LC, Burleigh BD, Dell A, Morris HR, Hartley BS. Primary structure of a chloramphenicol acetyltransferase specified by R plasmids. Nature 1979; 282: 870–872

24 Alton NK, Vapnek D. Nucleotide sequence analysis of the chloramphenicol resistance transposon Tn9. Nature 1979; 282: 864–869

25 Marcoli R, Iida S, Bickle TA. The DNA sequence of an IS1-flanked transposon coding for resistance to chloramphenicol and fusidic acid. FEBS Lett 1980; 110: 11–14

26 Horinouchi S, Weisblum B. Nucleotide sequence and functional map of pC194, a plasmid that specifies inducible chloramphenicol resistance. J Bacteriol 1982; 150: 815–825

27 Harwood CR, Williams DM, Lovett PS. Nucleotide sequence of a *Bacillus pumilus* gene specifying chloramphenicol acetyltransferase. Gene 1983; In press

28 Reeve ECR. Characteristics of some single-step mutants to chloramphenicol resistance in *Escherichia coli* K12 and their interactions with R-factor genes. Genet Res 1966; 7: 281–286

29 Foster TJ. R factor tetracycline and chloramphenicol resistance in *Escherichia coli* K_{12} *cmlB* mutants. J Gen Microbiol 1975; 90: 303–310

30 Chandler M, Boy de la Tour E, Willems D, Caro L. Some properties of the chloramphenicol resistance transposon Tn9. Mol Gen Genet 1979; 176: 221–231

31 Iida S, Arbor W. On the role of IS1 in the formation of hybrids between the bacteriophage P1 and the R plasmid NR1. Mol Gen Genet 1980; 177: 261–270

32 Iida S, Hänni C, Echarti C, Arber W. Is the IS1-flanked r-determinant of the R plasmid NR1 a transposon? J Gen Microbiol 1981; 126: 413–425

33 Shaw WV, Hopwood DA. Chloramphenicol acetylation in *Streptomyces*. J Gen Microbiol 1976; 94: 159–166

34 Hughes VM, Datta N. Conjugative plasmids in bacteria of the 'pre-antibiotic' era. Nature 1983; 302: 725–726

35 Shaw WV, Brodsky RF. Characterization of chloramphenicol acetyltransferase from chloramphenicol-resistant *Straphylococcus aureus*. J Bacteriol 1968; 95: 28–36

36 Courvalin PM, Shaw WV, Jacob AE. Plasmid-mediated mechanisms of resistance to aminoglycoside-aminocyclitol antibiotics and to chloramphenicol in Group D streptococci. Antimicrob Agents Chemother 1978; 13: 716–725

37 Dang-Van A, Tiraby G, Acar JF, Shaw WV, Bouanchand DH. Chloramphenicol resistance in *Streptococcus pneumoniae*: Enzymatic acetylation and possible plasmid linkage. Antimicrob Agents Chemother 1978; 13: 577–583

38 Williams DM, Duvall EJ, Lovett PS. Cloning restriction fragments that promote expression of a gene in *Bacillus subtilis*. J Bacteriol 1981; 146: 1162–1165

39 Duvall EJ, Williams DM, Lovett PS, Rudolph C, Vasantha N, Guyer M. Chloramphenicol inducible gene expression in *Bacillus subtilis*. Gene 1983; In press

40 Winshell E, Shaw WV. Kinetics of induction and purification of chloramphenicol acetyltransferase from chloramphenicol-resistant *Staphylococcus aureus*. J Bacteriol 1969; 98: 1248–1257

41 Skinner S. Studies on staphylococcal chloramphenicol resistance plasmids. PhD Thesis, University of Leicester, 1983

42 Yanofsky C. Attenuation in the control of expression of bacterial operons. Nature 1981; 289: 751–758

43 Kono M, O'Hara K. Mechanism of chloramphenicol resistance mediated by kR102 factor in *Pseudomonas aeruginosa*. J Antibiot 1976; 29: 176–180

44 Nagai Y, Mitsuhashi S. New type of R factors incapable of inactivating chloramphenicol. J Bacteriol 1972; 109: 1–7

45 Gaffney DF, Cundliffe E, Foster TJ. Chloramphenicol resistance that does not involve chloramphenicol acetyltransferase encoded by plasmids from gram-negative bacteria. J Gen Microbiol 1981; 125: 113–121

46 Dorman CJ, Foster TJ. Nonenzymatic chloramphenicol resistance determinants specified by plasmids R26 and R55-1 in *Escherichia coli* K-12 do not confer high-level resistance to fluorinated analogs. Antimicrob Agents Chemother 1982; 22: 912–914

47 Syriopoulou VP, Harding AL, Goldmann DA, Smith AL. *In vitro* antibacterial activity of fluorinated analogs of chloramphenicol and thiamphenicol. Antimicrob Agents Chemother 1981; 19: 294–297

48 Schafer TW, Moss EL Jr, Nagabhushan TL, Miller GH. Novel fluorine-containing analogs of chloramphenicol and thiamphenicol: anti-bacterial and biological properties. In: Nelson JD, Grassi C, eds. Current chemotherapy and infectious disease. Washington DC: American Society for Microbiology, 1980; 444–446

49 Neu HC, Fu KP, Kung K. Fluorinated chloramphenicol analogs active against bacteria resistant to chloramphenicol. In: Nelson JD, Grassi C, eds. Current chemotherapy and infectious disease. Washington DC: American Society for Microbiology, 1980; 446–447

50 van Klingeren B, van Embden JDA, Dessens-Kroon M. Plasmid-mediated chloramphenicol resistance in *Haemophilus influenzae*. Antimicrob Agents Chemother 1977; 11: 383–387

51 Jahn G, Laufs R, Kaulfers P-M, Kolenda H. Molecular nature of two *Haemophilus influenzae* R factors containing resistances and the multiple integration of drug resistance transposons. J Bacteriol 1979; 138: 584–597

52 Roberts M, Corney A, Shaw WV. Molecular characterization of three chloramphenicol acetyltransferases isolated from *Haemophilus influenzae*. J Bacteriol 1982; 151: 737–741

53 Turk DC. A comparison of chloramphenicol and ampicillin as bactericidal agents for *Haemophilus influenzae* type b. J Med Microbiol 1977; 10: 127–131

54 Rahal JJ Jr, Simberkoff MS. Bactericidal and bacteriostatic action of chloramphenicol against meningeal pathogens. Antimicrob Agents Chemother 1977; 16: 13–18

55 Feldman WE, Manning NS. Effect of growth phase on the bactericidal action of chloramphenicol against *Haemophilus influenzae* type b and *Escherichia coli* K-1. Antimicrob Agents Chemother 1983; 23: 551–554

56 Britz ML, Wilkinson RG. Chloramphenicol acetyltransferase of *Bacteroides fragilis*. Antimicrob Agents Chemother 1978; 14: 105–111

57 Tally FP, Cuchural GJ, Jacobus NV, *et al*. Susceptibility of the *Bacteroides fragilis* group in the United States in 1981. Antimicrob Agents Chemother 1983; 23: 536–540

British Medical Bulletin (1984) Vol. 40, No. 1, pp. 42–46

BACTERIAL RESISTANCE TO ANTIFOLATE CHEMOTHERAPEUTIC AGENTS MEDIATED BY PLASMIDS

J T SMITH BPharm PhD FPS

*Microbiology Section
Department of Pharmaceutics
The School of Pharmacy
University of London*

S G B AMYES BSc MSc PhD

*Department of Bacteriology
The Medical School
University of Edinburgh*

1 Alternative biochemical pathway
   a R-plasmid-determined by-pass resistance mechanisms
   b Different types of trimethoprim-resistant dihydrofolate reductase
2 Transposition
3 Sulphonamide resistance
   References

Resistance to antibiotics in bacteria has shown an explosive increase in recent years, which in some instances has more than kept pace with the commercial production and clinical use of antibiotics and chemotherapeutic agents.

Although it is known that bacteria can mutate to become drug-resistant, this process is generally not responsible for the resistance of clinical bacterial isolates to antibiotics. One reason for this is perhaps because such mutants often exhibit reduced pathogenicity.[1] Clinical antibiotic resistance is usually caused by the presence of antibiotic resistance plasmids (R plasmids) and hence, by definition, the presence of such R plasmids must have little or no deleterious effect on pathogenicity.

There have been many mechanisms proposed by which bacteria may resist antibacterial drugs.[2] The mechanisms most favoured by bacteria are lowering of the intracellular drug concentration (impermeability), destruction or modification of the drug to an inactive form, alteration of the target site of the drug so that it no longer binds the inhibitor, increasing the synthesis of the target enzyme in excess of the inhibitor or the production of an alternative biochemical pathway by-passing the drug-sensitive target site. Which of these mechanisms prevails is dependent on a number of factors. These include the nature of the antibacterial agent, its target site, the bacterial species and whether the resistance is mediated by the chromosome via mutation or by R plasmids. This paper describes how bacteria acquire drug resistance by possessing an alternative biochemical pathway to by-pass the effect of the inhibitory agent.

1 Alternative Biochemical Pathway

Bacteria rarely duplicate major biochemical pathways so inhibition of a single step in a vital pathway generally results in

complete cessation of metabolism. This probably stems from the fact that extensive duplication of biochemical pathways would result in an unacceptable drain on the cell's resources. There is one pathway, however, where duplication may not overburden the cell and that is the synthesis of tetrahydrofolic acid. Tetrahydrofolic acid derivatives are used in living cells to donate single carbon fragments in anabolic metabolism which result in the *de novo* biosynthesis of several amino acids for protein synthesis and of several nucleotides for DNA and RNA synthesis. The ability to synthesize tetrahydrofolic acid from basic constituents is, however, confined to bacteria. This pathway is shown in Fig. 1. The condensation of 2-amino-4-hydroxy-6-hydroxymethyl-pteridine with *p*-aminobenzoic acid (PABA) by dihydropteroate synthase and of the resultant dihydropteroic acid with glutamic acid by dihydrofolate synthase occurs only in bacteria. Mammalian cells, which also require folic acid derivatives, do not exhibit this *de novo* synthesis but utilize preformed folates which are obtained as the vitamin folic acid from the diet. Pathogenic bacteria, with the notable exception of *Streptococcus faecalis*, are unable to take up preformed folic acid derivatives. Both mammalian cells and bacteria reduce dihydrofolic acid to the activated tetrahydrofolate form by the enzyme dihydrofolate reductase. However, there are important differences between the dihydrofolate reductases of mammals and bacteria. Notably, the mammalian enzyme can reduce folic acid to dihydrofolic acid whereas the bacterial enzyme cannot accomplish this step (Fig. 1).

The production of tetrahydrofolic acid is inhibited by two groups of compounds, those that inhibit the enzyme dihydropteroate synthase and those that inhibit dihydrofolate reductase. Of the first group, the sulphonamides have the most widespread use. Early work by Brown[3] on the action of these drugs revealed that they are structural analogues of PABA and competitively inhibit dihydropteroate synthase. He also showed that sulphonamides could be incorporated into inactive folate-like molecules but only in the absence of PABA in a cell-free system. It was later shown that even in the presence of PABA, these folate-like inactive analogues could be synthesized by intact bacteria which excrete them into the medium.[4] It is possible that the consequential depletion of

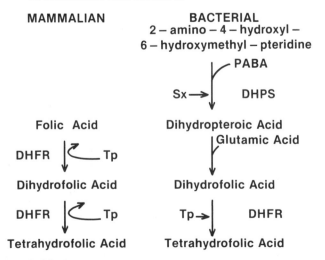

FIG 1. The tetrahydrofolic acid biosynthetic pathway in mammals and bacteria

DHPS: Dihydropteroate synthase; DHFR: Dihydrofolate reductase; Sx →: Sulphamethoxazole inhibits; Tp →: Trimethoprim inhibits; Tp ↄ: Trimethoprim does not inhibit

2-amino-4-hydroxy-6-hydroxymethyl pteridine reserves may contribute significantly to the antibacterial action of sulphonamides. Para-amino salycilic acid (PAS) used in the treatment of *Mycobacterium tuberculosis* infections is also incorporated into inactive folate-like analogues.[5]

There are two types of drug in the second group which inhibit dihydrofolate reductase. The first type consists of derivatives of 2,4-diaminopteridine which are close structural analogues of dihydrofolic acid and can bind in place of the substrate at the active site of most bacterial and mammalian dihydrofolate reductases.[6,7] The second type of drug, the 2,4-diaminopyrimidines, also competitively inhibit dihydrofolate reductases but, unlike 2,4-diaminopteridines, are much more species-specific in their activity.[8] Substitution on the diaminopyrimidine nucleus resulted in the synthesis of trimethoprim which is highly active against the bacterial enzyme and virtually without effect on the mammalian enzyme. This selectivity permitted the use of trimethoprim for the treatment of bacterial infections.

The success of inhibitors of folate metabolism in halting bacterial activities relies, in part, on the low concentrations of tetrahydrofolate present per cell. The inhibition of dihydrofolate reductase by the compounds is rapid with most bacterial enzymes. However, should a second inhibitor-resistant enzyme be produced in the cell, encoded in an acquired plasmid, the resultant functional diploid is able to metabolize tetrahydrofolates as though its sensitive chromosomally encoded enzyme did not exist. Thus inhibitors of folate metabolism are suitable candidates for a by-pass mechanism of resistance.

The only example of a chromosomally mediated by-pass mechanism was in a mutant of *Streptococcus faecalis* (SF/A), shown to produce two dihydrofolate reductases. One of them resembled the wild-type enzyme, possessing similar physical properties. The other had a lower molecular weight and turnover number.[9] When this strain was grown in the absence of methotrexate, tetrahydrofolate synthesis was governed by the normal dihydrofolate reductase; but as soon as the strain was challenged with methotrexate the resistant enzyme took over.

a R-Plasmid-Determined By-pass Resistance Mechanisms

The problems that R plasmids have in producing an efficient resistance mechanism, effective in a variety of different bacterial hosts, are severe. The inhibitors of enzymes involved in tetrahydrofolate synthesis are synthetic and not natural compounds so it is unlikely that specific enzymes could have evolved to inactivate these drugs. Indeed, an extensive search was made in the case of trimethoprim for specific modifying enzymes and also for a plasmid-determined mechanism that prevented uptake of the drug, but none could be found.[10]

When *E. coli* 114 harbouring the first R plasmid, R388, known to confer trimethoprim resistance,[11] was investigated for dihydrofolate reductase activity, it was found that the strain possessing the R plasmid seemed to exhibit the same level of activity as the host strain lacking the plasmid. Eighteen litre cultures of exponential phase bacteria were then harvested and cell extracts fractionated by ammonium sulphate precipitation. No significant activity could be found in the 0–50% saturation ammonium sulphate precipitate but 94% or more of the dihydrofolate reductase activity was found in the 50–80% saturation ammonium sulphate precipitate. When this precipitate was applied to Sephadex G-75, a single dihydrofolate reductase peak was eluted from both the R⁺ and R⁻ strains (Fig. 2). However, the peak from the plasmid-containing strain exhibited a shoulder on the higher-molecular-weight side. When the pooled Sephadex fractions from the R⁻ strain were

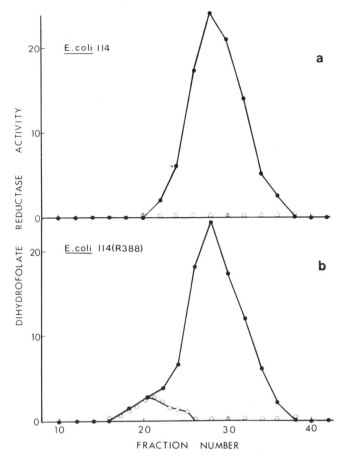

FIG 2. The elution of dihydrofolate reductase by gel filtration using Sephadex G-75

The dihydrofolate reductase assays were performed in both the absence (●—●) and presence (○—○) of 4 × 10⁻⁶ M trimethoprim. Figure 2a shows the R⁻ strain and figure 2b shows the R⁺ strain

assayed in increasing concentrations of trimethoprim, it was found that activity could be abolished completely with 4 × 10⁻⁶ M trimethoprim. Consequently, all the Sephadex fractions from the R⁺ strain were re-assayed in the presence of 4 × 10⁻⁶ M trimethoprim. This revealed a small peak of trimethoprim-resistant dihydrofolate reductase activity amounting to only 9.5% of the total (Fig. 2b). This small peak was situated within the shoulder observed when the R⁺ strain was fractionated by gel filtration and assayed in the absence of trimethoprim.[12]

The trimethoprim-resistant dihydrofolate reductase mediated by R388 possessed a higher molecular weight than the sensitive chromosomal enzyme. Repetition of gel filtration in the presence of standard marker proteins revealed the plasmid enzyme to be of molecular weight (mol.wt.) 35 000 compared with the *E. coli* chromosomal enzyme, of mol.wt. 21 000. The trimethoprim-resistant fractions were pooled and the concentration of trimethoprim required to inhibit the enzyme was determined. It was found that inhibition of the plasmid-mediated enzyme was linear with respect to logarithmic trimethoprim concentration while that of the chromosomal enzyme was not linear, suggesting the enzymes differ in their mechanism of trimethoprim binding. When the concentration of trimethoprim required to cause 50% inhibition was interpolated it was found that 22 000 times more drug was required to inhibit the plasmid enzyme than that required to inhibit the chromosomal enzyme. The concentration of trimethoprim required to prevent the growth of bacteria harbouring R388 was 15 000 times more than that needed to inhibit the strain lacking the plasmid, so these results were in agreement. Thus, for the first time, an R plasmid was shown to encode an insusceptible target enzyme that by-passed an inhibited step in the bacterium.[12] These discoveries were made despite the fact that other workers had claimed that R388 did not confer the synthesis of an additional dihydrofolate reductase.[13]

It seems unlikely that the plasmid-mediated dihydrofolate reductase could have arisen from an *E. coli* chromosomal trimethoprim-sensitive ancestral enzyme. From the molecular weights of dihydrofolate reductases reported in the literature, it would seem that the source of plasmid-mediated trimethoprim resistance could have been a bacteriophage. Mathews & Sutherland[14] have shown that the dihydrofolate reductase of bacteriophage T6 has a molecular weight of 31 000. In addition, mutants of another T even phage (T4) have been isolated which produce mutated dihydrofolate reductases exhibiting resistance to antifolate drugs.[15]

Subsequent to the discovery of the dihydrofolate reductase of R388, another plasmid conferring trimethoprim resistance, R483, was also shown to mediate the synthesis of an additional trimethoprim-resistant dihydrofolate reductase.[16] In this case, the R plasmid-encoded dihydrofolate reductase activity far exceeded that of the chromosomal enzyme, the specific activity of the plasmid-containing strain being about 10 times greater than that of the strain lacking the plasmid. This plasmid-determined dihydrofolate reductase was very sensitive to heat, far more so than the normal chromosomal enzyme. Again, in contrast to the chromosomal enzyme (mol.wt. 21 000), plasmid dihydrofolate reductases related to that of R483 are comprised of two identical subunits of mol.wt. 18 000 each.[17]

The separation of plasmid and chromosomal dihydrofolate reductases by gel filtration was not sufficient to produce plasmid enzyme free from that mediated by the chromosome. Therefore the 50–80% saturation ammonium sulphate precipitate of *E. coli* 114 (R388) was separated using DEAE cellulose ion-exchange chromatography.[18] We found a distinguishing feature of the plasmid-mediated enzyme was that it could not utilize NADH as hydrogen donor. The sensitive enzyme can utilize NADH instead of NADPH, albeit at a lower efficiency than NADPH. We further discovered that the plasmid-coded enzyme was not only highly resistant to trimethoprim but also to the 2,4-diaminopteridines methotrexate and aminopterin.[18] These compounds are close structural analogues of dihydrofolic acid and they inhibit the enzyme competitively, in the same way as trimethoprim. Unlike trimethoprim, these compounds can inhibit mammalian dihydrofolate reductase and it is surprising, therefore, that methotrexate was unable to inhibit the plasmid enzyme. Thus the R-plasmid dihydrofolate reductase has the ability to differentiate between the substrate and its close structural analogue. This may have some serious consequences in the search for new antibacterial inhibitors of dihydrofolate reductase. Any new drug that competitively inhibits dihydrofolate reductase would have to resemble the substrate more closely than methotrexate in order to penetrate the active site of the plasmid enzyme but, on the other hand, it must also be selective and only inhibit the bacterial enzyme.

The gene encoding the R388 dihydrofolate reductase was excised from its host plasmid by restriction endonuclease digestion and integrated into a multiple-copy derivative of plasmid ColE1.[19]

This step made possible the production of much larger quantities of the plasmid enzyme. The size of the DNA fragment encoding the R388 dihydrofolate reductase was 1770 base pairs (bp). This fragment could code for a protein of at most 13 000 daltons whereas the molecular weight estimation for the plasmid enzyme was 35 000 by Sephadex gel filtration.[12] Therefore the R plasmid dihydrofolate reductase must have been comprised of subunits, which were later shown to be identical, of mol.wt. 8300; hence, the R388 holoenzyme is tetrameric.[20] Other trimethoprim-resistant dihydrofolate reductases related to that of R388 have also been found to be tetrameric.[17,21]

b Different Types of Trimethoprim-Resistant Dihydrofolate Reductase

During the initial identification of R-plasmid-determined trimethoprim-resistant dihydrofolate reductases, the properties of the enzymes from different plasmids seemed to be similar. Their molecular weights, molecular charges and resistance profiles were all very similar.[22] However, the quantity of enzyme from the different plasmids varied considerably. A study of R plasmids conferring trimethoprim resistance in a French hospital revealed that some encoded a dihydrofolate reductase of different properties from those previously reported. The enzymes from such plasmids (R67, R67bis and R27) were produced in low quantities and were even less susceptible to trimethoprim than those plasmid enzymes previously reported.[23] The molecular weights of the former enzymes determined by Sephadex G-75 gel filtration were found to be 35 000 which was the same as those previously reported for earlier plasmid-mediated dihydrofolate reductases. Pattishall *et al.*[23] proposed that two (rather than one) types of R-plasmid dihydrofolate reductase existed; those of type 1 (exemplified by the dihydrofolate reductase from R483) produced in large quantities, heat-sensitive and less susceptible to trimethoprim than the chromosomal enzyme by four orders of magnitude, and those of type II (exemplified by R67) produced in low quantities, heat-resistant and virtually insusceptible to trimethoprim at any concentration.

Tennhamar-Ekman & Sköld[24] re-examined the properties of the dihydrofolate reductases encoded by three R plasmids, R751, R388 and R483. Each R-plasmid enzyme had slightly different migratory properties on polyacrylamide gel electrophoresis and the authors concluded that the three enzymes were distinct from one another. The dihydrofolate reductases from R388 and R751 were produced in low quantities, were much more heat-resistant than the R483 enzyme, and could be classified as similar to the type II enzyme.[23] However, they differed in their relative sensitivities to trimethoprim. The apparent confusion in the classification of these plasmid-determined dihydrofolate reductases required a more exacting technique. Broad & Smith[25] examined dihydrofolate reductases of type I and type II as well as those from R388 and R751 by isoelectric focusing. They found that type I enzymes exhibited isoelectric points (pI) of 6.4 while type II enzymes were of pI 5.5. As the dihydrofolate reductase of R388 also exhibited a pI of 5.5 it was clearly a type II rather than a type I enzyme. On the other hand, the enzyme mediated by R751 exhibited a unique isoelectric point (pI 7.2) and hence could constitute a third type. Nevertheless, as the enzymes of R751 and R388 are known to be serologically related,[17] perhaps the R751 enzyme should be regarded as a sub-group of type II rather than being of a completely separate type. Recently a new type of plasmid-mediated dihydrofolate reductase has been detected in a non-self-transmissible plasmid (p669) which conferred resistance to modest concentrations of trimethoprim (64 μg/ml).[26] In agreement with this was the finding that the ID$_{50}$ of trimethoprim for this enzyme was 1.5 µM compared with 60 µM for type I enzymes and 70000 µM for type II enzymes.[23] Moreover the molecular weight of the p669 enzyme was, unusually, found to be 16000–18000. The enzyme was also antigenically distinct from type I or II dihydrofolate reductases.

2 Transposition

With R-plasmid-mediated resistance to the β-lactam antibiotics it was found that, when the enzymological properties of the β-lactamases mediated by such R plasmids were analysed, an enzymic type termed TEM predominated, and it was concluded that 'the ubiquity of the structural gene for the TEM-like enzyme demonstrates its evolutionary success which probably results from its ability to be translocated from one replicon to another'.[27] The term *transposon* was proposed for such mobile R-plasmid antibiotic resistance genes.[28] Subsequently, the DNA segment containing the TEM β-lactamase gene (termed transposon A, but now called Tn*1*) was shown to be bounded by inverted repeated DNA sequences that possibly facilitate the exchange of this particular DNA molecule between R plasmids.[29] Other antibiotic resistance genes of R plasmids (such as tetracycline, chloramphenicol and kanamycin) have since been classified as transposons.[30] The spread of trimethoprim resistance between R plasmids has been rapid in France,[31] Italy,[32] England[25,33] and Scotland.[34] This suggests that the genes are being broadcast on transposons. Barth *et al.*[35] showed that one of the early trimethoprim R plasmids, R483, carried its trimethoprim resistance gene on an 8.7 megadalton fragment of DNA that is able to integrate into the chromosome as well as into other plasmids. This transposon also carries streptomycin and spectinomycin resistance and is known as transposon 7 (Tn*7*). R483 was the first plasmid shown to encode the type I dihydrofolate reductase and in almost every case where this enzyme has been identified it has been found to be associated with Tn*7*. Richards & Datta[36] found that Tn*7* was present in the majority of R-plasmid-mediated trimethoprim-resistant bacteria isolated from human infection in hospitals and in general practice patients. Other trimethoprim resistance transposons have since been found in clinical isolates.[37] Moreover, this study also showed that Tn*7* could be detected in the chromosome of some clinical strains which do not possess trimethoprim R plasmids. It is worrying to note that trimethoprim resistance in animal isolates is even more common than in human patients[38] and enzymological and resistance studies suggest that plasmids from these animal strains also possess Tn*7*.[25] It is hence possible that the source of trimethoprim resistance in humans could have arisen in animals and that transposition is the mechanism of spread of this resistance, not only within bacterial populations, but also between bacterial populations. However, as yet, transposons associated with a type II enzyme have not been described despite intensive searches.[20] It has been claimed that R751 contains a 5 megadalton transposon,[39] which solely confers trimethoprim resistance. However, as the trimethoprim-resistant dihydrofolate reductase of R751 has not yet been reported to be associated with any other R-plasmid, its trimethoprim resistance gene does not seem to undergo transposition in the clinical situation.

3 Sulphonamide Resistance

Most of the work on plasmid-mediated resistance to inhibitors of tetrahydrofolate biosynthesis has been on trimethoprim. Sulphonamide resistance has been a problem for much longer but far less is known about it. When R plasmids conferring sulphonamide resistance were first found, it was thought that the resistance mechanism was drug impermeability.[40] Indeed some sulphonamide resistant organisms do exhibit reduced uptake of radioactively labelled sulphonamide.[41] Following our elucidation of the mechanism of R-plasmid-mediated trimethoprim resistance,[12] a similar technique was applied to show that R-plasmid-mediated sulphonamide resistance operated by a similar mechanism.[42] Dihydropteroate synthase activity of bacteria with and without R-plasmids conferring sulphonamide resistance was separated by Sephadex gel exclusion chromatography and fractions assayed in the presence and absence of sulphathiazole. It was found that some, but not all, strains harbouring sulphonamide resistance plasmids contained an additional dihydropteroate synthase, resistant to sulphathiazole. In each case the sulphathiazole-resistant dihydropteroate synthase peak exhibited a slightly lower molecular weight than the chromosomal sulphonamide-sensitive enzyme. The chromosomal peak was eluted at a molecular weight of 49000 while the plasmid peak was at 45000 daltons. When inhibitor profiles were examined, the resistant enzyme was about three orders of magnitude less susceptible to sulphonamide inhibition than was the corresponding chromosomal enzyme. This was similar to the factor by which the plasmid of the resistant strains had increased the insusceptibility of its host to sulphonamides as judged by sensitivity testing. A further similarity to the trimethoprim resistance mechanism conferred by type I dihydrofolate reductases was that the sulphathiazole-resistant dihydropteroate synthases were more sensitive to thermal inactivation than the chromosomal enzyme.[42] Similar functional diploidy with respect to sulphathiazole-resistant dihydropteroate synthases was confirmed by Sköld.[43] Nagate *et al.*[44] studied in greater detail plasmids conferring sulphonamide resistance. They found that the molecular weight of the DNA of all those which mediated an additional sulphonamide-resistant dihydropteroate synthase was low and that large plasmids did not seem to confer an extra enzyme. It is possible that this result can be explained by the findings of Swedberg & Sköld[45] who showed that large, stringently controlled plasmids do mediate dihydropteroate synthase but it is present in such small amounts that it is undetectable in cell extracts. The presence of such an enzyme was rendered detectable by cloning the sulphonamide resistance gene on to the multi-copy plasmid, pBR322, when by virtue of gene dosage, detectable amounts of sulphonamide-resistant dihydropteroate synthase were produced. Using this gene amplification technique, Swedberg & Sköld[45] demonstrated that every plasmid tested conferring sulphonamide resistance produced a drug-resistant dihydropteroate synthase. Moreover they found, on the basis of restriction endonuclease digestion and hybridization with the sulphonamide resistance gene of R388, that two different dihydropteroate synthase genes exist which confer clinical sulphonamide resistance. It would be extremely interesting to know the origin of these dihydropteroate synthase genes.

REFERENCES

1 Knox, R, Smith JT. The nature of penicillin resistance in Staphylococci. Lancet 1961; 2: 520–522
2 Goldstein A, Aronow L, Kalman SM. In: Principles of drug action. The basis of pharmacology. New York: Harper and Row, 1968; 518–545
3 Brown GM. The biosynthesis of folic acid. Inhibition by sulfonamides. J Biol Chem 1962; 237: 536–540
4 Roland S, Ferone R, Harvey RJ, Styles VL, Morrison RW. The characteristics and significance of sulfonamides as substrates for *Escherichia coli* dihydropteroate synthase. J Biol Chem 1979; 254: 10337–10345

5 Wacker A, Grisebach H, Trebst A, Ebert M, Weygand F. Über den Wirkungsmechanismus der p-Aminosalicylsäure. Stoffwechseluntersuchen bei Mikroorganismen mit Hilferadioactiver Isotope IX. Agnew Chem 1954; 66: 712–713

6 Seeger DR, Smith JM Jr, Hultquist ME. Antagonist for pteroylglutamic acid. J Am Chem Soc 1947; 69: 2567

7 Hitchings GH, Burchall JJ. Inhibition of folate biosynthesis and function as a basis of chemotherapy. Adv Enzymol 1948; 27: 417–468

8 Burchall JJ, Hitchings GH. Inhibitor binding analysis of dihydrofolate reductases from various species. Mol Pharmacol 1965; 1: 126–136

9 Nixon PF, Blakley RL. Dihydrofolate reductase of *Streptococcus faecium*. II. Purification and some properties of two dihydrofolate reductases from the amethopterin-resistant mutant *Streptococcus faecium* var. *durans* strain A. J Biol Chem 1968; 243: 4722–4731

10 Amyes SGB. The susceptibility of Gram negative bacteria to antifolate chemotherapeutic agents. London: University of London, 1974: 132–145. PhD thesis

11 Datta N, Hedges RW. Trimethoprim resistance conferred by W plasmids in Enterobacteriaceae. J Gen Microbiol 1972; 72: 349–355

12 Amyes SGB, Smith JT. R-factor trimethoprim resistance mechanism: an insusceptible target site. Biochem Biophys Res Commun 1974; 58: 412–418

13 Datta N, Jobanputra RS. The epidemiology of R-factors conferring trimethoprim resistance. Prog Chemother 1974; 1: 29 34

14 Mathews CK, Sutherland KE. Comparative biochemistry of bacterial and phage-induced dihydrofolate reductases. J Biol Chem 1965; 240: 2142–2147

15 Johnson JR, Hall DW. Isolation and characterization of mutants of bacteriophage T4 resistant to folate analogs. Virology 1973; 53: 413–426

16 Sköld O, Widh A. A new dihydrofolate reductase with low trimethoprim sensitivity induced by an R factor mediating high resistance to trimethoprim. J Biol Chem 1974; 249: 4324–4325

17 Fling ME, Elwell LP. Protein expression in *Escherichia coli* minicells containing recombinant plasmids specifying trimethoprim-resistant dihydrofolate reductases. J Bacteriol 1980; 141: 779–785

18 Amyes SGB, Smith JT. The purification and properties of the trimethoprim-resistant dihydrofolate reductase mediated by the R-factor, R388. Eur J Biochem 1976; 61: 597–603

19 Zolg JW, Hänggi UJ, Zachau HG. Isolation of a small DNA fragment carrying the gene for a dihydrofolate reductase from a trimethoprim resistance factor. Mol Gen Genet 1978; 164: 15–29

20 Zolg JW, Hänggi UJ. Characterization of an R plasmid-associated, trimethoprim-resistant dihydrofolate reductase and determination of the nucleotide sequence of the reductase gene. Nucleic Acids Res 1981; 9: 697–710

21 Smith SL, Stone D, Novak P, Baccanari DP, Burchall JJ. R plasmid dihydrofolate reductase with subunit structure. J Biol Chem 1979; 254: 6222–6225

22 Amyes SGB, Smith JT. R-factor mediated dihydrofolate reductases which confer trimethoprim resistance. J Gen Microbiol 1978; 107: 263–271

23 Pattishall KH, Acar J, Burchall JJ, Goldstein FW, Harvey RJ. Two distinct types of trimethoprim-resistant dihydrofolate reductases specified by R-plasmids of different compatibility groups. J Biol Chem 1977; 252: 2319–2323

24 Tennhamar-Ekman B, Sköld O. Trimethoprim resistance plasmids of different origin encode different drug-resistant dihydrofolate reductases. Plasmid 1979; 2: 334–346

25 Broad DF, Smith JT. Classification of trimethoprim-resistant dihydrofolate reductases mediated by R-plasmids using isoelectric focussing. Eur J Biochem 1982; 125: 617–622

26 Fling ME, Walton L, Elwell LP. Monitoring of plasmid-encoded, trimethoprim-resistant dihydrofolate reductase genes: Detection of a new resistant enzyme. Antimicrob Agents Chemother 1982; 22: 882–888

27 Hedges RW, Datta N, Kontomichalou P, Smith JT. Molecular specificities of R factor-determined beta-lactamases: correlation with plasmid compatibility. J Bacteriol 1974; 117: 56–62

28 Hedges RW, Jacob AE. Transposition of ampicillin resistance from RP4 to other replicons. Mol Gen Genet 1974; 132: 31–40

29 Heffron F, Rubens C, Falkow S. Translocation of a plasmid DNA sequence which mediates ampicillin resistance: Molecular nature and specificity of insertion. Proc Natl Acad Sci USA 1975; 72: 3623–3627

30 Cohen SN. Transposable genetic elements and plasmid evolution. Nature 1976; 263: 731–738

31 Acar JF, Goldstein FW, Gerbaud GR, Chabbert YA. Plasmides de résistance au triméthoprime: transférabilité et groupes d'incompatibelité. Ann Inst Pasteur (Paris) 1977; 128A: 41–47

32 Romero E, Perduca M. Compatibility groups of R-factors for trimethoprim resistance isolated in Italy. J Antimicrob Chemother 1977; 3 (suppl C): 35–38

33 Amyes SGB, Emmerson AM, Smith JT. R-factor mediated trimethoprim resistance: result of two three-month clinical surveys. J Clin Pathol 1978; 31: 850–854

34 Amyes SGB, McMillan CJ, Drysdale JL. Transferable trimethoprim resistance amongst hospital isolates. In: Grassi GG, Sabath LD, eds. *New trends in antibiotics: Research and therapy*. New York: Elsevier/ North-Holland Biomedical Press, 1981; 325–327

35 Barth PT, Datta N, Hedges RW, Grinter NJ. Transposition of a deoxyribonucleic acid sequence encoding trimethoprim and streptomycin resistances from R483 to other replicons. J Bacteriol 1976; 125: 800–810

36 Richards H, Datta N. Transposons and trimethoprim resistance. Br Med J 1981; 282: 1118–1119

37 Amyes SGB, Drysdale JL, McMillan CJ, Young H-K. The diversity of trimethoprim resistance within hospital isolates. J Pharm Pharmacol 1982; 34: 60P

38 Smith HW. Antibiotic-resistant *Escherichia coli* in market pigs in 1956–1979: the emergence of organisms with plasmid-borne trimethoprim resistance. J Hyg 1980; 84: 467–477

39 Shapiro JA, Sporn P. Tn *402*: A new transposable element determining trimethoprim resistance that inserts in bacteriophage lambda. J Bacteriol 1977; 129: 1632–1635

40 Watanabe T. Infective heredity of multiple drug resistance in bacteria. Bacteriol Rev 1963; 27: 87–115

41 Akiba T, Yokota T. Studies on the mechanism of transfer of drug resistance in bacteria. 18. Incorporation of ^{35}S-sulphathiazole into cells of the multiply-resistant strain and artificial sulphonamide-resistant strain of *E. coli* Med Biol 1962; 63: 155–159

42 Wise EM Jr, Abou-Donia MM. Sulfonamide resistance mechanism in *Escherichia coli*: R plasmids can determine sulfonamide-resistant dihydropteroate synthases. Proc Natl Acad Sci USA 1975; 72: 2621–2625

43 Sköld O. R-factor-mediated resistance to sulfonamides by a plasmid-borne, drug-resistant dihydropteroate synthase. Antimicrob Agents Chemother 1976; 9: 49–54

44 Nagate T, Inoue M, Inoue K, Mitsuhashi S. Plasmid-mediated sulphanilamide resistance. Microb Immunol 1978; 22: 367–375

45 Swedberg G, Sköld O. Plasmid-borne sulphonamide resistance determinants studied by restriction enzyme analysis. J Bacteriol 1983; 153: 1228–1237

British Medical Bulletin (1984) Vol. 40, No. 1, pp. 47–53

INDUCIBLE ERYTHROMYCIN RESISTANCE IN BACTERIA

BERNARD WEISBLUM MD

Pharmacology Department
University of Wisconsin Medical School

1   Historical background
2   Inducibility of MLS resistance
3   23S ribosomal RNA methylation and MLS resistance
4   The search for the adenine methylase structural gene and its regulator
5   Plasmid pE194: a model system and its mutants
6   Induction of MLS resistance and inhibition of protein synthesis are inseparable properties of erythromycin
7   A molecular model for translational attenuation of MLS resistance
    a Structure and function of the pE194 MLS attenuator
    b Critical tests of the model
8   How can an inhibitor of protein synthesis induce by inhibiting translation?
9   Negative feedback components in the regulation of MLS resistance
10 Summing up
    References

Erythromycin belongs to the class of macrolides, a group of antibiotics which exert their inhibitory effect on bacterial growth by specifically binding to the 50S ribosome subunit and inhibiting protein synthesis. The introduction of erythromycin into medical practice[1] was followed by reports from France, UK, and USA during 1956–1957[2-4] of erythromycin-resistant *Staphylococcus aureus*. What appeared initially as uncomplicated resistance to erythromycin in gram-positive bacteria has actually been found to constitute a resistance syndrome, dependent upon biochemical modification of the 50S ribosome subunit which, in turn, confers resistance to three chemically distinct classes of antibiotics—the macrolides, lincosamides, and streptogramin type-B (MLS) antibiotics.

That expression of staphylococcal MLS resistance is inducible poses provocative questions in the research laboratory and potential problems in the clinic. In many, but not all, clinical isolates the gene which confers resistance is not expressed until the bacterium encounters subinhibitory concentrations of the drug. The chain of molecular events whereby *S. aureus* senses inducing concentrations of drug and specifically processes the information so as to render the cell phenotypically resistant will be the subject of this review.

1   Historical Background

It was already noted in the early clinical reports of erythromycin-resistant *S. aureus* that such strains were either co-resistant to other macrolides or that they could become so rapidly.[2-4] It was likewise noted that such strains were also, or could rapidly become, resistant to the streptogramin type-B antibiotics and to the lincosamides.[4-9]

In the light of subsequent findings based on tests involving selected antibiotics with different modes of action,[10] the state of affairs can be summarized as follows: *S. aureus* cells become resistant to erythromycin by a single biochemical alteration of the ribosome, as a result of which the affinity between drug and ribosome is reduced. By this single alteration, namely N[6]-methylation of adenine in 23S ribosomal RNA, a structural component of the 50S ribosome subunit, cells become more generally resistant to all of the MLS antibiotics. The MLS antibiotics comprise three of at least ten chemically distinct classes which inhibit protein synthesis by their action on the 50S ribosomal subunit. In view of the apparent functional relationship defined by observed co-resistance patterns, these three groups of inhibitors were designated collectively as the MLS antibiotics.[11]

MLS resistance in *S. aureus* can either be expressed constitutively or be inducible. In the latter case, erythromycin, but not most other MLS antibiotics, is highly active as inducer. Cells induced by erythromycin become resistant to all MLS antibiotics including those with low inducing (but high inhibitory) activity. Constitutively resistant mutants can be obtained from an inducible population by using MLS antibiotics with low inducing activity for selection, because in such mutants survival is based on the continuous synthesis of methylase. MLS resistance is not limited to *S. aureus* and occurs in other staphylococci including *S. epidermidis*[12] and *S. hycis*.[13]

The descriptive terminology used in early reports of MLS resistance in *S. aureus* included references to 'dissociated' and 'generalized' resistance as well as to an apparent 'antagonism' between erythromycin and other MLS antibiotics.[2,3,5,8] The terms 'dissociated' and 'double' resistance were used to describe strains which we have come to recognize as inducibly and constitutively resistant, respectively. The term 'dissociated' referred to the observation that test disks containing spiramycin, a macrolide, produced a large, clear inhibition zone, indicative of sensitivity, whereas disks containing an equivalent amount of erythromycin produced only a small inhibition zone, indicative of resistance. The term 'antagonism' referred to the distorted D-shaped (rather than circular) inhibition zone surrounding a spiramycin disk on a lawn of inducible *S. aureus* if an erythromycin disk which produced no significant inhibition itself was placed nearby. We now recognize that this phenomenon reflects induction of resistance by erythromycin to spiramycin in situ and that it can be demonstrated generally with any pair of MLS antibiotics of which one induces efficiently and the other does not. Although these designations provided accurate descriptions of aspects of induced MLS resistance at the cellular level, terminology descriptive of the induction mechanism at the molecular level required further biochemical analysis.

2   Inducibility of MLS Resistance

Weaver & Pattee,[14] using a turbidimetric assay of growth described time and concentration requirements for appearance of resistance in broth cultures and drew the important conclusion that expression of erythromycin resistance in the dissociated strains resembled expression of inducible enzymes. From the studies of Kono *et al.*[15] it became clearer that ribosomes from MLS-resistant staphylococci had a lower affinity for erythromycin than those from sensitive strains, and Nakajima *et al.*[16] noted that erythromycin remained unchanged after incubation with extracts of resistant cells. Together, these findings indicated that, unlike clinical resistance to penicillin, streptomycin, or chloramphenicol (for which conversion of the drug to an inactive derivative was responsible) MLS resistance involved a modification of the target of antibiotic action, the ribosome. This work provided a useful framework for further biochemical studies of MLS resistance.

Weisblum *et al.*[17] measured efficiency of plating (EOP) on medium incorporating erythromycin (5×10^{-5} M) a function of inducing conditions and correlated increased EOP with appearance of ribosomes incapable of binding erythromycin. Optimal induction of MLS resistance, whether tested by measurement of turbidity or of increased EOP (approximately 100% EOP), was attained if the culture was incubated for a period of one hour in medium containing erythromycin in the range 10^{-8} to 10^{-7} M. What structural modification of the ribosome occurs during one hour's incubation which results in 100% EOP? How does erythromycin at subinhibitory concentrations switch on expression of the gene(s) which confer resistance?

3 23S Ribosomal RNA Methylation and MLS Resistance

Studies of rRNA methylation provided part of the answer. 23S ribosomal RNA from induced or constitutively resistant cells was found to contain the modified base N^6,N^6-dimethylamino purine (N^6,N^6-dimethyl adenine, m_2^6A), absent from the 23S rRNA of sensitive or uninduced cells.[18,19] Induction provided a powerful biological handle for switching on the resistance phenotype in connection with analytical biochemical studies and ribosome reconstitution experiments.

That modification of 23S rRNA is both necessary and sufficient for the MLS resistance phenotype was demonstrated by experiments of Lai *et al.*[20] in which 23S rRNA from three sources, uninduced cells, induced cells, and constitutively resistant cells, was reconstituted in vitro with the total ribosomal protein fraction plus 5S rRNA from sensitive cells of *Bacillus stearothermophilus*. The resultant reconstituted 50S ribosome subunits, tested for antibiotic-resistant protein synthesis, were found to be resistant or sensitive according to the phenotype of the cells from which the 23S rRNA used for reconstitution was obtained.

4 The Search for the Adenine Methylase Structural Gene and its Regulator

For analysis of the mechanism of induction it was desirable to obtain a minimal DNA sequence which could specify inducible MLS resistance. Plasmid pE194 (molecular mass 2.4×10^{-6} daltons), discovered by Iordănescu[21] and described in further detail by Iordănescu & Surdeanu,[22] was found to specify inducible MLS resistance in *S. aureus* in a form indistinguishable from that reported in previous studies. We therefore posed the question: does plasmid pE194 alone confer inducible MLS resistance (or does it work in concert with specific functions determined by chromosomal genes or with genes associated with other plasmids)? This question was answered by showing that cells of *B. subtilis* into which pE194 was introduced by transformation showed the same inducible phenotype at the biochemical (adenine methylation) and microbiological level (inducible MLS resistance); plasmid pE194 worked alone.[23]

An upper limit to the DNA sequence length required for inducible MLS resistance was reduced from the full length of pE194 (3728 nucleotides) to the length of the largest of three pE194 subfragments, fragment A, (1442 nucleotides) obtained by digestion with *Taq*I restriction endonuclease, shown in Fig. 1. Transformant cells of *B. subtilis* into which pE194 *Taq*I fragment A was introduced cloned in a *Cla*I site of plasmid pC194[24] expressed inducible MLS resistance. The sequence of pE194 *Taq*I fragment

FIG. 1. Physical map of plasmid pE194

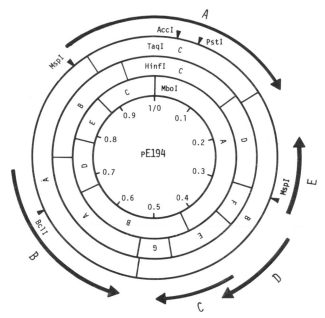

The map shows five open-reading frames and sites of cleavage by selected restriction endonucleases. Arrows indicate open-reading frames identified by computer-aided analysis of the DNA sequence and labelled alphabetically in order of decreasing size. The methylase structural gene is encoded by the open-reading frame labelled B and corresponds to the 29K protein referred to in Figs. 2 and 3.

A revealed one open-reading frame capable of specifying a protein with molecular mass 29000 daltons (29K),[25] suggesting that this was the methylase predicted by our earlier studies.

5 High Copy Mutants of Plasmid pE194

In parallel studies of pE194 in *B. subtilis*, we isolated a series of high-copy-number mutants of this plasmid.[23] *B. subtilis* CU403 is a strain with defective septation which, at cell division, produces minicells without chromosomal DNA.[26] One of the high-copy-number plasmids, cop-6, introduced into *B. subtilis* CU403, gave minicells with multiple copies of the plasmid. Using this strain, Shivakumar *et al.*[27] demonstrated that a 29K protein was synthesized in response to inducing concentrations of erythromycin, and that deletion mutations produced in vitro within the 29K determinant reduced the size and led to loss of erythromycin resistance. Moreover, Shivakumar *et al.*[28] made the interesting observation, to be discussed below, that such defective 29K protein was hyperinducible. From *B. subtilis* cells carrying the cop-6 mutant, Shivakumar & Dubnau[29] have partially purified the MLS methylase and studied some of the properties of the enzyme in vitro. Skinner & Cundliffe[30] have purified a cognate methylase from *Streptomyces erythreus* and shown that erythromycin-resistant ribosomes can be made in vitro by the action of the methylase on 23S rRNA followed by reconstitution into functional ribosomes.

6 Induction of MLS Resistance and Inhibition of Protein Synthesis are Inseparable Activities

Pestka *et al.*[31] compared activities for induction and inhibition in a series of 57 erythromycin derivatives and showed that the two activities were closely correlated. This provocative observation posed a paradox: how does one switch on protein synthesis using an inhibitor of protein synthesis? One simple (but incorrect) answer would be that a hypothetical regulator protein, e.g. repressor, could become fully saturated with inducer at concentrations which only partially saturate the ribosomes. In such an interaction the inducer would bind to the repressor with the same specificity with which it binds to the ribosome. Such a model would be consistent with the observation that erythromycin induces resistance optimally at subinhibitory concentrations but, to accord with the observations of Pestka *et al.*,[31] would require that a 'simple' regulatory molecule distinguish between inhibitors and non-inhibitors of protein synthesis with a degree of accuracy comparable to that of the ribosome. Moreover, if inhibition of protein synthesis is functionally correlated with induction, how can one account for an observed induction optimum 10^{-8} to 10^{-7} M, at least one order of magnitude lower than the threshold for inhibition of protein synthesis (10^{-7} to 10^{-6} M)?

The regulatory macromolecule with which erythromycin interacts during induction turns out to be the ribosome itself, as we shall discuss in further detail below. The similarity between induction of the operons for biosynthesis of amino acids (tryptophan, histidine, phenylalanine, threonine, and isoleucine-valine), and induction of MLS resistance should have been apparent since both are mediated by inductive stimuli dependent upon inhibition of protein synthesis. But even that perception would have provided only part of the solution. An explicit molecular model of induction could be made following DNA sequence analysis of the minimal 1442 nucleotide *Taq*I fragment A obtained from pE194 and critically tested by mapping nucleotide changes in constitutively resistant mutants.

Although Pestka's data showed a correlation between inhibitory activity and inducing activity in the erythromycin series, they did not explain why other MLS antibiotics whose inhibitory potency was comparable to that of erythromycin lacked demonstrable inducing activity in *S. aureus*. Thus at least two components appear to contribute to induction, a quantitative component, related to inhibitory potency which allows comparison within the erythromycin series, and a qualitative component distinguishing one subset of MLS antibiotics, members of which induce in a given system, from another subset, members of which do not.

7 A Molecular Model for Translational Attenuation Control of MLS Resistance

a *Structure and Function of the pE194 MLS Attenuator*

Mechanisms of gene regulation at the level of mRNA can be subdivided into three general classes, according to whether regulation affects the decision: (i) the start of synthesis of the specific mRNA, (ii) the termination of its synthesis or (iii) its utilization. The term 'attenuation' applied to gene regulation has

FIG. 2. Details of MLS control region and analysis of 11 mutants

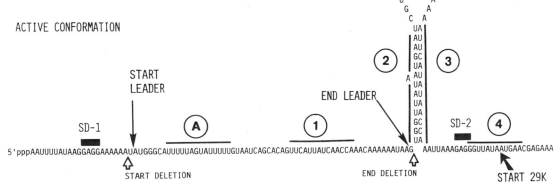

The sequence of the control region at the 5′ end of the adenine methylase mRNA, deduced from the DNA sequence, is shown in inactive and active conformations discussed in detail in the text. These correspond to conformations II and III, respectively, shown in Fig. 3. The mutations in 3 (C to A or U) or in 4 (G to A) are postulated to destabilize 3+4 directly, whereas mutations in 1 (C to A, or the deletion) are postulated to act indirectly by destabilizing 1+2, enabling 2 to preempt 3.

FIG. 3. Conformations of adenine methylase control region

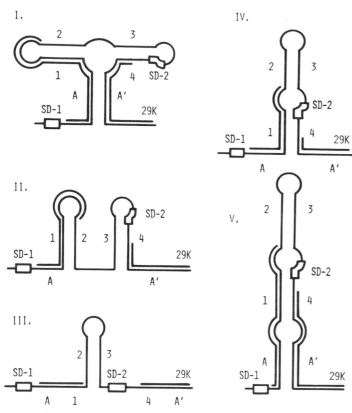

Five possible conformations of the methylase mRNA control region are shown. The free energies calculated for each of these conformations are: (kcal/mol) −30.4, −25.8, −14.2, −29.8, and −34.4 respectively. According to our model, activation of the nascent mRNA involves the transition I to II to III, whereas deactivation following removal of the inductive stimulus involves the transitions III to IV to V, rather than III to II to I. The double lines over sequences A, 1, 4, and A' indicate ability to code for polypeptide, and correspond respectively to the sequences which encode the control peptide and the N-terminal portion of adenine methylase.

largely been used for effects related to termination of transcription and its non-termination under inducing conditions, that is, with mechanism ii.[32-34] In view of structural and functional similarities between the regions which control amino-acid biosynthesis (by aborted transcription, mechanism ii) and MLS resistance (by arrested translation, mechanism iii), the control mechanism for MLS resistance can be referred to as 'translational attenuation'.

Functional mapping of the 1442 base-pair sequence from pE194 that encodes inducible MLS resistance identified the control sequence as a region comprising about 10% of the whole. On the basis of the DNA sequences which we determined for pE194 *Taq*I fragment A and for 11 constitutively resistant mutants, it was possible to propose tentatively an explicit model for regulation of MLS resistance falling into category iii above. This postulates that the methylase mRNA is synthesized in an inactive conformation and that the process of induction converts it to an active form (Figs. 2 and 3). A similar model has also been proposed by Gryczan *et al.*[35] and by Hahn *et al.*[36]

According to the model we proposed,[37,38] mRNA encoding the MLS methylase is synthesized constitutively in an inactive form. The 5' end of this mRNA contains a set of four inverted complementary repeat sequences capable of assuming alternative conformations. The four sequences, designated 1, 2, 3, and 4, can associate by virtue of their complementarity: as 1 + 2 and 3 + 4, or as 2 + 3. An additional set of inverted complementary repeat sequences, A and A', bearing no sequence similarity to 1, 2, 3, and 4, is also present (Fig. 2). The numbering scheme used for our model was chosen to facilitate comparison between inducible MLS resistance and the trp operon attenuator, discussed in further detail below.

We postulate further that the 1 + 2, 3 + 4 association pattern corresponds to the nascent inactive conformation of the control region. The messenger is inactive because the ribosome loading site for synthesis of the MLS methylase, labelled SD-2[39] is sequestered in the loop formed by the association of 3 + 4. Activation of the methylase mRNA is achieved by a conformational rearrangement of the inverted complementary sequences resulting in association of 2 + 3, thereby unmasking the sequestered ribosome loading site. The conformational rearrangement results from hindered translation of a 19 amino acid 'leader' or 'control' peptide utilizing SD-1 as its ribosome loading site and encoded by sequences A and 1; if the ribosomes stall during translation of these sequences, sequence 2 is freed from its pairing with sequence 1. The stalling required for induction is brought about by formation of a complex between erythromycin and ribosomes which load at SD-1.

The unmasking of SD-2 can occur either indirectly or directly— i.e., either as (i), in which dissociation of 1 + 2 allows 2 to preempt 3, freeing 4 or (ii), direct dissociation of 3 + 4 which can result from mutation in the sequence of 3 or 4, weakening their association so that spontaneous unmasking of SD-2 can occur with a higher degree of probability than in the wild-type inducible form. Basal level expression could occur (i) by spontaneous dissociation of 3 + 4, or (ii) by a potential conformation of the nascent methylase mRNA (not shown) deduced by Hahn *et al.*[36] from the DNA structure in which SD-2 is initially accessible to ribosomes for methylase synthesis.

The translational attenuation model for regulation of MLS resistance resembles the transcriptional attenuation models for control of amino-acid biosynthesis (reviewed by Yanofsky[33] and Kolter & Yanofsky[34]); in both, hindered ribosome function in the course of synthesis of a control peptide leads to a modification of the secondary structure of mRNA with predictable biological consequences.

We postulate that hindered translation of the MLS control peptide mediates the induction process for MLS resistance, but with two important features distinguishing this process from induction of the trp operon. (i) In the case of induced MLS resistance, ribosome function is hindered by the inducer, erythromycin, whereas in the case of the tryptophan operon, the ribosome is hindered by a deficiency of tryptophanyl tRNA (or histidinyl tRNA in the case of the histidine operon etc.). (ii) Reorientation of the MLS control region results in unmasking the sequestered ribosome loading site for synthesis of the MLS methylase, whereas reorientation of the attenuator regions associated with biosynthesis of tryptophan, histidine, phenylalanine, threonine, and isoleucine-valine, results in completion of the respective mRNAs otherwise prematurely terminated by the fact that the association of 3 + 4 (or its functional equivalent) supplies the signal for termination of mRNA synthesis.

b *Critical Test of the Model*

The proposed model predicts that mutation to constitute expression of MLS resistance would be most effective for nucleotide changes in sequences 1, 3, and 4, but *not* 2. Thus, nucleotide changes in 1 would weaken its association with 2 and favour preemptive association of 2 with 3. However, base alterations in 2 to weaken association with 1 would likewise weaken the association of 2 with 3, thereby reducing the efficiency of the 2 + 3 preemptive pairing reaction. Mutations which directly affect either 3 or 4 would reduce the energy of association of 3 with 4, bypassing the preemptive reaction.

In a test of this model, 11 independent constitutively resistant mutants were selected randomly and the DNA sequence of the MLS control region was determined. In agreement with predictions none of these 11 mutants involved sequence 2. Alterations in sequences 3 and 4 were found in nine of the mutants analysed (five in sequence 3, and four in sequence 4), as shown in Fig. 2.

Analysis of the remaining two mutants was particularly informative. One of these, three bases from the 5′ end of sequence 1, had a change from C to A. Insofar as this mutation would have a destabilizing effect on the pairing of the first two residues of sequence 1 (UU), as well as the third, we infer that a significant level of induction occurs when the control region is disrupted as far as the third of the 13 bases in sequence 1. In the work of Steitz,[40] ribosomes were found capable of protecting from ribonuclease digestion between 10 and 20 nucleotides at the 5′ end of RNA phage gene sequences. Thus a single stalled ribosome should be able, in principle, to cover sequence 1 entirely. We do not yet know the extent to which constitutive MLS resistance resulting from this point mutation is influenced by a change in the amino acid sequence of the putative control peptide, histidine (CAU) to asparagine (AAU), as distinct from the more direct impact on destabilization of 1 + 2. In the other constitutive mutant, 62 nucleotides which specify the control peptide (19 amino acids), including all of sequence 1, were excised leaving a control region containing intact sequences 2, 3, and 4. In the nascent methylase mRNA specified by this mutant, 2 + 3 would form as soon as sequence 3 was synthesized resulting in a fully active conformation of the message.

8 How can an Inhibitor of Protein Synthesis Induce by Inhibiting Translation?

Recalling the report of Pestka *et al.*,[31] that inhibitory and inducing activities in a set of erythromycin derivatives were inseparable, it is pertinent to ask: since induction requires an environment in which synthesis of the control peptide is inhibited, why is this same environment not equally inhibitory for synthesis of the methylase? To answer this question, we begin by assuming that ribosomes, during induction, fall into one of three classes: (i) sensitive ribosomes complexed with erythromycin, (ii) sensitive ribosomes uncomplexed with erythromycin, and (iii) resistant ribosomes containing specifically methylated 23S rRNA. Let us ask what might happen to ribosomes belonging to each of these classes during translation of the control peptide, and of the methylase structural gene.

Sensitive ribosomes complexed with erythromycin would stall in the control region and induce conformational realignment. Eventually, they would either complete synthesis of the control peptide, or release the partially completed control peptide. Sensitive ribosomes uncomplexed with erythromycin as well as resistant ribosomes would synthesize the control peptide without any marked effect on induction.

Following induction, sensitive ribosomes complexed with erythromycin would synthesize short peptides and release them. Sensitive ribosomes not complexed with erythromycin would synthesize methylase efficiently, as would resistant ribosomes. For induction to work effectively it is therefore necessary that the concentration of erythromycin used should not saturate the ribosomes. This would require that subinhibitory concentrations be used for induction, in accord with experimental observation.

Erythromycin appears to inhibit protein synthesis in a manner consistent with its ability to act as inducer. Pestka[31] and Tai *et al.*[41] concluded that (i) inhibition by erythromycin is limited to an early stage of protein synthesis after initiation but before extensive elongation has occurred, and (ii) inhibition results in polysome breakdown and release of short peptides (betwen 5 and 12 amino acids in length). Menninger & Otto[42] have examined biochemical aspects of macrolide action and they ascribe the inhibitory action of erythromycin, spiramycin, and carbomycin to their proposed ability to stimulate dissociation of peptidyl tRNA from ribosomes rather than to direct inhibition of peptide bond formation. This effect would not only inhibit protein synthesis overall, but would allow for synthesis of the methylase under inducing conditions, as described above.

9 Negative Feedback Components in the Regulation of MLS Resistance

Mechanisms of gene regulation which serve the cell optimally should contain negative feedback features which switch off gene expression when it is no longer required. The switch-off of gene expression can be in response either (i) to reduction in the original inductive stimulus, or (ii) to saturation of the cell with the products of induced synthesis. Optimal function of the latter mechanism should result in turning off gene expression even in the presence of continued inductive stimulation.

The translational attenuation model predicts that synthesis of methylase should eventually become self-limiting. Only sensitive ribosomes will stall in the control region, so when the level of resistant ribosomes reaches an (unspecified) critical level, the number of sensitive ribosomes remaining would not suffice to provide the amount of stall in sequence 1 needed to maintain a maximal level of methylase synthesis. Results which support of this aspect of the model were obtained by Shivakumar *et al.*[28] who reported that no induction was demonstrable in an oleandomycin resistant *B. subtilis* carrying a chromosomal mutation which affects a ribosomal protein constituent of the 50S subunit. Moreover, these authors showed that inactivation of the methylase structural gene by in-vitro deletion of an undetermined small portion of it yielded, in *B. subtilis*, an inactive methylase which appeared to be synthesized at an abnormally high rate following induction by erythromycin. This interesting phenomenon was ascribed to an intracellular maximal level of sensitive ribosomes resulting in turn in maximal expression of the induced phenotype.

10 Summing Up

In his early paper describing inducible erythromycin resistance, Garrod[3] stated, 'This is not an antagonism in the ordinary sense, but a kind of interaction of which, so far as I am aware, no previous example has been seen.' Indeed, post-synthetic modification of the antibiotic receptor remains one of the more exotic forms of clinical resistance.

In terms of its prevalence, however, the MLS-resistance phenotype occurs in a wide range of organisms. In streptococci, for example, it has been the subject of many papers, going back almost as far as the staphylococcus literature (see, e.g. Dixon & Lipinski,[43] Hyder & Streitfeld,[44] Malke.[45,46] Clewell[47] has reviewed the field of streptococcal plasmid research including coverage of numerous streptococcal MLS-determinant plasmids. By nucleic acid hybridization and direct sequence analysis the MLS determinants of *S. pyogenes*, *S. fecalis*, *S. pneumoniae*, and *S. sanguis* have been shown to be related to each other and to the MLS determinants of staphylococci.[47–50]

As we have searched for and characterized other examples, we have learned that the phenotype is so pervasive in certain organisms, e.g. *Streptomyces*, (see Cundliffe, pp. 61–67) that its absence in members of this group seems to be the exception. We have also described a wide variety of MLS resistance phenotypes in *Streptomyces* which differ with respect to (i) relative efficiencies of induction by a test panel of selected MLS antibiotics, and (ii) utilization of mono- or dimethylation (or both) as the biochemical alteration in resistant organisms responsible for the resistance phenotype.[50–53]

Clinical MLS-resistant isolates of *Clostridium perfringens*,[54] *Bacteroides fragilis*,[55] and *Corynebacterium diphtheriae*[56] have also been reported. In studies of *Mycoplasma pneumoniae*, Niitu *et al.*[57] have reported strains coresistant to erythromycin and lincomycin. Since streptogramin B-type antibiotics were not tested, MLS resistance in this medically important group of organisms remains presumptive.

A detailed understanding of the biochemistry and genetics of inducible MLS resistance is directly applicable to a wide range of medical, technological, as well as speculative questions. The work reviewed above helps us to understand how a *Staphylococcus* found resistant to erythromycin but sensitive to other MLS antibiotics might give the false impression that it was safe to use the MLS antibiotics to which the organism appeared sensitive. Studies of the MLS control region indicate how alteration of a single nucleotide can lead to constitutive synthesis of the methylase and coresistance to all MLS antibiotics. Reports of Desmyter & Reybrouck[6] and Watanakunakorn[58] suggest that this type of mutation to constitutive resistance has, in fact, occurred in the clinical setting.

Ironically, the same type of manipulation, namely selective pressure on an inducible strain of *Streptomyces* using a non-inducing MLS antibiotic, has been shown to select constitutive methylating strains.[53] Two of these strains, *S. fradiae* and *S. lincolnensis*, when tested for antibiotic production starting from a small inoculum were found to enter the phase of antibiotic production earlier and, in the case of *S. lincolnensis*, to produce several-fold higher levels of antibiotic than the wild-type inducible parent strain.[59]

ACKNOWLEDGEMENTS

This work was supported by research grants PCM-7719390 from The National Science Foundation and AI-18283 from The National Institutes of Health. Support from the research foundations of The Upjohn Company and of Eli Lilly and Company is gratefully acknowledged.

REFERENCES

1 McGuire JM, Bunch RL, Anderson RC *et al.* 'Ilotycin', a new antibiotic. Antibiot Chemother 1952; 2: 281–283

2 Chabbert Y. Antagonisme *in vitro* entre l'érythromycine et la spiramycine. Ann Inst Pasteur (Paris) 1956; 90: 787–790

3 Garrod LP. The erythromycin group of antibiotics. Br Med J 1957; 2: 57–63

4 Jones WF Jr, Nichols RL, Finland M. Development of resistance and cross-resistance *in vitro* to erythromycin, carbomycin, oleandomycin, and streptogramin. Proc Soc Exp Biol Med 1956; 93: 388–393

5 Barber M, Waterworth PM. Antibacterial activity of lincomycin and pristinamycin: a comparison with erythromycin. Br Med J 1964; 2: 603–606

6 Desmyter J, Reybrouck G. Lincomycin sensitivity of erythromycin-resistant staphylococci. Chemotherapia 1964; 9: 183–189

7 Griffith LJ, Ostrander WE, Mullins CG, Beswick DE. Drug antagonism between lincomycin and erythromycin. Science 1965; 147: 746–747

8 Bourse R, Monier J. Effet de l'érythromycin sur la croissance de *Staph. aureus* 'résistant dissocié' en bactériostase par un autre macrolide ou un antibiotique apparente. Ann Inst Pasteur (Paris) 1967; 113: 67–79

9 Goldmann SF, Heiss F. Untersuchungen zum Phänomen von Resistenz und Resistenzkoppelung gegenüber Erythromycin, Lincomycin, und Staphylomycin. Z Med Mikrobiol Immunobiol 1971; 156: 168–173

10 Weisblum B Demohn V. Erythromycin-inducible resistance in *Staphylococcus aureus*: survey of antibiotic classes involved. J Bacteriol 1969; 98: 447–452

11 Weisblum B. Altered methylation of ribosomal ribonucleic acid in erythromycin-resistant *Staphylococcus aureus*. In: Schlessinger D, (ed.) Microbiology—1974. Washington DC: ASM, 1975; 199–206

12 Parisi JT, Robbins J, Lampson BC, Hecht DW. Characterization of a macrolide, lincosamide, and streptogramin resistance plasmid in *Staphylococcus epidermidis*. J Bacteriol 1981; 148: 559–564

13 DeVriese LA. *In vitro* susceptibility and resistance of animal staphylococci to macrolide antibiotics and related compounds. Ann Rech Vet 1976; 7: 65–74

14 Weaver JR, Pattee PA. Inducible resistance to erythromycin in *Staphylococcus aureus*. J Bacteriol 1964; 88: 574–580

15 Kono M, Hashimoto H, Mitsuhashi S. Drug resistance of staphylococci. III. Resistance to some macrolide antibiotics and inducible system. Jpn J Microbiol 1966; 10: 59–66

16 Nakajima Y, Inoue M, Oka Y, Yamagishi S. A mode of resistance to macrolide antibiotics in *Staphylococcus aureus*. Jpn J Microbiol 1968; 12: 248–250

17 Weisblum B, Siddhikol C, Lai C-J, Demohn V. Erythromycin-inducible resistance in *Staphylococcus aureus*: requirements for induction. J Bacteriol 1971; 106: 835–847

18 Lai C-J, Weisblum B. Altered methylation of ribosomal RNA in an erythromycin-resistant strain of *Staphylococcus aureus*. Proc Natl Acad Sci USA 1971; 68: 856–860

19 Lai C-J, Dahlberg JE, Weisblum B. Structure of an inducibly methylatable nucleotide sequence in 23S ribosomal ribonucleic acid from erythromycin-resistant *Staphylococcus aureus*. Biochemistry 1973; 12: 457–460

20 Lai C-J, Weisblum B, Fahnestock SR, Nomura M. Alteration of 23S ribosomal RNA and erythromycin-induced resistance to lincomycin and spiramycin in *Staphylococcus aureus*. J Mol Biol 1973; 74: 67–72

21 Iordănescu S. Three distinct plasmids originating in the same *Staphylococcus aureus* strain. Arch Roum Pathol Exp Microbiol 1976; 35: 111–118

22 Iordănescu S, Surdeanu M. New incompatibility groups for *Staphylococcus aureus* plasmids. Plasmid 1980; 4: 256–260

23 Weisblum B, Graham MY, Gryczan T, Dubnau D. Plasmid copy number control: isolation and characterization of high-copy-number mutants of plasmid pE194. J Bacteriol 1979; 137: 635–643

24 Iordănescu S, Surdeanu M, Della Latta P, Novick R. Incompatibility and molecular relationships between small staphylococcal plasmids carrying the same resistance marker. Plasmid 1978; 1: 468–479

25 Horinouchi S, Weisblum B. Posttranscriptional modification of mRNA conformation: mechanism that regulates erythromycin-induced resistance. Proc Natl Acad Sci USA 1980; 77: 7079–7083

26 Mertens G, Reeve JN. Synthesis of cell envelope components by anucleate cells (minicells) of *Bacillus subtilis*. J Bacteriol 1977; 129: 1198–1207

27 Shivakumar AG, Hahn J, Dubnau D. Studies on the synthesis of plasmid-coded proteins and their control in *Bacillus subtilis* minicells. Plasmid 1979; 2: 279–289

28 Shivakumar AG, Hahn J, Grandi G, Kozlov Y, Dubnau D. Posttranscriptional regulation of an erythromycin resistance protein specified by plasmid pE194. Proc Natl Acad Sci USA 1980; 77: 3903–3907

29 Shivakumar AG, Dubnau D. Characterization of a plasmid-specified ribosome methylase associated with macrolide resistance. Nucleic Acids Res 1981; 9: 2549–2562

30 Skinner RH, Cundliffe E. Dimethylation of adenine and the resistance of *Streptomyces erythraeus* to erythromycin. J Gen Microbiol 1982; 128: 2411–2416

31 Pestka S, Vince R, LeMahieu R, Weiss F, Fern L, Unowsky J. Induction of erythromycin resistance in *Staphylococcus aureus* by erythromycin derivatives. Antimicrob Agents Chemother 1976; 9: 128–130

32 Kasai T. Regulation of the expression of the histidine operon in *Salmonella typhimurium*. Nature 1974; 249: 523–527

33 Yanofsky C. Attenuation in the control of expression of bacterial operons. Nature 1981; 289: 751–758

34 Kolter R, Yanofsky C. Attenuation in amino acid biosynthetic operons. Annu Rev Genet 1982; 16: 113–134

35 Gryczan TJ, Grandi G, Hahn J, Grandi R, Dubnau D. Conformational alteration of mRNA structure and the posttranscriptional regulation of erythromycin-induced drug resistance. Nucleic Acids Res 1980; 8: 6081–6097

36 Hahn J, Grandi G, Gryczan TJ, Dubnau D. Translational attenuation of *ermC*: a deletion analysis. Mol Gen Genet 1982; 186: 204–216

37 Horinouchi S, Weisblum B. The control region for erythromycin resistance: free energy changes related to induction and mutation to constitutive expression. Mol Gen Genet 1981; 182: 341–348

38 Horinouchi S, Weisblum B. Nucleotide sequence and functional map of pE194, a plasmid that specifies inducible resistance to macrolide, lincosamide, and streptogramin type B antibiotics. J Bacteriol 1982; 150: 804–814

39 Shine J, Dalgarno L. The 3′ terminal sequence of *Escherichia coli* 16S ribosomal RNA: complementarity to nonsense triplets and ribosome binding sites. Proc Natl Acad Sci USA 1974; 71: 1342–1346

40 Steitz JA. Polypeptide chain initiation: nucleoside sequences of the three ribosomal binding sites in bacteriophage R17 RNA. Nature 1969; 224: 957–964

41 Tai P-C, Wallace BJ, Davis BD. Selective action of erythromycin on initiating ribosomes. Biochemistry 1974; 13: 4653–4659

42 Menninger JR, Otto DP. Erythromycin, carbomycin, and spiramycin inhibit protein synthesis by stimulating the dissociation of peptidyl-tRNA from ribosomes. Antimicrob Agents Chemother 1982; 21: 811–818

43 Dixon MS, Lipinski AE. Infections with β-hemolytic streptococcus resistant to lincomycin and erythromycin and observations on zonal-pattern resistance to lincomycin. J Infect Dis 1974; 130: 351–356

44 Hyder SL, Streitfeld MM. Inducible and constitutive resistance to macrolide antibiotics and lincomycin in clinically isolated strains of *Streptococcus pyogenes*. Antimicrob Agents Chemother 1973; 4: 327–331

45 Malke H. Genetics of resistance to macrolide antibiotics and lincomycin in natural isolates of *Streptococcus pyogenes*. Mol Gen Genet 1974; 135. 349–367

46 Malke H, Reichardt W, Hartmann M, Walter F. Genetic study of plasmid-associated zonal resistance to lincomycin in *Streptococcus pyogenes*. Antimicrob Agents Chemother 1981; 19: 91–100

47 Clewell DB. Plasmids, drug resistance, and gene transfer in the genus *Streptococcus*. Microbiol Rev 1981; 45: 409–436

48 Weisblum B, Holder SB, Halling SM. Deoxyribonucleic acid sequence common to staphylococcal and streptococcal plasmids which specify erythromycin resistance. J Bacteriol 1979; 138: 990–998

49 Horinouchi S, Weisblum B. Amino acid sequence conservation in two MLS resistance determinants. In: Schlessinger D, ed. Microbiology— 1982. Washington DC: ASM, 1982; 159–161

50 Horinouchi S, Byeon W-H, Weisblum B. A complex attenuator regulates inducible resistance to macrolides, lincosamides, and streptogramin type B antibiotics in *Streptococcus sanguis*. J Bacteriol 1983; 154: 1252–1262

51 Graham MY, Weisblum B. Altered methylation of adenine in 23S ribosomal RNA associated with erythromycin resistance in *Streptomyces erythreus* and *Streptococcus fecalis*. Contrib Microbiol Immunol 1979; 6: 159–164

52 Graham MY, Weisblum B. 23S ribosomal ribonucleic acid of macrolide-producing streptomycetes contains methylated adenine. J Bacteriol 1979; 137: 1464–1467

53 Fujisawa Y, Weisblum B. A family of r-determinants in *Streptomyces* spp. that specifies inducible resistance to macrolide, lincosamide, and streptogramin type B antibiotics. J Bacteriol 1981; 146: 621–631

54 Brefort G, Magot M, Ionesco H, Seybald M. Characterization and transferability of *Clostridium perfringens* plasmids. Plasmid 1977; 1: 52–66

55 Privitera G, Dublanchet A, Sebald M. Transfer of multiple antibiotic resistance between subspecies of *Bacteroides fragilis*. J Infect Dis 1979; 139: 97–101

56 Coyle MB, Minshew BH, Bland JA, Hsu PC. Erythromycin and clindamycin resistance in *Corynebacterium diphtheriae* from skin lesions. Antimicrob Agents Chemother 1979; 16: 525–527

57 Niitu, Y, Hasegawa S, Kubota H. In vitro development of resistance to erythromycin, other macrolide antibiotics, and lincomycin in *Mycoplasma pneumoniae*. Antimicrob Agents Chemother 1974; 5: 513–519

58 Watanakunakorn C. Clindamycin therapy of *Staphylococcus aureus* endocarditis. Clinical relapse and development of resistance to clindamycin, lincomycin, and erythromycin. Am J Med 1976; 60: 419–425

59 Weisblum B. Method of increasing the antibiotic yield of producing organisms. US Patent 1983; 4,376,823

FIG. 1. Formation and resolution of plasmid cointegrates during transposition of Tn3

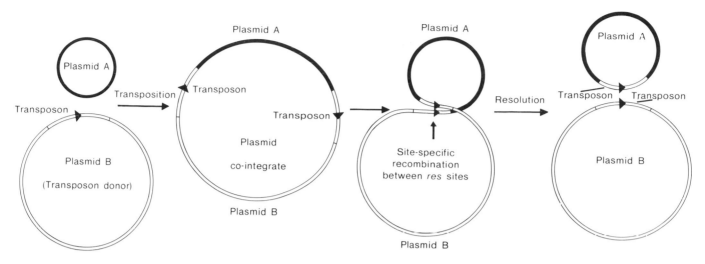

The diagram indicates the orientation of the DNA sequence of each copy of the transposon and position of *res* site.

FIG. 2. The genetic organization of Tn3

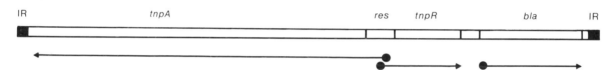

IR: 38bp inverted repeat sequence; *tnp*A: transposase gene; *res*: internal resolution site; *tnp*R: resolvase gene; *bla*: TEM-1 β-lactamase gene. Circles and arrows indicate the origin and direction of transcription respectively of the appropriate genes.

TABLE II. Some gram-negative pathogens specifying the TEM β-lactamase

Bacteria	Types of plasmid encoding β-lactamase		% Ampicillin-resistance transposon on plasmid
	Conjugative	Non-conjugative	
Escherichia coli	+	+	100
Klebsiella pneumoniae	+	−	100
Proteus rettgeri	+	−	100
Providencia sp.	+	−	100
Salmonella panama	−	+	100
Salmonella paratyphi	+	−	100
Shigella dysenteriae	−	+	100
Haemophilus influenzae	+	+	100 or 34
Haemophilus ducreyi	+	+	100 or 40
Haemophilus parainfluenzae	+	+	100 or 34
Neisseria gonorrhoeae	−	+	40
Neisseria meningitidis	−	+	40
Pseudomonas aeruginosa	+	−	100

Two variants of this β-lactamase differ slightly in biochemical properties. TEM-1 is determined by Tn2 and Tn3 and is the most widely distributed. TEM-2 is determined by Tn1. Where only part of the transposon is present the β-lactamase gene is not transposable.

insert efficiently into many sites on plasmids but into a single site on the chromosome of *E. coli* and other bacteria.[20]

Transposons probably account for the widespread distribution of certain resistance genes—such as that encoding the TEM β-lactamase—among unrelated bacteria and on different R plasmids (Table II).[1,5] It is possible for resistance transposons to be transferred to new species by 'hitch-hiking' on plasmid or phage

vector molecules. Where the vector cannot itself replicate and survive in a new host, the transposon may be rescued by transposition to an indigenous replicon such as a plasmid or the host chromosome.[1,21]

3   Genetic Transfer of Resistance

The ability of resistance genes to be shuffled between bacterial species is crucial to the evolution of resistant strains. Bacteria can possess three natural mechanisms for gene transfer; conjugation, transformation and transduction. Although bacteria exhibit various barriers to genetic exchange, certain genes may be transferred even between distantly related genera, albeit at very low frequency.

a *Conjugation*

Conjugation is a process requiring cell-to-cell contact whereby DNA is transferred from a donor bacterium to a recipient. The ability to conjugate is normally encoded by conjugative plasmids[2,3] or, less commonly, by conjugative transposons.[22] Such molecules determine the production of sex pili (surface hairs made of protein which are necessary for establishing and maintaining cell-to-cell contact) and the ability to mobilize DNA for transfer to recipients.[23,24] Many gram-negative and some gram-positive bacteria, notably streptococci, staphylococci and clostridia are able to conjugate. Plasmids that encode the apparatus for their own transfer by conjugation are termed conjugative, whereas those that

FIG. 3. Typical genetic organization of conjugative and non-conjugative R plasmids

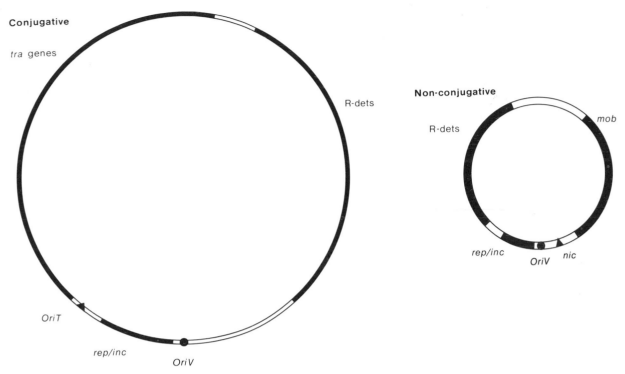

oriV: origin of vegetative replication; *oriT*: origin of transfer replication; *tra*: transfer genes; *mob*: mobility region; *nic*: nicking site for mobility proteins; r-det: resistance determinant; *rep*: replication genes; *inc*: incompatibility determinant

lack this ability are called non-conjugative. Conjugative plasmids are normally >30 kb in size to accommodate the large number of transfer (*tra*) genes required for conjugation. However, not all large plasmids are necessarily conjugative.

A large number of resistance plasmids, particularly those specifying multiple resistances, are conjugative with the resistance genes being covalently linked to the *tra* genes (Fig. 3). In some cases the *tra* genes are located in a single region on the plasmid, whereas in others they are scattered in several different regions.[24,25] The *tra* genes include those determining the production and assembly of the sex pilus. The sex pilus is characteristic of the type of plasmid involved and is often correlated with the incompatibility group.[26]

Although some resistance plasmids are non-conjugative they may often be transferred (mobilized) to a recipient provided they co-reside in a cell with a conjugative plasmid. Mobilization is characterized by lack of covalent union between the participating conjugative and non-conjugative plasmids. Hence, the two plasmids are not necessarily co-transferred to recipient cells. Furthermore the non-conjugative plasmid participates actively in the mobilization process. This can be deduced from the observation that about 30% of the genomes of ColE1 and related non-conjugative plasmids seem to be devoted to mobilization functions.[27] The *mob* (mobility) genes of ColE1 encode proteins that bind to a specific site on the ColE1 DNA molecule called *nic* (or *bom*) which is probably the origin of transfer (*oriT*) of the plasmid. The plasmid molecule is cleaved on one strand at *nic* by the mobilization proteins in order to initiate DNA transfer. A suitable co-resident conjugative plasmid provides the apparatus necessary for achieving mating contact between donor and

recipient, but triggering of transfer of the non-conjugative plasmid is probably determined by the mobilization proteins.[28] The precise details of the mobilization process are still not resolved but several molecular models have been proposed.[27,29]

In the absence of mobilization function, non-conjugative plasmids may be transferred by a less efficient process involving transient covalent union of the DNA of a non-conjugative and a conjugative plasmid.[30] This process can occur when a replicon fusion occurs in the donor cell between the participating plasmids either as a result of homologous recombination or by cointegrate formation during transposition of a transposon from one plasmid to another (Fig. 1). After transfer to the recipient, resolution of the cointegrate by a transposon-specified resolvase or by homologous (*rec*A-dependent) recombination would generate two separate molecules (Fig. 1). In contrast to mobilization, this process results inevitably in the recipient cell receiving both the conjugative and non-conjugative plasmid.

Conjugation is probably significant in the dissemination of resistance genes among bacteria that are normally found at high population density and hence are likely to come into frequent cellular contact with each other. It is hardly surprising therefore that both conjugative and mobilizable non-conjugative plasmids should be so common amongst the Enterobacteriaceae. Conjugative transfer of R plasmids between strains of *E. coli* has been demonstrated in the intestines of both humans and animals albeit at low frequencies.[31-34] The poor transferability of certain conjugative plasmids has been attributed to the unfavourable anaerobic conditions of the gut or to inhibitory effects of the intestinal microflora.[33,34] Recent experimental and mathematical models of transfer have, however, indicated that there is no apparent inhibition of conjugation in the gut.[35] The low frequencies of transfer reported are apparently due simply to using insufficiently sensitive assays to detect transconjugants (recipients that have received a plasmid by conjugation). Whatever the frequency of conjugation in the gut, enterobacteria are presented with numerous opportunities for extra-intestinal transfer of R plasmids (for example in sewage) which may also be significant in the spread of resistance. Less is known about the role of conjugative transfer in the spread of resistance in non-enteric pathogens. However, it has been shown that a non-conjugative β-lactamase plasmid may be mobilized by a conjugative plasmid between strains of *Neisseria gonorrhoeae* growing in guinea-pig tissue chambers.[36]

b Transformation

Transformation is a process whereby bacteria are able to take up naked DNA and incorporate it into their genome.[37] The process occurs naturally in some species but must be induced by artificial treatments in others. A variety of mechanisms are involved for transporting plasmid, bacteriophage or chromosomal DNA across the cell envelope.[37] In general, bacteria do not discriminate against foreign DNA during the uptake process. Thus transformation is potentially an ideal mechanism for transferring useful genes across generic boundaries. However, some bacteria such as *Haemophilus* spp. and *Neisseria* spp. will only take up homologous DNA efficiently. Discrimination against heterologous DNA is effected by envelope proteins that recognize specific nucleotide sequences present in homospecific DNA but lacking in other types of DNA.[37] This specificity severely limits the ability of *Haemophilus* and *Neisseria* to acquire genes from unrelated bacteria by transformation.

There is some evidence that gonococci, which are highly transformable, can become transformed simply by growing donor and recipient bacteria in mixed laboratory culture.[4] In this case, transforming chromosomal DNA is released when the donor gonococci lyse naturally during growth. However, there has been no convincing demonstration in any clinically important species that transformation plays a major role in the dissemination of resistance. Nevertheless it is conceivable that transformation may occasionally be the route by which resistance genes enter new species.

c Transduction

Transduction is the transfer of genes by bacteriophage particles. The process can only occur between donor and recipient bacteria that share appropriate cell surface receptors for the transducing phage. Transduction is therefore generally limited to related species and is relatively ineffectual as a means of intergeneric transfer.[38]

Bacteriophages may be virulent, in which case they kill the cell by lysing it at the end of a round of phage multiplication. Alternatively, they may be temperate, in which case they may either multiply and lyse the host or enter into a stable relationship with it. This involves maintenance as a prophage, either extrachromosomally like a plasmid or by insertion into the host genome. Induction of such a prophage by treatments such as ultraviolet irradiation that damage DNA initiates a lytic cycle. The result of a lytic burst is a population of bacteriophage particles, the vast majority of which contain phage DNA. However, a small proportion of particles (the transducing particles) erroneously contain bacterial DNA and can be used to transfer this DNA to other bacteria. There is considerable evidence that transduction

plays a significant role in the natural transmission of resistance genes and R plasmids between strains of *S. aureus*[39] and between strains of *Streptococcus pyogenes*.[40]

4 Plasmids in Bacterial Populations

The reported incidence of bacteria (predominantly enterobacteria) that harbour R plasmids is normally higher in countries where the use of antibiotics is not controlled.[41,42] Several studies in developed countries have shown that the incidence of resistant enterobacteria is higher in hospitals than in the community at large.[41–43] Fluctuations in the proportion of strains resistant to specific drugs can also be related to changes in antibiotic policy within hospitals.[44] These findings strongly suggest that there is a causal relationship between antibiotic use (and over-use) and the evolution of a resistant bacterial flora.

Relatively little is known about the overall behaviour of resistance genes in natural bacterial populations. However, much can be deduced by studying the molecular and genetic properties of R plasmids from defined clinical situations such as single wards or hospitals. The same plasmid(s) has/have been demonstrated in different strains or species associated, for example, with cross infections involving enterobacteria[5,45] or staphylococci.[46] Minor evolutionary changes such as the gain or loss of transposons by plasmids may also occur during the course of infections.[45,47] The ability of a plasmid to transfer to more than one bacterial species may play an important role in maintaining resistance genes within hospital environments. Thus R plasmids residing in the commensal flora of staff and patients could remain available for transfer to pathogenic species. Bacteria vary considerably in their ability to colonize and survive in their hosts. The persistence of a particular plasmid may therefore depend on its carriage by biotypes with particularly good survival characteristics.

Monitoring the spread of R plasmids on a global basis is problematical due to the sampling difficulties involved. However, it is evident that some R plasmids, such as the group of non-conjugative IncQ plasmids specifying streptomycin and sulphonamide resistance,[48] and notably some resistance transposons, such as the Tn*3* family, have become very widespread (see Table II). A good example of the evolutionary success of a particular class of plasmid may be found in the family of non-conjugative β-lactamase plasmids found in *Neisseria* and *Haemophilus*.[1] Despite the widespread occurrence of β-lactamase producing gonococci, only two types of closely related non-conjugative plasmids (both containing a non-transposing part of Tn*2*) of 4.7 and 6.8 kb have been found. The evidence suggests that gonococci acquired these plasmids (possibly from *Haemophilus* sp.) in only two separate evolutionary events in West Africa and the Far East respectively. Subsequently the host strains and hence their β-lactamase plasmids have been spread worldwide by travellers.

The evolutionary success of particular types of R plasmid is partly dependent on their host range. This is determined by the ability of a plasmid to be transferred to a particular species or biotype, to overcome barriers such as restriction endonucleases which degrade foreign DNA and to replicate in a novel environment. Some plasmids are limited to a single species or genus such as *Staphylococcus* or *Pseudomonas*, whereas others have a much broader host range. Conjugative plasmids of groups IncP, N and W and non-conjugative plasmids of group IncQ have a particularly wide host range and can be transferred to many different gram-negative bacteria. Such plasmids, particularly where they act as transposon donors, may therefore be responsible for much of the traffic in resistance genes between species.

Carriage of a plasmid normally imposes a physiological burden on host cells. Cells which accidentally lose their plasmids due to errors in plasmid replication and/or segregation may therefore be able to outgrow their plasmid-containing parents. Thus, in the absence of selection pressure imposed by antibiotics, there would be a tendency for R-plasmid-free cells to accumulate in populations. However, in practice, plasmid loss is counterbalanced by reacquisition of the plasmid through conjugative transfer or mobilization involving remaining plasmid-containing members of the population.

R plasmids may encode virulence determinants such as adhesins or toxins.[49] Such properties may therefore contribute to the stability of resistance genes in pathogenic species. The *tra*T protein of certain conjugative plasmids provides an interesting example of a plasmid character that incidentally contributes to virulence and stability. The *tra*T protein is a necessary part of the conjugative apparatus and is laid down in large quantities in the outer membrane of host *E. coli*.[24] Its presence in the membrane confers enhanced resistance to complement-mediated serum killing and phagocytosis.[50] This might thus indirectly provide a mechanism for maintenance of conjugative plasmids in human or animal pathogens.

5 The Origins of Resistance Genes

The rapidity with which different resistance genes, transposons and R plasmids have spread to various pathogens around the world demonstrates the powerful selective forces imposed by human use of antibiotics. There is, however, some evidence to suggest that resistance genes may have existed within the bacterial gene pool prior to man's introduction of chemotherapeutic antimicrobials. For example, resistant *E. coli* have been isolated from the faeces of primitive peoples who have not been administered antibiotics.[41] In addition, some enterobacteria lyophilized prior to the antibiotic era have been found to be resistant to drugs that had not been introduced at the time of storage.[51] However, a recent survey of over 400 enterobacteria collected and subsequently stored between 1917 and 1954 suggests that resistance was very uncommon in the pre-antibiotic era.[52] What little drug resistance that was found in this survey was probably chromosomally determined. Interestingly, however, 24% of this collection of strains carried conjugative plasmids as judged by their ability to mobilize non-conjugative test plasmids. This compares with surveys of healthy humans and animals carried out since the general introduction of antibiotics which indicated that 17–33% of faecal *E. coli* contained conjugative plasmids.[53,54] Such findings illustrate that the human bacterial flora had the potential to transfer genes long before resistance

became a problem. The resident plasmids of enterobacteria and indeed other species have thus probably provided core molecules on to which resistance genes have become grafted by transposition or other recombination events.

Whilst core plasmids that might act as progenitors of R plasmids do exist in clinically important bacteria, there is no evidence that the resistance genes themselves originate in such species. It is possible that resistance determinants could arise over a long period by mutation of existing chromosomal genes. For example, β-lactamases could have evolved by sequential mutations affecting one of the several penicillin-binding proteins (PBPs) that are present in the bacterial envelope. PBPs are the target sites for β-lactams and some of these proteins have weak β-lactamase activity.[55] It is unlikely, however, that all the resistance genes now extant could have evolved in human pathogens or commensals. The majority of R determinants must have been acquired from other bacterial species by gene transfer. One immediate source for the R plasmids in human strains may be the food chain, through contaminated meat and dairy products.[1,56] However, the ultimate sources of many resistance genes are likely to be the soil microorganisms that actually produce most antibiotics or that would be competing with such producers.[58] Since antibiotics are potentially toxic to the producing organism, it is hardly surprising that bacteria such as streptomycetes should possess resistance mechanisms to protect themselves from the antibiotics they produce. For example, *Streptomyces erythraeus* which produces erythromycin protects itself from the antibiotic by methylation of its 23S rRNA. Plasmid-mediated resistance to erythromycin and other members of the macrolide, lincosamide and streptogramin B (MLS) group of antibiotics in *S. aureus* and certain streptococci is apparently determined by a 23S rRNA methylase similar to that in *S. erythraeus*.[58] This suggests that there may be a common evolutionary origin for the genes encoding these enzymes.

The evolutionary route a resistance gene might take from its originating organism to present-day human pathogens would be an extremely tortuous one. It would require association of the gene, possibly after acquiring the ability to transpose, with a series of phage or plasmid vectors capable of transfer to successive bacterial species. Each individual transfer or transposition event in such an evolutionary chain would presumably occur with a very low probability. Rare though such events may be, they must occur with sufficient frequency to generate genetic diversity within bacterial populations. Bacterial clones acquiring novel combinations of genes would be continually tested against prevailing selective pressures and, if successful, would multiply. The antibiotic-resistant bacteria seen in hospitals today have largely resulted from this process of clonal selection operating on R plasmids and their hosts.

REFERENCES

1 Saunders JR. Human impact on microbial evolution. In: Bishop JA, Cook LM, eds. Genetic consequences of man-made change. London: Academic Press, 1981; 249–294

2 Broda P. Plasmids. San Francisco: Freeman, 1979

3 Hardy K. Bacterial plasmids. London: Nelson, 1981

4 Sparling PF. Antibiotic resistance in the gonococcus. In: Roberts RB, ed. The gonococcus. New York: Wiley, 1977; 111–135

5 Datta N, Richards H. Trimethoprim-resistant bacteria in hospital and in the community: spread of plasmids and transposons. In: Levy SB, Clowes RC, Koenig EL, eds. Molecular biology, pathogenicity, and ecology of bacterial plasmids. New York: Plenum Press, 1981, 21–30

6 Bird PI, Pittard J. Demonstration of a third incompatibility function on plasmids already incompatible with Group P and Group I plasmids. Plasmid 1983; 9: 191–200

7 Lacatena RM, Cesareni G. Base pairing of RNA I with its complementary sequence in the primer precursor inhibits ColE1 replication. Nature 1981; 294: 623–626

8 Tomizawa J-I, Itoh T, Selzer G, Som T. Inhibition of ColE1 RNA primer formation by a plasmid-specified small RNA. Proc Natl Acad Sci USA 1981; 78: 1421–1425

9 Cesareni G, Muesing MA, Polisky B. Control of ColE1 DNA replication: the *rop* gene product negatively affects transcription from the replication primer promoter. Proc Natl Acad Sci USA 1982; 79: 6313–6317

10 Light J, Molin S. Replication control functions of plasmid R1 act as inhibitors of expression of a gene required for replication. Mol Gen Genet 1981; 184: 56–61

11 Ogura T, Hiraga S. Partition mechanism of F plasmid: two plasmid

gene-encoded products and a cis-acting region are involved in partition. Cell 1983; 32: 351–360

12 Meacock PA, Cohen SB. Partitioning of bacterial plasmids during cell division: a *cis*-acting locus that accomplishes stable plasmid inheritance. Cell 1980; 20: 529–542

13 Summers DK, Sherratt D. The stability of ColE1-related plasmid in *Escherichia coli*. Cell 1984; In press

14 Kleckner N. Transposable elements in prokaryotes. Ann Rev Genet 1981; 15: 341–404

15 Shapiro JA, ed. Mobile genetic elements. London, Academic Press 1983

16 Galas DJ, Chandler M. On the molecular mechanisms of transposition. Proc Natl Acad Sci USA 1981; 78: 4858–4862

17 Grindley NDF. Transposition of Tn3 and related transposons. Cell 1983; 32: 3–5

18 Heffron F, McCarthy J, Ohtsubo H, Ohtsubo E. DNA sequence analysis of the transposon Tn3: three genes and three sites involved in transposition of Tn3. Cell 1979; 18: 1153–1163

19 Kitts P, Symington L, Burke M, Reed R, Sherratt D. Transposon-specified site-specific recombination. Proc Natl Acad Sci USA 1982; 79: 46–50

20 Barth PT, Datta N, Hedges, RW, Grinter NJ. Transposition of a deoxyribonucleic acid sequence encoding trimethoprim and streptomycin resistances from R483 to other replicons. J Bacteriol 1976; 125: 800–810

21 Saunders JR, Elwell LP, Falkow S, Sykes RB, Richmond MH. Beta-lactamases and R-plasmids in *Haemophilus influenzae*. Scand J Infect Dis 1978 (Suppl 13) 16–22

22 Franke AE, Clewell DB. Evidence for a chromosome-borne resistance transposon Tn*916* in *Streptococcus faecalis* that is capable of "conjugal" transfer in the absence of a conjugative plasmid. J Bacteriol 1981; 145: 494–502

23 Manning PA, Achtman M. Cell-to-cell interactions in conjugating *Escherichia coli*: the involvement of the cell envelope. In: M Inouye, ed. Bacterial outer membrane. Biogenesis and functions. New York: Wiley, 1979; 407–449

24 Willetts N, Skurray R. The conjugation system of F-like plasmids. Ann Rev Genet 1980; 14: 41–76

25 Thomas CM. Molecular genetics of broad host range plasmid RK2. Plasmid 1980; 5: 10–19

26 Bradley DE. Morphological and serological relationships of conjugative pili. Plasmid 1980; 4: 155–169

27 Warren GJ, Saul MW, Sherratt DJ. ColE1 plasmid mobility: essential and conditional functions. Mol Gen Genet 1979; 170: 103–107

28 Willetts N. Sites and systems for conjugal DNA transfer in bacteria. In: Levy SB, Clowes RC, Koenig EL, eds. Molecular biology, pathogenicity, and ecology of bacterial plasmids. New York: Plenum Press, 1981: 207–215

29 Nordheim A, Hashimoto-Gotoh T, Timmis KN. Location of two relaxation nick sites in R6K and single sites in pSC101 and RSF1010 close to origins of vegetative replication: Implication for conjugal transfer of plasmid deoxyribonucleic acid. J Bacteriol 1980; 144: 923–932

30 Clark AJ, Warren GJ. Conjugal transmission of plasmids. Ann Rev Genet 1979; 13: 99–125

31 Anderson ES. Viability of, and transfer of a plasmid from, *E. coli* K12 in the human intestine. Nature 1975; 255: 502–504

32 Smith HW. Transfer of antibiotic resistance from animal and human strains of *Escherichia coli* to resident *E. coli* in the alimentary tract of man. Lancet 1969; i: 1174–1176

33 Smith MG. Transfer of R factors from *Escherichia coli* to Salmonellas in the rumen of sheep. J Med Microbiol 1977; 10: 29–35

34 Anderson JD. Factors that may prevent transfer of antibiotic resistance between Gram-negative bacteria in the gut. J Med Microbiol 1975; 8: 83–88

35 Freter R, Freter RR, Brickner H. Experimental and mathematical models of *Escherichia coli* plasmid transfer *in vitro* and *in vivo*. Infect Immun 1983; 39: 60–84

36 Roberts M, Falkow S. *In vivo* conjugal transfer of R plasmids in *Neisseria gonorrhoeae*. Infect Immun 1979; 24: 982–984

37 Smith HO, Danner DB, Deich RA. Genetic transformation. Ann Rev Biochem 1981; 50: 41–68

38 Reanney D. Extrachromosomal elements as possible agents of adaptation and development. Bacteriol Rev 1976; 40: 552–590

39 Lacey RW. Antibiotic resistance plasmids of *Staphylococcus aureus* and their clinical importance. Bacteriol Rev 1975; 39: 1–32

40 Hyder SL, Streitfeld MM. Transfer of erythromycin resistance from clinically isolated lysogenic strains of *Streptococcus pyogenes* via their endogenous phage. J Infect Dis 1978; 138: 281–286

41 Falkow S. Infectious multiple drug resistance. London: Pion, 1975

42 Datta N. Drug resistance and R factors in the bowel bacteria of London patients before and after admission to hospital. Br Med J 1969; 2: 407–411

43 Linton KB, Richmond MH, Bevan R, Gillespie WA. Antibiotic resistance and R factors in coliform bacilli isolated from hospital and domestic sewage. J Med Microbiol 1974; 7: 91–103

44 Buckwold FJ, Ronald AR. Antimicrobial misuse—effects and suggestions for control. J Antimicrob Chemother 1979; 5: 129–136

45 Datta N, Dacey S, Hughes V *et al*. Distribution of genes for trimethoprim and gentamicin resistance in bacteria and their plasmids in a general hospital. J Gen Microbiol 1980; 118: 495–508

46 Cohen ML, Wong ES, Falkow S. Common R-plasmids in *Staphylococcus aureus* and *Staphylococcus epidermidis* during a nosocomial *Staphylococcus aureus* outbreak. Antimicrob Agents Chemother 1982; 21: 210–215

47 Datta N, Hughes VM, Nugent ME, Richards H. Plasmids and transposons and their stability and mutability in bacteria isolated during an outbreak of hospital infection. Plasmid 1979; 2: 182–196

48 Grinter NJ, Barth PT. Characterization of SmSu plasmids by restriction endonuclease cleavage and compatibility testing. J Bacteriol 1976; 128: 394–400

49 Elwell LP, Shipley PL. Plasmid-mediated factors associated with virulence of bacteria to animals. Ann Rev Microbiol 1980; 34: 465–496

50 Agüero ME, De Luca AG, Timmis KN, Cabello FC. A plasmid encoded outer membrane protein, *traT*, enhances resistance to phagocytosis and *E. coli* virulence. Infect Immun 1983; In press

51 Smith DH. R factor infection of *Escherichia coli* lyophilized in 1946. J Bacteriol 1967; 94: 2071–2072

52 Hughes VM, Datta N. Conjugative plasmids in bacteria of the 'pre-antibiotic' era. Nature 1983; 302: 725–726

53 Lewis MJ. Transferable drug resistance and other transferable agents in strains of *Escherichia coli* from two human populations. Lancet 1968; i: 1389–1393

54 Smith HW, Lingwood MA. Transfer factors in *Escherichia coli* with particular regard to their incidence in enteropathogenic strains. J Gen Microbiol 1970; 62: 287–299

55 Spratt BG. Penicillin-binding proteins and the future of β-lactam antibiotics. J Gen Microbiol 1983; 129: 1247–1260

56 Linton AH. Antibiotic resistance. The present situation reviewed. Vet Rec 1977; 100: 354–360

57 Cundliffe E. Br Med Bull 1984; 40: 61–67

58 Weisblum B, Holder SB, Halling SM. Deoxyribonucleic acid sequence common to staphylococcal and streptococcal plasmids which specify erythromycin resistance. J Bacteriol 1979; 138: 990–998

British Medical Bulletin (1984) Vol. 40, No. 1, pp. 61-67

SELF DEFENCE IN ANTIBIOTIC-PRODUCING ORGANISMS

ERIC CUNDLIFFE MA PhD

Department of Biochemistry
University of Leicester

1   Resistance involving inactivation of antibiotics
    a Viomycin and capreomycin
    b Streptomycin
    c Other aminoglycoside–aminocyclitols
2   Resistance due to modification of antibiotic target-sites
    a Thiostrepton
    b Erythromycin
3   Discussion
    References

The survival strategies adopted by antibiotic-producing organisms in order to avoid self intoxication have been the subject of stimulating reviews.[1,2] Leaving aside important considerations such as inducibility or constitutive expression there are, broadly speaking, three resistance mechanisms which could be effective against extra-cellular drug: (i) The intracellular target to which the drug normally binds might be modified and thereby rendered unavailable. (ii) Antibiotic entering the cell might be inactivated. (iii) Entry of the active compound into the cell might be blocked. Clearly, the first of these mechanisms could render an organism totally insensitive to the action of specific antibiotics, as could the latter process provided exclusion were total. Otherwise, a partially effective permeability barrier would be adequate for resistance if coupled with an antibiotic-inactivation system to deal with small amounts of drug reaching the cytoplasm. However, in high-level producers, one might not expect antibiotic-inactivation to represent the sole means of self protection. In the absence of a reasonably effective permeability barrier, such organisms would need to inactivate the bulk of the antibiotic produced which, in addition to precluding their status as high-level producers, might be energetically unfeasible.

In addition to withstanding the effects of extracellular drug, producing organisms must also protect themselves against intracellular metabolites during antibiotic biosynthesis. Obviously, those which indulge in target-site modification face no such problem but others must either confine their toxic products within discrete subcellular compartments or produce them as inert derivatives to be activated during or following export. The latter procedure is probably quite common as, for example, in the biosynthesis of streptomycin (see below) and this raises certain problems when antibiotic-modifying enzymes are identified in extracts of producing organisms. In the intact cell, such an enzyme might normally act early in the biosynthetic route to the drug and might not constitute the principal mechanism of resistance to extracellular drug. Given such considerations, the physiological roles of antibiotic-inactivating enzymes should not lightly be assumed particularly when, as is usually the case, the relevant permeability properties of the cell surface are not known.

Whether or not a given antibiotic-modifying enzyme contributes to the resistance phenotype of a given organism can be established only by experimentation and not by sophistry or downright wishful thinking! The most unequivocal way to address this question is to use recombinant DNA methodology in order to examine the properties of putative resistance determinants in a 'clean' background. In practice, this will usually involve 'shotgun cloning' of DNA fragments from antibiotic producers in non-producing hosts, followed by selection for the resistance phenotype and biochemical characterization of resistance mechanisms in the clones. Since few such investigations have been reported, there are not many instances in which antibiotic-modifying enzymes can, confidently, be held responsible for the resistance of producing organisms. Which is not to say that more examples will not be forthcoming.

Whenever an organism possesses an altered drug-target site (e.g. an abnormal ribosome), this should be relatively easy to detect. In such cases, in-vitro studies (amounting to complementation analysis) must be carried out if a causal connection is to be established between the inability of the target (be it enzyme or organelle) to bind or respond to the drug and any structural change or modification process allegedly responsible for resistance. Alternatively (perferably in addition), the presence of specifically altered (and resistant) target sites could be sought in antibiotic-resistant clones. Two examples of the application of these criteria are discussed in detail below.

1.   Resistance Involving Inactivation of Antibiotics

Despite the caveats presented above, it seems probable that the ability to inactivate their antibiotic products is crucial to the survival of quite a few organisms. Table I lists some examples of modifying enzymes present in producers and active upon the endogenous antibiotics. Some of these enzymes have been implicated in resistance although, since aminoglycoside-modifying enzymes are present in many organisms which do not produce aminoglycosides, the mere presence of such an enzyme does not necessarily imply such a role.

a *Viomycin and Capreomycin*

Viomycin and the capreomycins are structurally related cyclic peptides, active against gram-positive bacteria, which inhibit protein synthesis by binding directly to ribosomes. Capreomycin is a complex of four components, predominantly capreomycins IA and IB, produced by *Streptomyces capreolus* whereas viomycin is synthesized as a single molecular species by *Streptomyces vinaceus*.

Like many other antibiotic producers, *S. vinaceus* and *S. capreolus* are highly resistant to their own products and this is evident throughout the growth cycle. Moreover, *S. capreolus* is cross-resistant to viomycin, whereas *S. vinaceus* is partially resistant to capreomycin IA but sensitive to capreomycin IB. When cell extracts were examined, ribosomes from either strain proved to be fully sensitive to the action of either drug.[3] However, viomycin and capreomycin were each inactivated when incubated with postribosomal supernatant from their respective producers. In extracts of *S. vinaceus*, viomycin was inactivated by a phosphotransferase enzyme and capreomycins IA and IIA (but not IB and IIB) were also phosphorylated (Table II). A similar pattern of phosphorylation was observed in extracts of *S. capreolus* and, again, both viomycin and capreomycin IA were shown to be inactivated.[3] Effects of phosphorylation upon the activity of

TABLE I. Antibiotic-modifying enzymes present in producers and active upon the endogenous antibiotic

Strain	Antibiotic produced	Modifying enzyme(s)
Streptomyces griseus	Streptomycin	APH(6)
S. bikiniensis	Streptomycin	APH(6)
S. glaucescens	Hydroxystreptomycin	APH(6)
S. fradiae	Neomycin	APH(3') + AAC(3)
S. lividus	Lividomycin	APH(3') + AAC(3)
S. ribosidificus	Ribostamycin	APH(3') + AAC(3)
S. kanamyceticus	Kanamycin	AAC(6')
*S. tenebrarius**	Tobramycin	AAC(6') + AAC(2')
S. hygroscopicus	Hygromycin B	Phosphotransferase
S. vinaceus	Viomycin	VPH
S. capreolus	Capreomycin	Phosphotransferase Acetyltransferase(s)

Abbreviations: APH: aminoglycoside phosphotransferase; AAC: aminoglycoside acetyltransferase; VPH: viomycin phosphotransferase
* Produces the nebramycin complex of which tobramycin is one component. Also possesses resistant ribosomes (see text).

TABLE II. Substrate specificities of antibiotic-modifying activities in extracts of *S. vinaceus* and *S. capreolus*

(data from Skinner & Cundliffe[3])

Substrate (600 pmol)	Phosphotransferase activity*		Acetyltransferase activity† *S. capreolus* extract
	S. vinaceus extract	*S. capreolus* extract	
Viomycin	76	455	7
Capreomycin IA	293	604	29
Capreomycin IB	1	2	49
Capreomycin IIA	287	488	27
Capreomycin IIB	0	8	61

* pmol [^{32}P] phosphoryl groups transferred from [γ-^{32}P] ATP
† pmol [^{14}C] acetyl groups transferred from [1-^{14}C] acetyl CoA

capreomycin IIA were not sought. Although these data do not prove that a single phosphotransferase was responsible, the presence of such activity (perhaps in association with an appropriate permeability barrier, as discussed above) could obviously account for the resistance of *S. vinaceus* to viomycin and capreomycin IA. It could not, however, be responsible for the resistance of *S. capreolus* to capreomycins IB and IIB, hence the presence in that organism of another inactivating enzyme was suspected. As shown in Table II, extracts of *S. capreolus* were capable of acetylating all the capreomycins (using acetyl-CoA as cofactor) and, at least for capreomycins IA and IB, this resulted in their inactivation.[3]

To characterize the viomycin-resistance mechanism further, DNA fragments from *S. vinaceus* were introduced into *Streptomyces lividans* and several viomycin-resistant clones were examined.[4] Most of them exhibited high-level resistance to viomycin, were cross-resistant to capreomycin IA (but not to capreomycin IB) and contained phosphotransferase activity similar to that previously found in *S. vinaceus*. The remainder were resistant only to low levels of viomycin, were sensitive to capreomycin IA and lacked viomycin phosphotransferase activity. These data suggest that a single enzyme, present in *S. vinaceus* and designated viomycin phosphotransferase (VPH), phosphorylates and inactivates both viomycin and capreomycin IA. Since the gene encoding VPH confers resistance to these compounds in *S. lividans*, it presumably could do so in *S. vinaceus* as well. Significantly, however, although both drugs are excellent substrates for VPH in vitro, capreomycin IA is distinctly more active than viomycin against *S. vinaceus*.[3] This differential could be accounted for if, of the two, viomycin were the more efficiently excluded from *S. vinaceus*. Possibly, those *S. lividans* clones which exhibited low-level resistance to viomycin had acquired a partially effective permeability barrier, but not VPH. If so, the resistance of *S. vinaceus* to viomycin would be seen to result from a combination of causes. As yet, capreomycin-resistant clones have not been characterized and the possible contributions of phosphotransferase and acetyltransferase activities to the resistance phenotype of *S. capreolus* cannot be assessed.

b *Streptomycin*

Streptomycin-producing strains of *Streptomyces griseus* and *Streptomyces bikiniensis* are normally sensitive to the drug during exponential growth but develop a high level of tolerance by the time antibiotic is produced. Such resistance is not simply due to total abolition of drug uptake, although this does decline in both

organisms during the stationary phase.[5,6] However, since sensitive and resistant strains of *S. bikiniensis* exhibited similar changes in the level of uptake,[6] this effect alone cannot determine resistance. Nor can resistance be attributed to modification of the normal antibiotic target-site, since ribosomes from streptomycin producers remain sensitive to the drug throughout the growth cycle.[5-8] Rather, as streptomycin enters stationary-phase mycelium, it is converted to the 6-phosphoryl derivative and thereby inactivated.[5,9] The enzyme responsible, known variously as streptomycin 6-kinase or aminoglycoside 6-phosphotransferase (APH(6)), is inducible in producing strains and is present at high levels during streptomycin production.[10,11] Accordingly, most investigations of resistance in *S. griseus* and *S. bikiniensis* have concentrated upon the function(s) of the APH(6) enzyme.

Studies of the biosynthesis of streptomycin have given rise to an attractive model of how metabolic shielding can be employed to allow production of a toxic metabolite. Streptomycin is made from myo-inositol via streptidine and it seems likely that the latter and all subsequent intermediates in the pathway are phosphorylated and are biologically inert.[10] The final reaction involves dephosphorylation during (or even after) transport through the membrane so that active drug is excreted.[12,13] Consistent with this scheme are the observations that phosphorylated streptomycin is produced when inorganic phosphate is added to the fermentation medium[14] or when the pH is manipulated.[15] The enzyme that phosphorylates streptidine is APH(6), which can presumably 'salvage' for drug production any intermediates which might otherwise be dephosphorylated and channelled elsewhere.[10] Thus, according to this model, APH(6) protects *S. griseus* and *S. bikiniensis* during the antibiotic-production phase by arranging for the synthesis of an inactive precursor, 6-phosphorylstreptomycin, within the cell. Certainly, a role for APH(6) in the production of streptomycin was indicated by the observation that strains of *S. griseus* or *S. bikiniensis* lacking the enzyme were invariably non-producers.[6,16] Usually, but curiously not always,[16] such strains were sensitive to streptomycin throughout the growth cycle, as were APH-minus mutants of *Streptomyces glaucescens* which produces hydroxystreptomycin.[17] It therefore seems likely that APH(6) additionally protects streptomycin producers by inactivating the drug if it gets back into the cell. This hypothesis could be tested directly, and possible contributions of enzyme and membrane to the resistance phenotype could perhaps be assessed, by cloning the streptomycin-resistance determinant(s) from a producer in a non-producing host.

c *Other Aminoglycoside-Aminocyclitols*

Several strains which produce aminoglycosides also produce enzymes capable of modifying such compounds (Table I). Since some such enzymes also inactivate their substrates, some authors have concluded that it is their presence which determines resistance. However, most of the aminoglycoside producers yet studied in detail possess more than one enzyme capable of modifying the endogenous antibiotic. To say the least, this complicates analysis of the functions of such enzymes and the results of recent studies[4] involving *Streptomyces fradiae* (the producer of neomycin) may serve as a cautionary tale. This organism, which contains neomycin-sensitive ribosomes, possesses two aminoglycoside-modifying enzymes, a phosphotransferase (APH) and an acetyltransferase (AAC). From their sites of action, these enzymes are designated APH(3′) and AAC(3) respectively[18] and both readily inactivate neomycin in vitro.[4] Accordingly, when *S. fradiae* DNA was cloned in *S. lividans* and neomycin-resistant clones selected, it was not altogether surprising that some contained APH activity and others AAC activity. What *was* surprising was that all such clones displayed only low-level resistance to neomycin, despite the fact that those with APH activity produced large amounts of the enzyme. High-level resistance (as in *S. fradiae*) was observed only when APH clones were crossed with AAC clones and was associated (as in *S. fradiae*) with the presence of both enzymes.[4] While the full implications of these findings are not at all obvious, one thing at least is clear. The genes encoding APH(3′) and AAC(3) do not separately function as efficient resistance determinants in all organisms. Thus, we can rationalize, if not explain, the presence of both genes in *S. fradiae*. The moral appears to be that the presence of multiple antibiotic-inactivating enzymes in a given producing organism does not necessarily imply that Nature believes in overkill.

2 Resistance due to Modification of Antibiotic Target-Sites

The normal target for drug action is known to be refractory to the endogenous antibiotic in various producing organisms although, in most cases, the basis of such resistance has not been further determined. For example, RNA polymerase of *Nocardia* (previously called *Streptomyces*) *mediterranei* is resistant to rifampicin[19] and isoleucyl-tRNA synthase from *Pseudomonas fluorescens* binds pseudomonic acid relatively weakly.[20] In extracts of *Streptoverticillium mobaraense,* the protein elongation factor Tu is sometimes recovered as aggregates of undefined physiological status; perhaps significantly, such aggregates are resistant to the action of pulvomycin.[21] Among eukaryotes, the fungus *Myrothecium verrucaria* (which produces T-2 toxin) possesses ribosomes resistant to this and other trichothecenes;[22] also RNA polymerase II from the carpophores of *Amanita* species which produce α-amanitin is notably resistant to that drug.[23] More generally, 'ribosome-inactivating proteins' of catalytic action, which are present in a wide range of plants, may discriminate between ribosomes of the producers and those from other plants.[24]

Resistant ribosomes are found in some actinomycetes which produce aminoglycosides, e.g. *Streptomyces tenjimariensis* which makes istamycin[25] and *Micromonospora purpurea*, the gentamicin producer.[26] Moreover, although ribosomes from both strains are resistant to a range of aminoglycosides, it is evident that *S. tenjimariensis* and *M. purpurea* do not employ identical defence mechanisms since their ribosomes differ in response to gentamicin. In the case of *Streptomyces tenebrarius*, the situation is more complicated. This organism produces the nebramycin complex which includes kanamycin B and derivatives thereof, most notably tobramycin. Ribosomes from *S. tenebrarius* are resistant to kanamycin B (indeed, their resistance profile resembles that of *M. purpurea* ribosomes) and this drug is also a substrate for acetyltransferase activity present in the same organism.[27] However, the response of *S. tenebrarius* ribosomes to the novel aminoglycoside apramycin (factor 2 of the nebramycin complex) has not been reported nor has apramycin yet been shown to be a substrate for any of the aminoglycoside-modifying enzymes so far characterized in *S. tenebrarius*.[28]

As yet, there are only two mechanisms of self protection, involving modification of antibiotic target-sites, which have been fully characterized. Both involve inhibitors of protein synthesis (namely, thiostrepton and erythromycin) and both involve specific methylation of rRNA. These are discussed below.

a *Thiostrepton*

Thiostrepton is a modified peptide produced by *Streptomyces azureus*. Normally, it binds very tightly to a single site on the larger (50S) subunit of the bacterial ribosome and thereby inhibits protein synthesis. Although, in general, *Streptomyces* are quite sensitive to thiostrepton, *S. azureus* is totally unaffected by the drug and this character is reflected in the properties of its ribosomes. This is due to the possession by *S. azureus* of a methylase enzyme, which acts in vitro upon ribosomal RNA from other bacteria,[29] and introduces a single methyl group into residue 1067 of *E. coli* 23S rRNA.[30] The product of methylation is 2′-O-methyladenosine and ribosomes containing such modified RNA do not bind thiostrepton.[31] Studies of the function of the 'thiostrepton-resistance methylase' were complicated by the fact that the enzyme acts only upon naked 23S rRNA and not upon intact ribosomes.[32] Hence, in order to demonstrate a causal connection between methylation and resistance, it was necessary to subject rRNA to the action of the enzyme in vitro and then to reconstitute ribosomes containing such RNA in order that their response to thiostrepton could be examined. The most convenient assay for the action of thiostrepton involves the inhibition of GTP hydrolysis catalysed jointly by the ribosome and the protein known as elongation factor G (factor EF G). Normally, during protein synthesis, GTP is hydrolysed in a strictly controlled manner but, in the absence of other components required for protein synthesis, the ribosome and factor EF G catalyse 'uncoupled' hydrolysis of GTP. This is powerfully inhibited by thiostrepton (reviewed in reference 33). In the critical experiment, when *E. coli* ribosomes containing RNA modified due to the action of the *S. azureus* methylase were re-assembled in vitro, they were found to be insensitive to thiostrepton (Table III). Moreover, when fragments of DNA from *S. azureus* were subsequently cloned in *S. lividans*, resistance to thiostrepton was invariably associated with the presence of RNA-pentose methylase activity as in *S. azureus*.[4]

Unlike some of the aminoglycoside-modifying enzymes, the thiostrepton-resistance methylase appears not to be widespread among actinomycetes. It has so far been found only in organisms which produce thiostrepton or antibiotics very closely related to it in structure and/or in function. Presumably, in *S. azureus* where it is apparently produced constitutively, the methylase acts upon rRNA at an early stage during or following transcription but prior to ribosome assembly. The site of methylation (Fig. 1) probably pinpoints the binding site for thiostrepton since the drug is known to bind directly to 23S rRNA. Moreover, in view of the mode of action of thiostrepton, it seems clear that this site lies within the ribosomal GTP hydrolysis centre. Clearly, enzymes such as the thiostrepton-resistance methylase are potentially useful probes of functional sites within the ribosome. The gene encoding the methylase also has its uses; it now provides the prime selectable marker on various recombinant plasmids developed as vectors for cloning in *Streptomyces*.[34]

TABLE III. Properties of *E. coli* ribosomes containing 23S RNA modified by the methylase purified from *S. azureus*

State of RNA in reconstituted ribosomes	Thiostrepton added[*]	GTP hydrolysis[†]
Unmethylated	0	170
Unmethylated	3	24
Methylated	0	185
Methylated	30	175

[*] molar excess over reconstituted ribosomes
[†] pmol GTP hydrolysed per min per pmol reconstituted ribosomes

b *Erythromycin*

The erythromycin-producer, *Streptomyces erythraeus*, also modifies ribosomal RNA as a means of self defence. Normally, erythromycin inhibits bacterial protein synthesis by binding to 50S ribosomal subunits but those from *S. erythraeus* do not bind the drug[35] and are insensitive to its action. The mechanism of resistance is now known and is closely similar to that first observed in clinical isolates of staphylococci possessing the so-called MLS resistance-phenotype (see Weisblum, pp. 47–53). In such strains, resistance to macrolides (such as erythromycin and spiramycin), to lincosamides (lincomycin and clindamycin) and to streptogramin B-group antibiotics (including virginiamycin S) is induced by erythromycin and is due to the action of a plasmid-encoded methylase upon 23S rRNA.[36,37] The product of methylation is N[6]-dimethyl-adenine and its presence in 23S rRNA from *S. erythraeus* first prompted the speculation that the mechanism of resistance in the erythromycin-producer might resemble that in staphylococci.[38] The validity of that hypothesis has since been established.[39] A methylase, purified from *S. erythraeus*, introduced two methyl groups into 23S rRNA from *Bacillus stearothermophilus* and produced a single residue of N[6]-dimethyladenine. As with the thiostrepton-resistance methylase, intact ribosomes were not substrates for the enzyme so that the functional significance of

this methylation could only be established using 50S ribosomal particles reconstituted in vitro. As shown in Table IV, when such particles contained RNA previously subjected to the action of the methylase from *S. erythraeus*, they were resistant to MLS antibiotics such as spiramycin and lincomycin. (Their response to erythromycin could not be assessed in these experiments since that drug is a poor inhibitor of cell-free protein synthesis directed by polyU.) Recently, the site of action of the 'erythromycin-resistance methylase' from *S. erythraeus* within *B. stearothermophilus* 23S RNA was determined and was shown to correspond to residue 2058 in *E. coli* 23S RNA (Fig. 2) although, for some reason, the latter was not a good substrate for the enzyme.[40] The extensive sequence homologies which exist between rRNA molecules from different prokaryotes, which allowed the above correspondence to be established, extend to mitochondrial rRNA. Hence, it has also been possible to identify in *E. coli* 23S RNA the site corresponding to that at which a single base change in yeast mitochondrial rRNA is associated with resistance to erythromycin. Adenosine-2058 is again involved,[41] which seems to confirm the critical role for this site in the binding of erythromycin to the ribosome. Presumably, substitution or dimethylation of residue 2058 in *E. coli* 23S RNA would render ribosomes resistant to the drug.

Also indicated in Fig. 2 are four sites within 23S RNA of *E. coli* which correspond to those at which single base changes have been detected in rRNA from mitochondria resistant to chloramphenicol.[42,43] The fact that all four sites are close to residue 2058 in models of the secondary structure of 23S RNA is presumably related to the fact that chloramphenicol competes with erythromycin (and other MLS antibiotics) for binding to the ribosome. Although these data do not necessarily imply that these antibiotics bind directly to RNA in the ribosome (although any of them might well do so), it seems inescapable that a limited region of 23S RNA is common to their binding sites. Since chloramphenicol and some of the macrolides inhibit peptide bond formation *per se* (see reference 33), that portion of 23S RNA shown in Fig. 2 may well be present in the peptidyltransferase centre of the ribosome.

FIG. 1. Site of action of the thiostrepton-resistance methylase of *S. azureus* within *E. coli* 23S rRNA

From Thompson *et al.*[30]

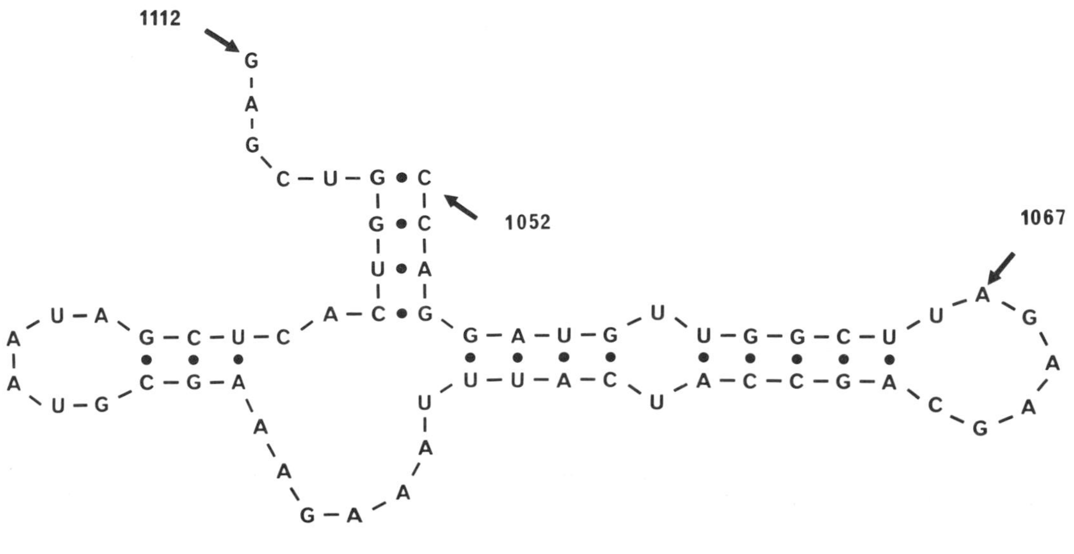

TABLE IV. Properties of *B. stearothermophilus* ribosomes containing 23S RNA modified by the methylase purified from *S. erythraeus*

State of RNA in reconstituted ribosomes	Activity in protein synthesis* (normalized)		
	Control	Plus spiramycin	Plus lincomycin
Unmethylated	100	8	5
Methylated	100	64	44

* Synthesis of polyphenylalanine directed by polyuridylic acid

The mechanisms of resistance in streptomycetes which produce MLS antibiotics other than erythromycin still remain conjectural. In some such organisms, induction of resistance is circumstantially associated with the appearance of mono- or di-methylated adenine within 23S rRNA[44] and, while no causal connection has been established between these events, there is obviously a case for closer inspection. If, as suggested by Fujisawa & Weisblum,[44] a hierarchy of rRNA methylases can render ribosomes resistant to specific groups of MLS antibiotics, it will be important, not only in the context of antibiotic action and resistance but also for our knowledge of ribosomal structure and function, to determine their sites of action.

3 Discussion

Two conceptually different survival strategies have been described and it might be asked which one is better or preferable from the viewpoint of an antibiotic-producing organism. Certainly, target-site modification is capable of rendering cells totally resistant to drugs and it may be that, in general, this mechanism is more efficient than antibiotic modification if levels of resistance are the sole criterion. However, such considerations ignore the reason(s) why antibiotics are produced in the first place (for reviews, see references 45, 46). Obviously, some of them may be weapons, although direct evidence that antibiotic production confers a competitive advantage is not abundant. Some may be involved in the regulation of cell growth, of differentiation (e.g. sporulation) or of spore germination so that the producers may need to be at least partially sensitive to their products at some stage(s) of the growth cycle. Under such circumstances, total resistance would obviously be undesirable and this might dictate the 'choice' of defence mechanism actually employed. There might also be more obvious constraints governing that choice since some antibiotics presumably do not have vital groups which can readily be modified and some target sites may prove impossible to blockade without undesirable perturbation of their function.

The possibility that enzymes involved in resistance mechanisms might fulfil additional roles in producing organisms should also be considered. As documented above for streptomycin synthesis, some antibiotic-modifying enzymes may participate in the production of drug percursors which can be activated by other enzymes during export. Such reasoning would be consistent with the presence in *Streptomyces kanamyceticus* (the kanamycin producer) of both AAC(6') and acetylkanamycin hydrolase activities.[47] Possibly, *S. vinaceus* employs VPH to produce viomycin in phosphorylated form, in which case one might predict the occurrence of a phosphoviomycin phosphatase in that organism. Perhaps significantly, the presence of inorganic phosphate in the fermentation medium inhibits viomycin production,[48] possibly by inhibiting the putative phosphatase. It would therefore be

FIG. 2. Site of action of the erythromycin-resistance methylase of *S. erythraeus*

From Skinner *et al.*[40]

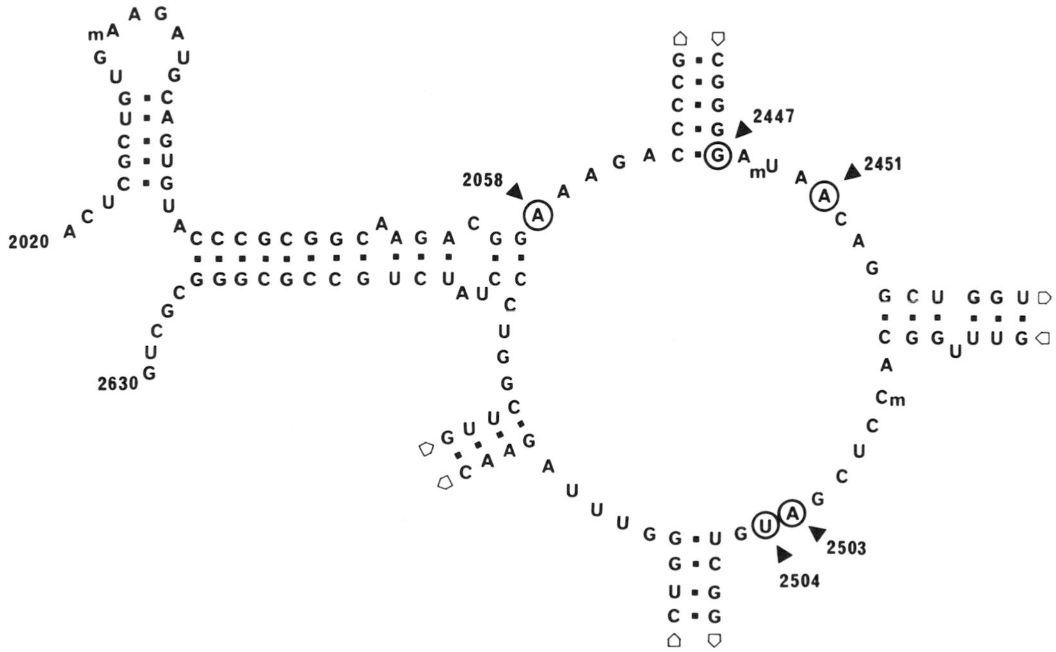

Possible secondary structure of part of *E. coli* 23S rRNA. Transposed on to this model are the site of action of the *S. erythraeus* methylase within *B. stearothermophilus* rRNA and the sites of alterations of rRNA in chloramphenicol-resistant mitochondria (residues 2447, 2451, 2503 and 2504).

interesting to know whether phosphoviomycin is excreted as is phosphostreptomycin under similar circumstances.

The possibility that enzymes involved in target-site modification might also have alternative functions is less easy to assess. The thiostrepton-resistance methylase seems unlikely to be involved in drug production and there is no reason to suspect that it and thiostrepton would recognize each other. Nor is it evident that *S. azureus* would benefit from constitutive expression of the methylase gene were it not a thiostrepton producer. Indeed, there is something of a chicken-and-egg paradox about how the genes for thiostrepton production and resistance came to congregate in the same cell. The puzzle applies also to other cases where enzymes involved in the modification of antibiotic target-sites are not also involved in drug production. To suggest that genes encoding such enzymes might have been acquired together with genes for antibiotic production as packages, all encoded together on plasmids, does nothing to resolve the problem but does raise a question concerning the possible involvement of plasmids in these processes.

This is not the place (nor this the author) for a detailed discussion of the genetics of antibiotic production, except to say that plasmids seem to be involved in the biosynthesis, or in regulation of the biosynthesis, of a number of antibiotics (for a definitive review, see reference 49). There is also unequivocal evidence for the involvement of a plasmid in the resistance of at least one producing organism. Thus, in *Streptomyces coelicolor*, plasmid SCP 1 carries genes required for methylenomycin production and for methylenomycin resistance.[50] (In the present context, it is a pity that neither the mode of action of methylenomycin nor the mechanism of resistance is known.) Otherwise, in a very few cases, there is strong circumstantial evidence linking the loss of plasmids to the loss of resistance, e.g. in *Streptomyces reticuli,* which produces leucomycin.[51]

It would also be interesting to know whether enzymes of similar activity (such as the phosphotransferases in *S. vinaceus* and *S. capreolus* or the methylases present in *S. azureus* and other thiostrepton producers) are homologous proteins, i.e., whether their genes are derived from common ancestors. This raises the broader question of the origin(s) of antibiotic resistance determinants in general. The proposition that producing organisms might represent the source of (at least some of) the resistance determinants commonly encountered in clinical isolates followed the observation that streptomycin was inactivated by phosphorylation both in *S. bikiniensis* and in bacteria harbouring R plasmids.[52] Subsequently, a number of aminoglycoside-modifying enzymes similar to those encoded on R plasmids were found in actinomycetes which produce aminoglycosides.[18,53] Although the occurrence of such enzymes is not restricted to producers of aminoglycosides, the hypothesis still has far-reaching implications. More importantly, there is now direct evidence in favour of it. Recent analysis of the nucleotide sequences of genes encoding APH (3′) from *S. fradiae, Staphylococcus aureus* and transposons Tn5 and Tn903 has revealed significant homologies (Thompson & Gray[54]; J Davies, personal communication).

In conclusion, it may be seen that studies of antibiotic resistance in producing strains have a potentially useful predictive aspect in addition to their more arcane attraction. Novel resistance mechanisms may be characterized prior to their emergence in clinical situations and, in some cases, possibly circumvented by strategic modification of native antibiotic structures.

ACKNOWLEDGEMENTS

Work in the author's laboratory is supported by the Medical Research Council and by the Science and Engineering Research Council.

REFERENCES

1 Demain AL. How do antibiotic-producing microorganisms avoid suicide? Ann NY Acad Sci 1974; 235: 601–612

2 Vining LC. Antibiotic tolerance in producer organisms. Adv Appl Microbiol 1979; 25: 147–168

3 Skinner RH, Cundliffe E. Resistance to the antibiotics viomycin and capreomycin in the *Streptomyces* species which produce them. J Gen Microbiol 1980; 120: 95—104

4 Thompson CJ, Skinner RH, Thompson J, Ward JM, Hopwood DA, Cundliffe E. Biochemical characterization of resistance determinants cloned from antibiotic-producing streptomycetes. J Bacteriol 1982; 151: 678–685

5 Cella R, Vining LC. Resistance to streptomycin in a producing strain of *Streptomyces griseus.* Canad J Microbiol 1975; 21: 463–472

6 Piwowarski JM, Shaw PD. Streptomycin resistance in a streptomycin-producing microorganism. Antimicrob Agents Chemother 1979; 16: 176–182

7 Hotta K, Yamamoto H, Okami Y, Umezawa H. Resistance mechanisms of kanamycin-, neomycin-, and streptomycin-producing streptomycetes to aminoglycoside antibiotics. J Antibiot 1981; 34: 1175–1182

8 Sugiyama M, Mochizuki H, Nimi O, Nomi R. Assessment of competitive action of streptomycin 6-kinase and streptomycin 6-phosphatase in the *in vitro* protein synthesis of a streptomycin-producing microorganism. FEBS Lett 1982; 139: 331–333

9 Nimi O, Sugiyama M, Kameoka H, Tomoeda H, Ono K, Nomi R. Fate of streptomycin in mycelium of the producer organism. Biotech Lett 1981; 3: 239–244

10 Miller AL, Walker JB. Enzymatic phosphorylation of streptomycin by extracts of streptomycin-producing strains of *Streptomyces.* J Bacteriol 1969; 99: 401–405

11 Nimi O, Ito G, Sueda S, Nomi R. Phosphorylation of streptomycin at C_6-OH of streptidine moiety by an intracellular enzyme of *Streptomyces griseus.* Agric Biol Chem 1971; 35: 848–855

12 Nomi R, Nimi O, Miyazaki T, Matsuo A, Kiyohara H. Biosynthesis of Streptomycin Part III. Liberation of inorganic phosphate from a natural precursor in transformation of the precursor to streptomycin. Agric Biol Chem 1967; 31: 973–978

13 Walker MS, Walker JB. Streptomycin biosynthesis. Separation and substrate specificities of phosphatases acting on guanidino-deoxy-*scyllo*-inositol phosphate and streptomycin-(*streptidino*) phosphate. J Biol Chem 1971; 246: 7034–7040

14 Miller AL, Walker JB. Accumulation of streptomycin-phosphate in cultures of streptomycin producers grown on a high-phosphate medium. J Bacteriol 1970; 104: 8–12

15 Nomi R, Nimi, R, Kado T. Biosynthesis of streptomycin IV. Accumulation of a streptomycin precursor in the culture broth and partial purification of the precursor. Agric Biol Chem 1968; 32: 1256–1260

16 Nimi O, Ito G, Ohata Y, Funayama S, Nomi R. Streptomycin-phosphorylating enzyme produced by *Streptomyces griseus.* Agric Biol Chem 1971; 35: 856–861

17 Ono H, Crameri R, Hintermann G, Hütter R. Hydroxystreptomycin production and resistance in *Streptomyces glaucescens.* J Gen Microbiol 1983; 129: 529–537

18 Davies J, Houk C, Yagisawa M, White TJ. Occurrence and function of aminoglycoside-modifying enzymes. In: Sebek OK, Laskin AI, eds. Genetics of Industrial Microorganisms. Washington DC: American Society for Microbiology, 1979; 166–169

19 Watanabe S, Tanaka K. Effect of rifampicin on *in vitro* RNA synthesis of *Streptomyces mediterranei.* Biochem Biophys Res Commun 1976; 72: 522–529

20 Hughes J, Mellows G, Soughton S. How does *Pseudomonas fluorescens,* the producing organism of the antibiotic pseudomonic acid A, avoid suicide? FEBS Lett 1980; 122: 322–324

21 Glöckner C, Wörner W, Wolf H. Kirromycin-resistant elongation factor Tu from pulvomycin-producing wild-type of *Streptoverticillium mobaraense.* Biochem Biophys Res Commun 1982; 107: 959–965

22 Hobden AN, Cundliffe E. Ribosomal resistance to the 12,13-epoxytrichothecene antibiotics in the producing organism *Myrothecium verrucaria*. Biochem J 1980; 190: 765–770

23 Johnson BC, Preston III JF. α-Amanitin-resistant RNA polymerase II from carpophores of *Amanita* species accumulating amatoxins. Biochim Biophys Acta 1980; 607: 102–114

24 Stirpe F. On the action of ribosome-inactivating proteins: are plant ribosomes species-specific? Biochem J 1982; 202: 279–280

25 Yamamoto H, Hotta K, Okami Y, Umezawa H. Ribosomal resistance of an istamycin producer, *Streptomyces tenjimariensis*, to aminoglycoside antibiotics. Biochem Biophys Res Commun 1981; 100: 1396–1401

26 Piendl W, Böck A. Ribosomal resistance in the gentamicin producer organism *Micromonospora purpurea*. Antimicrob Agents Chemother 1982; 22: 231–236

27 Yamamoto H, Hotta K, Okami Y, Umezawa H. Mechanism of resistance to aminoglycoside antibiotics in nebramycin-producing *Streptomyces tenebrarius*. J Antibiot 1982; 35: 1020–1025

28 Davies J. Enzymes modifying aminocyclitol antibiotics and their roles in resistance determination and biosynthesis. In: Rinehart KL Jr, Suami T, eds. Aminocyclitol antibiotics. Washington DC: American Chemical Society, 1980: 323–334

29 Cundliffe E. Mechanism of resistance to thiostrepton in the producing organism *Streptomyces azureus*. Nature 1978; 272: 792–795

30 Thompson J, Schmidt FJ, Cundliffe E. Site of action of a ribosomal RNA methylase conferring resistance to thiostrepton. J Biol Chem 1982; 257: 7915–7917

31 Cundliffe E, Thompson J. Ribose methylation and resistance to thiostrepton. Nature 1979; 278: 859–861

32 Thompson J, Cundliffe E. Purification and properties of an RNA methylase produced by *Streptomyces azureus* and involved in resistance to thiostrepton. J Gen Microbiol 1981; 124: 291–297

33 Gale EF, Cundliffe E, Reynolds PE, Richmond MH, Waring MJ. The molecular basis of antibiotic action, 2nd ed. London: Wiley, 1981

34 Thompson CJ, Kieser T, Ward JM, Hopwood DA. Physical analysis of antibiotic-resistance genes from *Streptomyces* and their use in vector construction. Gene 1983; 20: 51–62

35 Teraoka H, Tanaka K. Properties of ribosomes from *Streptomyces erythreus* and *Streptomyces griseus*. J Bacteriol 1974; 120: 316–321

36 Lai CJ, Weisblum B. Altered methylation of ribosomal RNA in an erythromycin-resistant strain of *Staphylococcus aureus*. Proc Natl Acad Sci USA 1971; 68: 856–860

37 Lai CJ, Weisblum, B, Fahnestock SR, Nomura M. Alteration of 23S ribosomal RNA and erythromycin-induced resistance to lincomycin and spiramycin in *Staphylococcus aureus*. J Mol Biol 1973; 74: 67–72

38 Graham MY, Weisblum B. 23S ribosomal ribonucleic acid of macrolide-producing streptomycetes contains methylated adenine. J Bacteriol 1979; 137: 1464–1467

39 Skinner RH, Cundliffe E. Dimethylation of adenine and the resistance of *Streptomyces erythraeus* to erythromycin. J Gen Microbiol 1982; 128: 2411–2416

40 Skinner RH, Cundliffe E, Schmidt FJ. Site of action of a ribosomal RNA methylase responsible for resistance to erythromycin and other antibiotics. J Biol Chem 1983; In press

41 Sor F, Fukuhara H. Identification of two erythromycin resistance mutations in the mitochondrial gene coding for the large ribosomal RNA in yeast. Nucleic Acids Res 1982; 10: 6571–6577

42 Dujon B. Sequence of the intron and flanking exons of the mitochondrial 21S RNA gene of yeast strains having different alleles at the W and rib-1 loci. Cell 1980; 20: 185–197

43 Kearsey SE, Craig IW. Altered ribosomal RNA genes in mitochondria from mammalian cells with chloramphenicol resistance. Nature 1981; 290: 607–608

44 Fujisawa Y, Weisblum B. A family of r-determinants in *Streptomyces* spp that specifies inducible resistance to macrolide, lincosamide, and streptogramin type B antibiotics. J Bacteriol 1981; 146: 621–631

45 Woodruff HB. The physiology of antibiotic production: the role of the producing organism. In Newton BA, Reynolds PE, eds. Biochemical studies of antimicrobial drugs. Cambridge: Cambridge University Press, 1966; 22–46

46 Demain AL, Piret JM. Why secondary metabolism? In Schlessinger D, ed. Microbiology—1981. Washington DC: American Society for Microbiology, 1981; 363–366

47 Satoh A, Ogawa H, Satomura Y. Regulation of N-acetylkanamycin amidohydrolase in the idiophase in kanamycin fermentation. Agric Biol Chem 1976; 40: 191–196

48 Pass L, Raczynska-Bojanowska K. On the inhibition mechanisms of viomycin synthesis by inorganic phosphate. Acta Biochim Pol 1968; 15: 355–367

49 Hopwood DA. Extrachromosomally determined antibiotic production. Ann Rev Microbiol 1978; 32: 373–392

50 Kirby R, Wright LF, Hopwood DA. Plasmid-determined antibiotic synthesis and resistance in *Streptomyces coelicolor*. Nature 1975; 254: 265–267

51 Schrempf H. Plasmid loss and changes within the chromosomal DNA of *Streptomyces reticuli*. J Bacteriol 1982; 151: 701–707

52 Walker MS, Walker JB. Enzymatic phosphorylation of dihydrostreptobiosamine moieties of dihydrostreptomycin-(*streptidino*) phosphate and dihydrostreptomycin by *Streptomyces* extracts. J Biol Chem 1970; 245: 6683–6689

53 Benveniste R, Davies J. Aminoglycoside antibiotic-inactivating enzymes in actinomycetes similar to those present in clinical isolates of antibiotic-resistant bacteria. Proc Natl Acad Sci USA 1973, 70: 2276–2280

54 Thompson CJ, Gray GS. The nucleotide sequence of a streptomycete aminoglycoside phosphotransferase gene and its relationship to phosphotransferases encoded by resistance plasmids. Proc Natl Acad Sci USA 1983; In press

British Medical Bulletin (1984) Vol. 40, No. 1, pp. 68–76

DRUG RESISTANCE IN GRAM-NEGATIVE AEROBIC BACILLI

B ROWE MA MB FRCPath

E J THRELFALL BSc PhD

Division of Enteric Pathogens
Central Public Health Laboratory
London

1   Resistance acquisition in animals
    a Multiple drug resistance in *Salmonella typhimurium* in Britain
    b Trimethoprim resistance
    c Gentamicin resistance
2   Resistance acquisition in humans
    a Salmonella typhi
    b Other salmonella serotypes
    c Shigellae
    d Escherichia coli
    e Vibrio cholera 01
    f Opportunist pathogens
3   Conclusions
    References

Some aerobic gram-negative bacteria, such as salmonellae other than *Salmonella typhi* and *S. paratyphi B*, have their main ecological reservoir in animals and are usually spread to humans through the food chain or, less frequently, by the ingestion of contaminated water. Others, such as *S. typhi*, *Vibrio cholerae* 01 and *Shigella*, are essentially human pathogens. Whilst these may be spread by contaminated food or water, person-to-person spread is also important, particularly in *Shigella* and *S. typhi*. A third group includes opportunist pathogens such as *Klebsiella*, *Proteus*, *Pseudomonas* and *Serratia* and these are particularly important in hospital infections.

In all instances, the acquisition of antimicrobial drug resistance results from antibiotic pressures to which the organism is exposed. Nevertheless, for an overall appreciation, the epidemiology of the organism must be understood. This review will consider resistance in strains of epidemiological importance and attempt to assess the factors involved in the acquisition of resistance.

1   Resistance Acquisition in Animals

In Britain, salmonella infections, excluding those with *S. typhi* and *S. paratyphi B*, are primarily zoonoses. The most important salmonella serotype in human food poisoning is *S. typhimurium* and infections with this serotype comprise 25–30% of all salmonella infections each year.[1–3] *S. typhimurium* is also the serotype in which drug resistance is most common, in strains from both animals and humans. Important food-animal reservoirs of *S. typhimurium* are poultry and cattle and changes in eating habits over the last 15 years have resulted in an increase in the number of salmonella infections. Probably the two most important factors are the increased consumption of poultry instead of red meat and the increased tendency to eat out or to purchase food from 'fast-food' establishments.

S. typhimurium is subdivided by phage typing[4,5] and long-term studies have demonstrated the association of certain phage types with poultry and other types with cattle. The poultry-associated phage types are mainly drug-sensitive, whereas the bovine-associated types are more likely to be resistant, frequently to several antibiotics. It is thought that this dichotomy may have resulted from differences in antibiotic usage in cattle and poultry.[6]

a   *Multiple Drug Resistance in* Salmonella typhimurium *in Britain*

Before 1963, less than 3% of *S. typhimurium* isolated in Britain from humans and food animals were drug-resistant.[7] Between 1963 and 1969, the incidence of multiply-resistant strains increased as a result of the dissemination in calves of a drug-resistant strain of phage type 29.[8] In 1965, over 70% of animal strains and 20% of human strains were multiply resistant. By 1970, type 29 had disappeared from bovine animals in Britain and, for the next six years, less than 8% of strains from cattle and 3% of strains from humans were multiply-resistant. Isolations of type 29 were at a low level before the enactment of the Swann recommendations[9] and factors other than restrictions on the use of antibiotics as feed additives probably contributed to the disappearance of this multiresistant strain.

Since 1974, resistant strains of new phage types have emerged and spread in calves and caused human infections, some of which were fatal. Particularly since 1976, the incidence of multiresistant *S. typhimurium* has increased in cattle and humans but, because of the importance of drug-sensitive, poultry-associated phage types in food-poisoning outbreaks, this increase has not been as pronounced in humans as in cattle.[6] Nevertheless, in humans the incidence of multiresistant *S. typhimurium* has increased from about 1% in 1971 and 1972, to 10% in 1978 and 9% in 1979 and, since 1980, multiresistant strains have comprised almost 8% of isolations. In cattle, about 35–40% of strains isolated since 1977 have been multiresistant. Strains have been resistant to ampicillin (A), chloramphenicol (C), neomycin–kanamycin (K), streptomycin (S), sulphonamides (Su), tetracyclines (T) and trimethoprim (Tm), either individually or in combinations. Some strains have been resistant to all these antibiotics (R-type ACKSSuTTm) and resistances have been specified by plasmids. Strains with plasmid-encoded resistance to gentamicin have recently been isolated from pigs[10] and cattle.

Of particular importance have been a series of related strains belonging to phage types 204, 193, 204a and 204c (Table I). Since 1977, multiresistant strains in this series have caused widespread outbreaks in calf herds. Mortality has been high and economic losses considerable. In these strains, the sequential acquisition of resistance plasmids, transposons and carried phages has resulted in changes in both the phage type and resistance spectrum and this has caused complications in strain discrimination.[11–14]

TABLE I. *Salmonella typhimurium* phage type 204 and related types in Britain, 1974–1982

Phage type	R-type	Plasmid-encoded drug resistances	Date of appearance
204	SuT	Su, T	1974 January
	CSSuT	Su, T, CSSuT	1977 January
193	ACKSSuT	Su, T, CSSuT, AKS	1977 December
204a	SuT	Su, T	1978 October
	CKSSuT	Su, T, CKSSuT	1980 March
204c	CSSuTTm	Su, T, CSSuTTm	1979 March
	ACKSSuTTm	Su, T, CSSuTTm, AK	1979 October

Resistance symbols: A: ampicillin; C: chloramphenicol; K: neomycin–kanamycin; S: streptomycin; Su: sulphonamides; T: tetracyclines; Tm: trimethoprim

FIG. 1. Occurrence of *Salmonella typhimurium* phage types 204, 193, 204a and 204c in cattle, 1977–1982

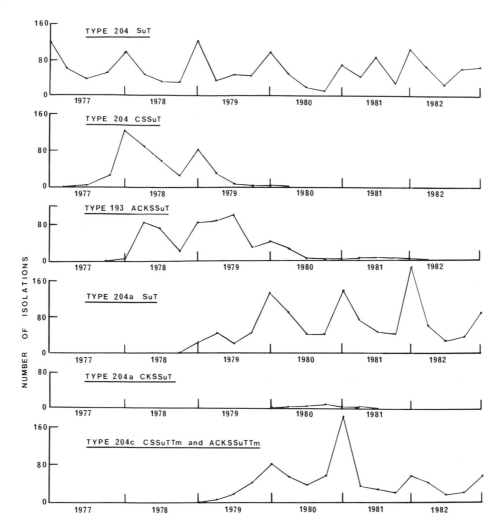

The occurrence in cattle of these related types from 1977 to 1982 is shown in Fig. 1. It is noticeable how the fall in prevalence of strains of R-type CSSuT coincided with the appearance and spread of strains of R-type ACKSSuT. The decline in isolations of this type coincided with the appearance of strains resistant to trimethoprim (R-types CSSuTTm and ACSSuTTm). It is possible that the rise and subsequent fall in the prevalence of these multiresistant strains may be related to changes in selective pressures brought about by the successive use of different antimicrobials for the therapy and prophylaxis of salmonellosis in calves. Once a multiresistant strain has become established in a calf herd, the mixing of batches of calves during marketing has ensured its rapid dissemination over a wide area.

In humans, 611 infections with multiresistant strains of types 204, 193, 204a and 204c have been recognized since the appearance of multiple resistance in type 204, in 1976 (Table II). The majority of patients suffered from mild to moderate enteritis but several persons developed severe diarrhoea which persisted for several weeks. Three died of enteritis and there was extra-intestinal spread in at least a further twelve persons. One child died of

TABLE II. Human infections with multiresistant *Salmonella typhimurium* of phage types 204, 193, 204a and 204c, 1977–1982

| Year | Type 204 CSSuT | Type 193 ACKSSuT | Type 204c | | Type 204a CKSSuT | Totals | Per cent* |
			CSSuTTm and ACKSSuTTm	SSuTTm			
1977	37	4	0	0	0	41	1.7
1978	51	89	0	0	0	140	4.5
1979	15	94	20	0	0	129	3.5
1980	0	29	102	16	48	195	4.8
1981	0	0	63	2	5	70	1.4
1982	0	6	30	0	0	36	0.6
Totals	103	222	215	18	53	611	2.5

Source: Strains referred to the Division of Enteric Pathogens, Central Public Health Laboratory, London
* Percentage of strains received

septicaemia resulting from infection with a strain of type 193 of R-type ACKSSuT and a male patient died of salmonella meningitis following infection with a multiresistant strain of type 204c.

b *Trimethoprim Resistance*

Since 1979, there has been a substantial increase in isolations of trimethoprim-resistant salmonellae in Britain (Fig. 2). This increase has been particularly evident in *S. typhimurium* and has resulted mainly from the appearance and spread of trimethoprim-resistant strains of three phage types: types 18, 170 and 204c.[15] Between 1979 and 1982, 832 human infections caused by trimethoprim-resistant strains of these three phage types were recognized. These accounted for 4.5% of *S. typhimurium* isolated from humans since 1979 (Table III).

Characterization of the plasmids conferring resistance to trimethoprim in phage types 18, 170 and 204c has demonstrated that this resistance originated in strains from cattle.[16] Because of

FIG. 2. Incidence of trimethoprim resistance in salmonellae isolated in Britain, 1974–1981

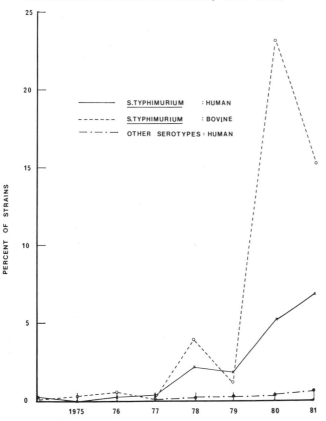

TABLE III. Infections with trimethoprim-resistant *Salmonella typhimurium* of phage types 18, 170 and 204c, 1979–1982

Year	No. of Infections			Totals	Per cent*
	Type 18	Type 170	Type 204c		
1979	47	0	20	67	1.8
1980	67	0	118	185	4.5
1981	67	150	65	282	5.8
1982	86	182	30	298	4.9
Totals	267	332	233	832	4.5

Source: as Table II
* Percentage of strains received

the proliferation of these resistant strains, the value of trimethoprim in Britain for the treatment of systemic salmonella infections is much reduced.

c *Gentamicin Resistance*

Until 1981, most gentamicin-resistant salmonellae isolated from humans in Britain were from patients who had either acquired their infections abroad or had been in contact with persons from countries in South-East Asia where gentamicin-resistant strains are endemic.[17] In salmonellae from food animals in Britain, gentamicin resistance was first reported in 1982, after a strain of *S. typhimurium* isolated from a four-week-old pig had been observed to carry plasmid-encoded resistance to gentamicin and also to ampicillin, chloramphenicol, neomycin–kanamycin, streptomycin, sulphonamides and tetracyclines.[10] Subsequently, gentamicin-resistant *S. typhimurium* have been isolated from calves in Britain but as yet the strains have not become established in calf herds.

In 1981 and 1982, gentamicin resistance was observed in strains of *S. typhimurium* isolated from chickens from a large integrated poultry company in Scotland. The strains were of two closely related phage types, types 80 and 160 and were resistant to gentamicin and streptomycin, the minimum inhibitory concentration (MIC) of gentamicin being 16μg/ml. Subsequently strains of phage type 160 resistant to gentamicin and streptomycin (GS) have been isolated from cases of enteritis in humans. These strains were indistinguishable from those from chickens. The occurrence of gentamicin resistance in chicken-associated *S. typhimurium* is particularly disturbing because of the importance of poultry in food poisoning in Britain.

d *Multiple Drug Resistance in Salmonellae in Other European Countries*

In Belgium, France and the Netherlands, multiple antibiotic resistance has been observed in *S. typhimurium* and in other salmonella serotypes with animal reservoirs. For example, since 1975, an increasing number of multiply-resistant *S. dublin* have been isolated from calves in the Netherlands and have caused infections in humans.[18] Similar increases in the isolation of multiresistant *S. dublin* have been observed in France[19] and Belgium.[20] In contrast, since 1975, there has been an overall decrease in isolations of multiply-resistant *S. typhimurium* and *S. panama* in the Netherlands. This decrease has been attributed to legislation prohibiting the use of tetracyclines for growth promotion in food animals.[18] However, since 1978, multiply-resistant strains of *S. typhimurium* phage types 204 and 193 have been spread to Europe by the export of infected calves from Britain.[21] These strains have caused outbreaks in calf herds both in Belgium[22] and the Netherlands.[18]

2   Resistance Acquisition in Humans

S. typhi and *S. paratyphi*, *Shigella*, *Vibrio cholerae* 01 and certain serotypes of *Escherichia coli* are human pathogens. These organisms may cause epidemics and are spread from person to person or by contaminated food or water. In addition, in some developing countries, salmonella serotypes such as *S. typhimurium*, *S. wien*, *S. saintpaul* and *S. oranienburg* have undergone changes in their epidemiology and in their clinical disease. In Britain, infections caused by these serotypes are usually zoonotic and the clinical presentation is that of mild to moderate enteritis. In developing countries, strains of these serotypes have caused outbreaks, frequently over wide areas, without any evidence of animal reservoirs. The main method of transmission seems to be person-to-person spread, the food chain not being involved and the clinical presentation frequently being a systemic infection rather than enteritis.

Over the last decade, multiple antibiotic resistance, frequently plasmid-encoded, has been acquired by all the 'human-specific' pathogens listed above. In many instances, the resistant strains have caused epidemics and the range of antibiotics available for treatment has been diminished.

a *Salmonella Typhi*

Before 1970, drug resistance in *S. typhi* was uncommon.[23-25] The few resistant strains isolated had not caused outbreaks and were epidemiologically unimportant. Nevertheless, the appearance of chloramphenicol resistance in *S. typhi* was anticipated with trepidation. Fears were justified in 1972, when there was a major outbreak in Mexico of chloramphenicol-resistant *S. typhi* which continued until 1973.[25,26] Contaminated water supplies were a suggested method of spread.[27] At about the same time, there was a substantial outbreak in Kerala, India.[28] In both outbreaks mortality was high. Subsequently, chloramphenicol-resistant strains have become endemic in Vietnam and Thailand and sporadic isolations have been reported from Chile and several countries in South-East Asia (Table IV). Chloramphenicol-resistant strains have also been isolated from persons returning to England, Switzerland and USA after travelling in countries where outbreaks have occurred.[29,30]

The strain which caused the outbreak in Mexico in 1972–73 was of a degraded Vi-phage type and carried a plasmid of compatibility group H_1 which coded for the complete resistance spectrum of the host strain, CSSuT. Isolations of chloramphenicol-resistant *S. typhi* from India, other countries in South-East Asia and Chile have been of a variety of Vi-phage types but, in all instances, resistance to chloramphenicol has been mediated by a group H_1 plasmid. Plasmids of this group transfer at high frequency when crosses are incubated at 28°C, but at low frequency at 37°C[31] and appear to have a particular affinity for *S. typhi*.

Chloramphenicol-resistant strains of *S. typhi* are rarely isolated in Britain and, when encountered, are almost invariably confined to persons returning from South-East Asia or the Indian subcontinent. However, the in-vivo acquisition of resistance by *S. typhi* can occur and has been documented on at least three occasions. During the course of the disease, an Australian patient infected in 1978 with a drug-sensitive strain of Vi-phage type E1 acquired a plasmid which coded for ACSSuT. Details of antibiotic treatment were not available.[32] Resistance plasmid acquisition in response to antibiotic therapy was demonstrated in a British patient who was infected with a drug-sensitive strain of Vi-phage

type A. The patient was treated first with chloramphenicol and then with co-trimoxazole and the strain acquired plasmids which conferred resistance to these drugs and changed the phage type to that of a degraded Vi-type.[33] Similarly, a South African patient infected with a drug-sensitive strain of Vi-type A was treated with chloramphenicol and the strain acquired a plasmid which conferred resistance to ampicillin, chloramphenicol and tetracyclines.[34,35] These examples demonstrate that the in-vivo acquisition of resistance plasmids from non-pathogenic intestinal flora can occur. Such acquisition of resistance could affect the efficacy of the drugs used for treatment.

b *Other Salmonella Serotypes*

Since 1970, multiply-resistant salmonellae have caused extensive outbreaks in many countries, particularly in the developing world. The common pattern has been for several hospitals, often situated many miles apart, to be involved. Many outbreaks have occurred in neonatal and paediatric wards but, in some hospitals, older children and adults have been affected. In some countries, there have been community outbreaks in villages and small towns. These may have resulted from cross-infection after the return of a patient from hospital. The clinical disease has been severe, with enteritis frequently accompanied by septicaemia. Mortality has been high—up to 30% in some outbreaks in South America and the Middle East. In all instances, the strains have been resistant to at least six antibiotics and resistances have been plasmid-encoded.

Serotypes involved include *S. typhimurium* in many countries in South America,[36] the Middle East,[37] Africa[38,39] and the Indian subcontinent,[40] *S. wien* in North Africa and Southern Europe,[41] *S. ordonez* in Senegal,[42] *S. oranienburg* in Brazil[43] and Indonesia, *S. saintpaul* in Venezuela, *S. johannesburg* in Hong Kong[44] and *S. newport* in India.[45]

An example of the type of epidemic caused by multiresistant salmonellae is that which has occurred in India since late 1977. Outbreaks caused by multiresistant *S. typhimurium* have occurred in cites as widely separated as Trivandrum in the south and Ludhiana in the far north. Hospitals in Delhi, Bombay, Poona and Bangalore have also been affected. The rate of infection in neonates was particularly high although older children and some adults were also affected. The most common presentation was severe enteritis although there were some cases of septicaemia, and mortality was high in at least three outbreaks.[40] The strains were of phage type 66/122 or were untypable; it was demonstrated that the untypable strains had been derived from type 66/122 by the acquisition of temperate bacteriophages.[17] All strains carried a plasmid of the F_1me compatibility group which coded for ACGKSSuTTm. Other plasmids identified included a non-conjugative plasmid which coded for streptomycin–sulphonamide (SSu), a conjugative group I_2 plasmid which did not specify drug resistance and an unclassified R factor which coded for KSSu. These plasmids were present in some but not all of the strains. Type 66/122 strains or untypable strains with a similar plasmid content to those from India have subsequently been identified in an outbreak in Saudi Arabia and have caused sporadic infections in Britain among persons who had either been infected in India or had been in contact with Indian families.

F_1me plasmids similar to those in the Indian *S. typhimurium* strains, and which specify resistance to up to eight drugs, have previously been identified in the strain of *S. wien* which spread from North Africa to Southern Europe in the early 1970s,[46] in *S. typhimurium* types 208 and untypable from the Middle East,[47] in *S. johannesburg* from Hong Kong[48] and in other salmonellae which have caused outbreaks in various parts of the world (Table V).

TABLE IV. Chloramphenicol-resistant *Salmonella typhi*

Year	Country	Resistance	Plasmid type
1972–73	Mexico*	CSSuT	H_1
1972	India*	CSSuT	H_1
1972–74	Vietnam†	CSSuT	H_1
1972–75	Korea‡	CSSuT	H_1
1973–74	Thailand†	CSSuT	H_1
1973–74	Formosa†	CSSuT	H_1
1974–82	India†	CSSuT	H_1
1976	Chile‡	CSSuT	H_1
1981	Bangladesh‡	CSSuT	H_1

* Outbreak
† Endemic
‡ Sporadic

TABLE V. F$_I$*me* plasmids—distribution in salmonellae

Country/Area	Serotype	Year	Resistances specified
Middle East*†	*S. typhimurium* 208	1974–82	ACSSuT ACKSSuT ACGKSSuTTm
N. Africa* S. Europe* India*	*S. wien*	1970–80	ACSSuT ACSSuTTm
India*†	*S. typhimurium* 66/122	1978–82	ACGKSSuTTm
S. Africa* Hong Kong*	*S. johannesburg*	1974–78	ACKSSuT
Chile‡	*S. newington*	1976	ACSSuT
Indonesia‡	*S. oranienburg*	1974–80	ACKSSuT
Kenya*	*S. typhimurium* NC	1974–76	ACSSuT
Liberia*	*S. typhimurium* Untypable	1976–80	ACKSSuT

* Outbreak
† Endemic
‡ Sporadic
G: gentamicin

Most outbreaks caused by these strains have been characterized by their unusual severity. It may be relevant that group F$_I$ plasmids and other plasmids related to those of the F$_I$*me* group have been shown to be involved in the adherence and invasive properties of *S. typhimurium* in tissue culture tests,[49] in the iron uptake system of invasive strains of *E. coli*[50] and to be necessary for the virulence of *S. sonnei*[51] and *S. flexneri*.[52] Thus it is possible that, in addition to coding for resistance to a range of antibiotics and to possessing the ability to become established in different bacterial vectors, F$_I$*me* plasmids also enhance the virulence of carrier strains. This hypothesis awaits experimental verification.

c *Shigellae*

i *In Britain*

In a survey of the resistance to 12 antibiotics of strains of *S. dysenteriae*, *S. flexneri* and *S. boydii* isolated in England and Wales from 1974–1978, it was reported that 80% of strains were resistant to one or more drugs, with resistance to sulphonamides occurring most frequently.[53] During the period of the survey, resistance to streptomycin, tetracyclines, ampicillin and chloramphenicol increased, as did the incidence of multiple resistance. As can be seen from Fig. 3, this increase has been maintained. In many strains, resistances were plasmid-encoded.[54]

S. dysenteriae, *S. flexneri* and *S. boydii* are not indigenous to England and Wales and most infections caused by these serotypes are contracted abroad, particularly in the Indian subcontinent.[55] Thus, resistance in these serotypes does not reflect antibiotic usage in Britain. In *S. sonnei*, which is indigenous to the British Isles, a different picture has emerged. In this serotype, multiple resistance decreased from 38% in 1972 to 8% in 1977.[53]

ii *Outside Britain*

Since 1969, multiresistant strains of *S. dysenteriae* 1 (Shiga's bacillus) have caused extensive outbreaks in several countries. The first was that which occurred in Central America from 1969 to 1972.[56] In the first 10 months of 1969, this outbreak caused 8300 deaths among 112000 cases in Guatemala alone. Although not of the same scale, there have subsequently been outbreaks in Mexico (1972),[57] Bangladesh (1972),[58] India (1976)[59] and Sri Lanka (1976, 1978).[60,61] In all these outbreaks, symptoms were severe and mortality was high. The Central American strain was of R-type CSSuT and these resistances were transferred as a single linkage group of a plasmid by compatibility group B.[62] In the 1972 outbreaks in Mexico City, the strain carried a group B plasmid indistinguishable from that in the Central American strain and had also acquired an additional plasmid which coded for ampicillin resistance.[57] The strains from India, Bangladesh and Sri Lanka carried group B plasmids which coded for resistance to chloramphenicol and tetracyclines, and independent non-conjugative SSu plasmids.[63]

Since 1979, a multiresistant strain of *S. dysenteriae* 1 has caused an extensive outbreak of Shiga dysentery in north-east Zaire and has spread to the neighbouring states of Rwanda and Burundi. Nearly 13000 cases were registered in the Katana region of Eastern Zaire between April 1981 and July 1982. An attack rate of 6.4% and a case fatality of 2.4% was reported and adults were affected more frequently than children. There were 1782 deaths in the Watsa region between May and December 1980.[64] The strain was of R-type ACSSuT and carried two resistance plasmids, a plasmid of compatibility group X which coded for ACT and an independent non-conjugative SSu plasmid.[63]

Because the strain was resistant to tetracyclines, treatment with this antibiotic was ineffective and was discontinued early in 1981 in favour of co-trimoxazole, with encouraging results. However, by August 1981, resistance to trimethoprim had appeared, presumably in response to selective pressures imposed by the use of co-trimoxazole. Genetic studies showed that, in addition to the group X and SSu plasmids, the epidemic strain had acquired an additional plasmid of compatibility group I$_1$ which coded for the complete resistance spectrum, ACSSuTTm.[65]

With the appearance of trimethoprim resistance, no suitable drug was available to treat persons infected with strains of R-type ACSSuTTm and there was an immediate increase in the case fatality rate from 2.4% to 4.6%. By November 1981, nalidixic acid had become available and the use of this antibiotic resulted in a drop in the case fatality rate to 2.0%. By June 1982, occasional strains resistant to nalidixic acid had emerged but the impact of this on case fatality has not yet been evaluated.

The presence of group X plasmids and the absence of group B plasmids in isolations from this outbreak demonstrated that a Central American or Asian origin was unlikely. It is possible that the strain was spread to Zaire from Somalia, since *S. dysenteriae* 1

FIG. 3. Shigella drug resistance, 1974–1982

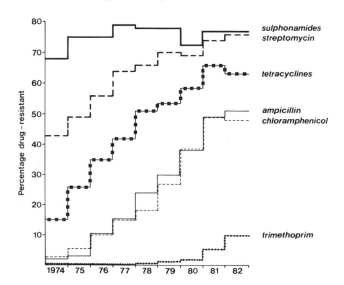

with an indistinguishable plasmid content to that of the Central African strain were isolated in 1976 from an outbreak in Somalia.[63]

d *Escherichia coli*

E. coli strains that cause diarrhoea in humans have been grouped according to their pathogenic mechanisms. In general, infantile enteropathogenic *E. coli* (EPEC) do not produce detectable enterotoxins in laboratory tests and have been identified by epidemiological studies using serotyping for strain discrimination. A range of serogroups have been identified and these have caused numerous outbreaks throughout the world. Over the last 10 years, such outbreaks have occurred only infrequently in North-West Europe and North America, although sporadic cases and small outbreaks have been reported. However, EPEC remain an important cause of infant mortality in tropical countries. Enterotoxigenic *E. coli* (ETEC) produce heat-labile and heat-stable toxins detectable by laboratory tests. Like EPEC, these strains are particularly important as a cause of enteritis and infant mortality in tropical and semi-tropical countries. A third group of pathogenic *E. coli* cause disease by invading the intestinal mucosa. These enteroinvasive *E. coli* (EIEC) resemble shigellae in their pathogenesis. This group will not be discussed further because of the paucity of information about drug resistance.

Although outbreaks caused by EPEC strains have been rarely reported in Britain over the last 10 years, there have been sporadic cases and the occasional institutional outbreak. A survey of the resistance to 10 antibiotics of EPEC strains isolated in Britain during 1980 and 1981 has demonstrated that over 50% of strains were resistant with resistance to sulphonamides, streptomycin, tetracyclines and ampicillin occurring most frequently.[66] Resistances were plasmid-mediated in 63% of resistant strains and a variety of plasmid compatibility groups were identified. Antimicrobial therapy is rarely necessary to treat infants with *E. coli* diarrhoea, but concern was expressed that, when antibiotics are indicated for the treatment of prolonged or severe illness, the choice has become limited.

In a study of drug resistance amongst toxin-producing strains isolated in the Far East, 72% of strains were reported to be drug-resistant and 44% were multiply-resistant.[67] Of 31 strains tested, 80% possessed transferable resistance and, in 35% of these strains, the ability to produce enterotoxins was also transferable. In a similar survey of ETEC strains from 14 countries, 24% of strains were found to be resistant and, in 3 strains, the ability to produce toxin was associated with the transfer or mobilization of resistance.[68] In one strain, the genes coding for ampicillin resistance had become transposed on to a conjugative plasmid which coded for the production of both heat-stable (ST) and heat-labile toxin (LT).[69] Linkage between ampicillin resistance and ST on a conjugative plasmid has also been reported[70] and the co-transfer of antibiotic resistance and enterotoxigenicity was observed in 20% of ETEC strains studied by Wachsmuth.[71] Thus, the selective pressures imposed by the injudicious use of antibiotics for the treatment or prophylaxis of ETEC diarrhoea can result in the appearance of strains able to co-transfer both antibiotic resistance and enterotoxigenicity. The use of antibiotics in the treatment of ETEC diarrhoea is questionable since this disease is usually self-limiting and in many cases rehydration therapy may be a more appropriate form of treatment.

e *Vibrio cholerae 01*

Although sporadic isolations of drug-resistant *V. cholerae* 01 biotype El Tor had been reported earlier, the first protracted outbreak was that which began in Tanzania in 1977.[72] The strain was of R-type ACKSSuT and the appearance of resistance was ascribed to the extensive use in Tanzania of tetracyclines for cholera prophylaxis. Subsequently, resistant strains of *V. cholerae* biotype El Tor have caused outbreaks in Bangladesh in 1979–80[73] and in 1981,[74] in Zaire in 1982–83 and in Tanzania in 1983. In the outbreak in Bangladesh in 1979–80, the predominant R-type was that of AKSTSuTm but other R-types were also identified. In the 1981 outbreak, resistant strains had acquired additional resistance to gentamicin. In Zaire, strains of R-types CSSu and ACGSuTm were identified. In Tanzania, strains were of R-type ACSSuTTm but the level of tetracycline resistance was not clinically significant. In all resistant strains from outbreaks in Asia and Africa, the complete resistance spectrum was invariably encoded by conjugative plasmids of compatibility group C. Plasmids of this compatibility group seem to have an affinity for *V. cholerae* similar to that shown by group H_1 plasmids for *S. typhi* (see above).

When antibiotic therapy is indicated for the treatment of cholera, tetracyclines are the drug of choice. Clinical trials have demonstrated that when patients are treated with tetracyclines there is a significant reduction both in stool volume and in the duration of purging.[75] The occurrence of strains resistant to tetracyclines and to many other antibiotics is concerning, particularly in countries with low standards of hygiene where there is considerable opportunity for epidemic spread. Reappraisal of the use of antibiotics for cholera prophylaxis may be necessary in countries where drug-resistant strains have caused outbreaks.

f *Opportunist Pathogens*

Since the 1950s, gram-negative bacteria have become increasingly important as opportunist pathogens in septic infections in hospitals and outbreaks have been reported in many countries. These opportunist pathogens are frequently resistant to antibiotics and the use of antibiotics in the hospital environment has contributed to their infective success. Of particular importance in Britain have been strains of *Klebsiella*[76–80] and *Pseudomonas aeruginosa*,[81,82] but outbreaks with multiply-resistant strains of *Serratia*,[83] *Enterobacter*,[84] *Proteus mirabilis*,[85] *E. coli*[86] and *Acinetobacter calcoaceticus*[87] have been reported. These strains have caused bronchopulmonary, urinary tract, septicaemic and meningeal infections and have been especially troublesome in urological, paediatric, geriatric and surgical wards, in intensive treatment units and burns units. *E. coli* of serotypes different from those found in enteritis outbreaks are also one of the most common causes of meningitis in neonates.[88] In a survey of *E. coli* isolated between 1975 and 1981 from the cerebrospinal fluid of patients in UK, resistance was reported in 49% of strains, with resistance to ampicillin, sulphonamides, streptomycin and tetracyclines occurring most frequently.[89] This can result in problems in clinical management, since prompt antibiotic treatment is essential in the treatment of meningeal infections and is frequently initiated before the isolation of the causative organism and identification of the spectrum of resistance.

Under the pressure of antibiotics, strains such as those described above have become resistant to drugs of therapeutic importance, probably by the acquisition of plasmids and transposons from the non-pathogenic bacterial flora.[90,91] The spread of plasmids to different serotypes and genera can then occur.[90,92,93] In one hospital in USA, a common resistance plasmid was identified in six species of gram-negative pathogens.[94] In another hospital, a plasmid which coded for the adenylation of gentamicin, tobramycin and kanamycin spread from *Klebsiella pneumoniae* to other *Klebsiella* biotypes, to *Serratia*, *E. coli*, *Citrobacter* and *Proteus morganii*.[95] Thus, in a hospital, epidemics caused by multiresistant opportunist pathogens can result from the transmission of strains from person to person or ward to ward, or from the spread of an 'epidemic' plasmid from strain to strain. This can result in the appearance of multiple resistance in several species, many of which have the capability of causing disease.

The use of antibiotics, particularly for prophylactic purposes, provides gram-negative opportunist pathogens with a selective advantage. Without this support, these pathogens have difficulty in competing with the normal bacterial flora and may disappear from the patient or from the hospital environment. An example of this was described in 1970, when an outbreak of *K. aerogenes* in a neurosurgical unit in Scotland was controlled by the withdrawal of antibiotics from the unit.[76] Similarly, gram-negative bacteria carrying an R factor which transferred resistance to carbenicillin, tetracyclines, kanamycin, ampicillin and cephaloridine to *Pseudomonas aeroginosa* in a burns unit, were eliminated by imposing a policy which restricted the use of these five antibiotics.[81] However, restrictive antibiotic policies can have limitations in the overall hospital environment[96] and the adoption of antibiotic policies for individual units rather than the entire hospital has been recommended.[84] When these are coupled with stringent infection control measures and, whenever possible, the isolation of infected patients, then limitation of the spread of resistant strains and of plasmids which specify resistance may be possible within the hospital environment.

3 CONCLUSIONS

Antimicrobial drug resistance is an unwelcome but inevitable consequence of the use of antibiotics in human and veterinary medicine. In Britain, the initial appearance of resistant strains of salmonellae is mostly a result of the use of antibiotics for therapy and prophylaxis in calf husbandry. The subsequent dissemination of resistant strains has mainly resulted from cross-infection after the distribution of infected calves; the use of antibiotics in attempts to combat stress-induced diarrhoea has provided an environment conducive to this process. This spread of resistant strains would be limited if use were made of the powers to reduce movement of infected animals as allowed by existing legislation. Consideration might even be given to introduce legislation to limit the number of times an animal could be moved between premises in the first three months of life. However, it must be emphasized that it is the use of antibiotics which has not only resulted in the appearance of resistant strains but also enhanced their persistence.

Because of the widespread dissemination of multiresistant strains in developing countries, many antibiotics have become virtually ineffective for the treatment of intestinal infections. In this respect the appearance of multiresistant strains of *S. typhi*, particularly in South-East Asia, *S. dysenteriae* 1 in Central Africa and *S. typhimurium* in South America, India and the Middle East, present special problems. In many developing countries, antibiotics are available without prescription and are widely used without professional supervision. Governments of developing countries should be encouraged to control the availability of antibiotics and, particularly, their prophylactic use.

Thus, antibiotic resistance in gram-negative aerobic bacteria of importance to public health can only be controlled if co-ordinated and concerted efforts are made on both a national and international scale to limit the unnecessary use of antibiotics in both human and veterinary medicine.

REFERENCES

1 Vernon E. Food poisoning and salmonella infections in England and Wales, 1973–1975. Public Health 1977; 91: 225–235

2 Hepner E. Food poisoning and salmonella infections in England and Wales, 1976–1978. Public Health 1980; 94: 337–349

3 Anonymous. Food poisoning and salmonellosis surveillance in England and Wales: 1981. Br Med J 1982; 185: 1127–1128

4 Callow BR. A new phage-typing scheme for *Salmonella typhimurium*. J Hyg 1959; 57: 346–359

5 Anderson ES. The phage typing of salmonellae other than *S. typhi*. In: Van Oye E, ed. The world problem of salmonellosis. The Hague: Dr W Junk, 1964; 89–110

6 Rowe B, Threlfall EJ. Multiply-resistant clones of *Salmonella typhimurium* in Britain: epidemiological and laboratory aspects. In: Levy SB, Clowes RC, Koenig EL, eds. Molecular biology, pathogenicity, and ecology of bacterial plasmids. New York: Plenum Press, 1981, 567–573

7 Anderson ES. The ecology of transferable drug resistance in the enterobacteria. Ann Rev Microbiol 1968; 22: 131–80

8 Anderson ES. Drug resistance in *Salmonella typhimurium* and its implications. Br Med J 1968; 3: 333–339

9 Report of the joint committee on the use of antibiotics in animal husbandry and veterinary medicine. London: HMSO, 1969

10 Sojka WJ, Wray C, Pritchard GC, Hedges RW. Gentamicin-resistant salmonella. Vet Rec 1982; 111: 512

11 Threlfall EJ, Ward LR, Rowe B. Epidemic spread of a chloramphenicol-resistant strain of *Salmonella typhimurium* phage type 204 in bovine animals in Britain. Vet Rec 1978; 103: 438–440

12 Threlfall EJ, Ward LR, Rowe B. Spread of multiresistant strains of *Salmonella typhimurium* phage types 204 and 193 in Britain. Br Med J 1978; ii: 997

13 Threlfall EJ, Ward LR, Ashley AS, Rowe B. Plasmid-encoded trimethoprim resistance in multiresistant epidemic *Salmonella typhimurium* phage types 204 and 193 in Britain. Br Med J 1980; 280: 1210–1211

14 Threlfall EJ. Multiresistant epidemic strains of *Salmonella typhimurium* in Britain. In: Pohl P, Leunen J, eds. Resistance and pathogenic plasmids. CEC seminar. Brussels: National Institute for Veterinary Research, 1982, 103–14

15 Ward LR, Rowe B, Threlfall EJ. Incidence of trimethoprim resistance in salmonellae isolated in Britain: a twelve year study. Lancet 1982; ii: 705–706

16 Threlfall EJ, Frost JA, King HC, Rowe B. Plasmid-encoded trimethoprim resistance in salmonellas isolated in Britain between 1970 and 1981. J Hyg 1983; 90: 55–60

17 Frost JA, Rowe B, Ward LR, Threlfall EJ. Characterization of resistance plasmids and carried phages in an epidemic clone of multiresistant *Salmonella typhimurium* in India. J Hyg 1982; 88: 193–204

18 Leeuwen WJ, van Embden J., Guinée P et al. Decrease of drug resistance in *Salmonella* in The Netherlands. Antimicrob Agents Chemother 1979; 16: 237–239

19 Gledel J, Pantaleon J, Corbion B. Etude de l'antiborésistance de 3600 souches de *salmonella* d'origine animale (1974–1975). Rec Med Vet 1977; 153: 109–118

20 Pohl P, Thomas J, Laub R, Hermans F. Evolution des salmonelloses bovines en Belgique. Aspects clinique, bactériologique et épidémiologique. Ann Med Vet 1974; 118: 325–336

21 Rowe B, Threlfall EJ, Ward LR, Ashley AS. International spread of multiresistant strains of *Salmonella typhimurium* phage types 204 and 193 from Britain to Europe. Vet Rec 1979; 105: 468–469

22 Pohl P, Thomas J. Salmonella résistantes au trimethoprime. II. Transfert des résistances. Ann Med Vet 1979; 123: 361–336

23 Manten A, Guinée PAM, Kampelmacher EH. Incidence of resistance to tetracycline and chloramphenicol among *Salmonella* bacteria found in the Netherlands in 1963 and in 1964. Zentral Bakteriol Mikrobiol Hyg [A] 1969; 200: 13-20

24 Voogd CE, van Leeuwen WJ, Guinée PAM, Manten A, Valkenburg JJ. Incidence of resistance to ampicillin, chloramphenicol, kanamycin and tetracycline among *Salmonella* species isolated in the Netherlands in 1972, 1973 and 1974. Antonie van Leeuwenhoek 1977; 43: 269–281

25 Anderson ES, Smith HR. Chloramphenicol resistance in the typhoid bacillus. Br Med J 1972; iii: 329–331

26 Olarte J, Galindo E. *Salmonella typhi* resistant to chloramphenicol, ampicillin and other antimicrobial agents: strains isolated during an extensive typhoid fever epidemic in Mexico. Antimicrob Agents Chemother 1973; 4: 597–601

27 Gonzalez-Cortes A, Bessudo D, Sanchez-Leyva R, Fragoso R, Hinojosa M, Beceril P. Water-borne transmission of chloramphenicol-resistant *Salmonella typhi* in Mexico. Lancet 1973; ii: 605–607

28 Paniker CK, Vimala KN. Transferable chloramphenicol resistance in *Salmonella typhi*. Nature 1972; 239: 109–110

29 Anderson ES. The problem and implications of chloramphenicol resistance in the typhoid bacillus. J Hyg 1975; 74: 289–299

30 Herzog C. New trends in the chemotherapy of typhoid fever. Acta Tropica 1980; 37: 275–280

31 Smith HW. Thermosensitive transfer factors in chloramphenicol-resistant strains of *Salmonella typhi*. Lancet 1974; ii: 281–282

32 Anonymous. Chloramphenicol-resistant *Salmonella typhi* Vi-phage type E1. WHO Wkly Epidem Rec 1980; 55: 81

33 Datta N, Richards H, Datta C. *Salmonella typhi* in vivo acquires resistance to both chloramphenicol and co-trimoxazole. Lancet 1981; i: 1181–1183

34 Robins-Browne RM, Bhamjee A, Kharsany A, Simje AE. Acquisition of resistance by *Salmonella typhi* in vivo. Lancet 1981; ii: 148

35 Threlfall EJ, Ward LR, Rowe B, Robins-Browne R. Acquisition of resistance by *Salmonella typhi* in vivo: the importance of plasmid characterisation. Lancet 1982; i: 740

36 Anonymous. Transferable drug resistance in salmonella in South and Central America. WHO Wkly Epidem Rec 1974; 8: 65–69

37 Anderson ES, Threlfall EJ, Carr JM, McConnell MM, Smith HR. Clonal distribution of resistance plasmid-carrying *Salmonella typhimurium*, mainly in the Middle East. J Hyg 1977; 79: 429–448

38 Robins-Browne RM, Rowe B, Ramsaroop R et al. A hospital outbreak of multiresistant *Salmonella typhimurium* belonging to phage type 193. J Infect Dis 1983; 147: 210–216

39 Threlfall EJ, Hall MLM, Rowe B. Lactose-fermenting salmonellae in Britain. FEMS Microbiol Lett 1983; 17: 127–130

40 Rowe B, Frost JA, Threlfall EJ, Ward LR. Spread of a multiresistant clone of *Salmonella typhimurium* phage type 66/122 in South-East Asia and the Middle East. Lancet 1980; i: 1070–1071

41 Le Minor S. Apparition en France d'une epidemie à *Salmonella wien*. Med Mal Infect 1972; 2: 441–448

42 Sarrat H, Le Minor L, Le Minor S, Lafaix C, Maydat L. Etude d'une épidémie due à "*Salmonella ordonez*" dans la région de Dakar (Sénégal). Pathol Biol (Paris) 1972; 20: 577–582

43 Le Minor L, Coynault C, Pessoa G. Déterminisme plasmidique du caractère atypique "lactose positif" de souches de *S. typhimurium* et de *S. oranienburg* isolées au Brésil lors d'épidémies de 1971 à 1973. Ann Microbiol (Paris) 1974; 125A: 261–285

44 Chau PY, Wong WT, Fok YP. Resistance to chloramphenicol and ampicillin in *Salmonella johannesburg* in Honk Kong: observations over a five-year period 1973–1977. J Hyg 1978; 81: 343–351

45 Sharma KB, Bheem Bhat M, Asha P, Diwan N, Vaze S. Multi-drug resistant *Salmonella newport* in Delhi during the years 1975–77. Ind J Med Res 1979; 69: 720–725

46 McConnell MM, Smith HR, Leonardopoulos J, Anderson ES. The value of plasmid studies in the epidemiology of infections due to drug-resistant *Salmonella wien*. J Inf Dis 1979; 139: 178–190

47 Threlfall EJ, Carr JM, Anderson ES. Compatibility relations of resistance plasmids in *Salmonella typhimurium* of Middle Eastern origin. Proc Soc Gen Microbiol 1976; 3: 88

48 Chau PY, Ling J, Threlfall EJ, Im SWK. Genetic instability of R plasmids in relation to the shift of drug resistance patterns in *Salmonella johannesburg*. J Gen Microbiol 1982; 128: 239–245

49 Jones GW, Robert DK, Svinarich DM, Whitfield HJ. Association of adhesive, invasive, and virulent phenotypes of *Salmonella typhimurium* with autonomous 60-megadalton plasmids. Infect Immun 1982; 38: 476–486

50 Williams PH, Warner PH. ColV plasmid-mediated, colicin V-independent iron uptake system of invasive strains of *Escherichia coli*. Infect Immun 1980; 29: 411–416

51 Sansonetti PJ, Kopecko DJ, Formal SB. *Shigella sonnei* plasmids: evidence that a large plasmid is necessary for virulence. Infect Immun 1981; 34: 75–83

52 Sansonetti PJ, Kopecko DJ, Formal SB. Involvement of a plasmid in the invasive activity of *Shigella flexneri*. Infect Immun 1982; 35: 852–860

53 Gross RJ, Rowe B, Cheasty T, Thomas LV. Increase in drug resistance among *Shigella dysenteriae*, *Sh. flexneri* and *Sh. boydii*. Br Med J 1981; 283: 575

54 Frost JA, Rowe B. Plasmid-determined antibiotic resistance in *Shigella flexneri* isolated in England and Wales between 1974 and 1978. J Hyg 1983; 90: 27–32

55 Gross RJ, Thomas LV, Rowe B. *Shigella dysenteriae*, *Sh. flexneri* and *Sh. boydii* infections in England and Wales: the importance of foreign travel. Br Med J 1979; 2: 744

56 Mata LJ, Gangarosa EJ, Caceres A, Perera DR, Mejicanos ML. Epidemic Shiga bacillus dysentery in Central America. I. Etiologic investigations in Guatemala, 1969. J Infect Dis 1970; 122: 170–180

57 Olarte J, Filloy L, Galindo E. Resistance of *Shigella dysenteriae* type 1 to ampicillin and other antimicrobial agents: strains isolated during a dysentery outbreak in a hospital in Mexico City. J Infect Dis 1976; 133: 572–575

58 Rahaman MM, Huq I, Dey CR, Kibriya AKMG, Curlin G. Ampicillin-resistant Shiga bacillus in Bangladesh. Lancet 1974; i: 406–407

59 Rahaman MM, Kahn MM, Aziz KMS, Islam MS, Kibriya AKMG. An outbreak of dysentery caused by *Shigella dysenteriae* type 1 on a coral island in the Bay of Bengal. J Infect Dis 1975; 132: 15–19

60 Anonymous. Surveillance of Shigella. WHO Wkly Epidemiol Rec 1978; 28: 208

61 Anonymous. Resistance of *Shigella dysenteriae* I to antibiotics. WHO Wkly Epidemiol Rec 1979; 21: 167

62 Grindley NDF, Grindley JN, Anderson ES. R factor compatibility groups. Mol Gen Genet 1972; 119: 287–297

63 Frost JA, Rowe B, Vandepitte J, Threlfall EJ. Plasmid characterisation in the investigation of an epidemic caused by multiply resistant *Shigella dysenteriae* type 1 in Central Africa. Lancet 1981; ii: 1074–1076

64 Malengreau M, Molima-Kaba, Gillieaux M, De Feyter M, Kyele-Duibone, Mukolo-Ndjolo. Outbreak of *Shigella dysentery* in Eastern Zaire, 1980–1982. Ann Soc Belge Med Trop 1983; 63: 59–67

65 Frost JA, Rowe B, Vandepitte J. Acquisition of trimethoprim resistance in epidemic strains of *Shigella dysenteriae* type 1 from Zaire. Lancet 1982; i: 963

66 Gross RJ, Ward LR, Threlfall EJ, King H, Rowe B. Drug resistance among infantile enteropathogenic *Escherichia coli* strains isolated in the United Kingdom. Br Med J 1982; 285: 472–473

67 Echeverria P, Verhaert L, Ulyangco CV et al. Antimicrobial resistance and enterotoxin production among isolates of *Escherichia coli* in the Far East. Lancet 1978; ii: 589–592

68 Scotland SM, Gross RJ, Cheasty T, Rowe B. The occurrence of plasmids carrying genes for both enterotoxin production and drug resistance in *Escherichia coli* of human origin. J Hyg 1979; 83: 531–538

69 McConnell MM, Willshaw GA, Smith HR, Scotland SM, Rowe B. Transposition of ampicillin resistance to an enterotoxin plasmid in an *Escherichia coli* strain of human origin. J Bact 1979; 139: 346–355

70 Stieglitz H, Fonesca R, Olarte J, Kupersztoch-Portnoy YM. Linkage of heat-stable enterotoxin activity and ampicillin resistance in a plasmid isolation from an *Escherichia coli* of human origin. Infect Immun 1980; 30: 617–620

71 Wachsmuth K, DeBoy J, Birkness K, Sack D, Wells J. Genetic transfer of antimicrobial resistance and enterotoxigenicity among *Escherichia coli* strains. Antimicrob Agents Chemother 1983; 23: 278–283

72 Mhalu FS, Mmari PW, Ijumba J. Rapid emergence of El Tor *Vibrio cholerae* resistant to antimicrobial agents during first of fourth cholera epidemic in Tanzania. Lancet 1979; i: 345–347

73 Huq MI, Alim ARMA, Mutanda LN, Yunus M, Khan MU. Multiply antibiotic-resistant O-group 1 *Vibrio cholerae*. Bangladesh. Morb Mortal Wkly Rep 1980; 29: 109–110

74 Threlfall EJ, Rowe B. *Vibrio cholerae* El Tor acquires plasmid-encoded resistance to gentamicin. Lancet 1982; i: 42

75 Glass RI, Huq I, Alim ARMA, Yunus M. Emergence of multiply antibiotic-resistant *Vibrio cholerae* in Bangladesh. J Inf Dis 1980; 142: 939–942

76 Price DJE, Sleigh JD. Control of infection due to *Klebsiella aerogenes* in a neurosurgical unit by withdrawal of all antibiotics. *Lancet* 1970; ii: 1213–1215

77 Casewell MW, Dalton MT, Webster M, Phillips I. Gentamicin-resistant *Klebsiella aerogenes* in a urological ward. Lancet 1977; ii: 444–446

78 Curie K, Speller DCE, Simpson RA, Stephens M, Cooke DI. A hospital epidemic caused by a gentamicin-resistant *Klebsiella aerogenes*. J Hyg 1978; 80: 115–123

79 Gordon AM. Gentamicin-resistant Klebsiella strains in a hospital. Br Med J 1980; 280: 722–723

80 Hart CA. Nosocomial gentamicin- and multiply-resistant enterobacteria at one hospital. 1. Description of an outbreak. J Hosp Inf 1982; 3: 15–28

81 Lowbury EJL, Babb JR, Roe E. Clearance from a hospital of gram-negative bacilli that transfer carbenicillin-resistance to *Pseudomonas aeruginosa*. Lancet 1972; ii: 941–945

82 Bridges, K, Kidson, A, Lowbury EJL, Wilkins MD. Gentamicin- and silver-resistant pseudomonas in a burns unit. Br Med J 1979; i: 446–449

83 Meers PD, Foster CS, Churcher GM. Cross-infection with *Serratia marcescens*. Br Med J 1978; i: 238–239

84 Speller DEC. Hospital infection by multi-resistant Gram-negative bacilli. J Antimicrob Chemother 1980; 6: 168–170

85 Shafi MS, Datta N. Infection caused by *Proteus mirabilis* strains with transferable gentamicin-resistance factors. Lancet 1975; i: 1355–1357

86 Grüneberg RN, Bendall MJ. Hospital outbreak of trimethoprim resistance in pathogenic coliform bacteria. Br Med J 1979; ii: 7–9

87 Lowes JA, Smith J, Tabaqchali S, Shaw EJ. Outbreak of infection in a urological ward. Br Med J 1980; 280: 722

88 Christie AB. Infectious diseases: epidemiology and clinical practice. 3rd edn. Edinburgh: Churchill Livingstone, 1980

89 Gross RJ, Ward LR, Threlfall EJ, Cheasty T, Rowe B. Drug resistance among *Escherichia coli* strains isolated from cerebrospinal fluid. J Hyg 1983; 90: 195–198

90 Datta N, Dacey S, Hughes V *et al.* Distribution of genes for trimethoprim and gentamicin resistance in bacteria and their plasmids in a general hospital. J Gen Microbiol 1980; 118: 495–508

91 Datta N, Richards H. Trimethoprim-resistant bacteria in hospital and the community: spread of plasmids and transposons. In: Levy SB, Clowes RC, Koenig EL eds. Molecular biology, pathogenicity and ecology of bacterial plasmids. New York: Plenum Press, 1981; 21–30

92 Elwell LP, Inamine JM, Minshew BH. Common plasmid specifying tobramycin resistance found in two enteric bacteria isolated from burn patients. Antimicrob Agents Chemother 1978; 13: 312–317

93 Datta N, Hughes VM, Nugent ME, Richards H. Plasmids and transposons and their stability and mutability in bacteria isolated during an outbreak of hospital infection. Plasmid 1979; 2: 182–196

94 Tompkins LS, Plorde JJ, Falkow S. Molecular analysis of R-factors from multiresistant nosocomial isolates. J Inf Dis 1980; 141: 625–36

95 O'Brien TF, Ross DG, Guzman MA, Medeiros AA, Hedges RW, Botstein D. Dissemination of an antibiotic resistance plasmid in hospital patient flora. Antimicrob Agents Chemother 1980; 17: 537–543

96 Jackson GG. Antibiotic policies, practices and pressures. J Antimicrob Chemother 1979; 5: 1–4

British Medical Bulletin (1984) Vol. 40, No. 1, pp. 77–83

ANTIBIOTIC RESISTANCE IN *STAPHYLOCOCCUS AUREUS* AND STREPTOCOCCI

R W LACEY MD PhD MRCPath

Department of Microbiology
University of Leeds

1 Distribution of DNA in *Staphylococcus aureus*
2 Mutation to antibiotic resistance in *Staphylococcus aureus*
3 Origin of staphylococcal plasmids
4 β-Lactam resistance in *Staphylococcus aureus*
5 Relationship of antibiotic resistance to virulence in *Staphylococcus aureus*
6 Macrolide resistance in *Staphylococcus aureus*
7 Why do so many staphylococci produce penicillinase?
8 Antibiotic resistance in streptococci
9 Resistance transfer in group D streptococci
10 Group A streptococci
11 Pneumococci
12 Origins of antibiotic resistance in streptococci
13 Conclusions
     References

In normal health, *Staphylococcus aureus* is a commensal of the anterior nares, moist skin, and the intestine, and streptococci are found in the respiratory, intestinal and genital tracts. Infection represents an uncommon migration from these habitats. Exposure of both the commensal organism and the pathogen to antibiotics can select resistance. The former may be more important than the latter.

Although gain of antibiotic resistance may be the most obvious way in which staphylococci and some streptococci have altered over the last forty years, other properties of the organisms and of their hosts have also varied. Some of these changes—notably prophage carriage in *S. aureus*—are closely involved with antibiotic resistance. In this brief review I shall discuss the way in which these organisms have acquired resistance and, to a certain extent, lost it, and also make some comments that relate to chemotherapy and laboratory sensitivity testing.

1 Distribution of DNA in *Staphylococcus Aureus*

The bulk of the cellular DNA in *S. aureus* is assumed to consist of a single chromosome, although there has been no formal proof of this. The molecular weight of this structure is uncertain because of clumping of the organism that makes definition of an individual cell difficult; a figure of about 3×10^9 daltons is probable. In addition to the chromosome, cultures of staphylococci may contain plasmids that vary in size from less than 2 million to more than 30 daltons (Table I). Most of these are present in multiple copies, particularly the smaller plasmids which may be present in up to 40 copies/cell,[1] although this is not always so. Small staphylococcal plasmids determine resistance to single antibiotics and the larger plasmids may either determine resistance to single antibiotics or perhaps two, three or very occasionally four (Table I). Strains that are resistant to several antibiotics characteristically harbour

TABLE I. Examples of some recently characterized staphylococcal plasmids

Reference	Antibiotic resistance coded	Comments
2	Tobramycin, gentamicin, streptogramins	Evidence for spread within the 'methicillin resistance clone'
3	Gentamicin, sometimes with β-lactamase	Similar plasmids found in both *S. aureus* and *S epidermidis* in one environment
4	Cadmium ions	Unusually small size (3.2 kb) and not conferring resistance to other heavy metals
5	Erythromycin	Small sizes, mol. wt. 0.85–2.4 $\times 10^6$ daltons
6	Cadmium, neomycin, streptomycin, β-lactamase	mol. wt. 21 $\times 10^6$ daltons

several different plasmids, all of which are compatible with each other. Few pairs of staphylococcal plasmids are incompatible, except some of the penicillinase plasmids.[7] Some staphyloccal plasmids determine toxins, for example the exfoliative toxin (ET) or resistance to heavy metals such as cadmium ions. The presence of different plasmids in one staphylococcal cell suggest that plasmid transfer may have occurred under natural conditions. There is indeed strong epidemiological evidence for this.[8]

In vitro plasmids can be released or extracted form a donor cell and incorporated into a recipient by transduction,[9] conjugation[10] and transformation.[11] In transduction—usually generalized transduction—during lysis of the donor cell, a bacteriophage occasionally incorporates plasmid genome into its protein coat instead of some or all of its own genome. Under appropriate conditions the plasmid is inserted into the recipient from this defective bacteriophage. For transduction to be accomplished successfully in vitro, care must be taken to protect the recipient from destruction by 'normal' phage particles and the process requires death of the donor cell. Transduction is not likely to occur in nature commonly unless a plasmid becomes incorporated at a very high frequency into a bacteriophage so the probability of a plasmid transfer outweighs the probability of the recipient being destroyed by 'normal' phage particles.

Transfer of plasmids between cells is more likely to occur under natural conditions by a process referred to as 'phage-mediated conjugation'. Here, the presence of a bacteriophage in either the donor or the recipient permits a high frequency of plasmid transfer—up to 1 in 10 recipients can acquire a new plasmid in a mixed culture—without death of the donor or the risk of the recipient being lysed by 'normal' phage particles.[10] The detailed mechanism of this transfer is not known; however, high cell density and calcium or magnesium ions are necessary and plasmids cannot be established in recipients from cell-free filtrates, unless enclosed in bacteriophage coats. The importance of cell aggregation in conjugation is difficult to define because of the tendency of cells of *S. aureus* to clump. We have recently identified prophage genes in either the donor or the recipient that facilitate plasmid transfer. These genes are distinct from those conferring lysogenic immunity. Finally, transformation can occur in vitro under certain conditions, although the presence of nucleases will reduce the likelihood of this in nature.

Although multi-resistant staphylococci isolated recently from Ireland[12] and Australia[13] contain relatively few plasmids, these clones have probably become resistant through acquisition of plasmids, to be followed by the transition of some of the genes coding for antibiotic resistance into the chromosome. When a cell is constructed in vitro to contain a large number of plasmids, some are unstable,[14] so the transition of resistance genes into the chromosome in multi-resistant cells might provide an advantage for the cell. It is therefore surprising that the genes determining β-lactamase in *S. aureus* are so rarely chromosomal.

Most of the interactions between genes recognized in other bacterial species have been shown to occur in *S. aureus*. An important series of papers by Novick and co-workers demonstrate transposition of plasmid genes to the chromosome and *vice versa*; [15-17] recombination can occur between plasmids and both these processes are controlled by specific sequences of DNA.[18,19] Staphylococcal plasmids give characteristic fragments following digestion by restriction endonucleases and are amenable to analysis by hybridization, heteroduplex formation and sequence techniques.[20] The order of genes in parts of the chromosome is now established, as is that of some of the DNA bases. These studies have been useful in refuting the suggestion that methicillin resistance is linked to the plasmid genes that determine production of β-lactamase and Enterotoxin B.[21,22]

2 Mutation to Antibiotic Resistance in *Staphylococcus Aureus*

During the 1940s and 1950s, antibiotic resistance in *S. aureus* was thought to have arisen by mutation; that is, a minority of cells in a culture were assumed to possess point changes in their DNA that conferred resistance to an antibiotic, notably to streptomycin. The use of the antibiotic selected resistant mutants at the expense of the predominant sensitive cells. Subsequent work has shown that most clinically important antibiotic resistance is determined by plasmids and has not arisen by mutation. However, resistance to streptomycin, novobiocin, rifampicin and fusidic acid can arise by mutation during therapy. Resistance to both streptomycin and fusidic acid are probably more frequently determined by plasmids than by chromosomal mutation and, as novobiocin is little used therapeutically, the most important risk of resistance arising by mutation concerns the use of rifampicin. Prior to exposure to rifampicin, most cultures of *S. aureus* contain about 1 in 10^8 cells that are resistant. The resistant cells appear normal in general properties, including growth rate, and can be assumed to be pathogenic. Indeed, I have studied a patient who died of staphylococcal pneumonia whilst being treated with rifampicin for tuberculosis. The resistance of the staphylococcus to rifampicin was determined by a chromosomal gene and presumably had been selected in vivo. This antibiotic should be used with extreme caution for treating serious staphylococcal infections.

3 Origin of Staphylococcal Plasmids

The DNA sequences of regions of several staphylococcal plasmids have been elucidated;[3,23,24] some of these are similar to parts of plasmids of other species such as *S. epidermidis*.[3] Surprisingly, a sequence of DNA of a staphylococcal plasmid that codes for neomycin resistance is almost identical to that of a plasmid harboured by a soil bacillus.[24] The identification of plasmids with similar DNA sequences in a variety of different strains or species has been explained by transfer of those plasmids between cultures in the recent past under natural conditions.[8] However, similar sequences are being found in an increasing variety of plasmids in very differing hosts between which it is not possible to transfer the plasmid in vitro by conventional techniques.[24] This raises doubt as to whether the inference of transfer in nature is valid. Two other general explanations should be considered. First, the differentiation of a gram-positive bacteria into a new species, with retention of a plasmid by a minority of the cells of each new species. Secondly, convergent

evolution may have occurred. The presence of similar determinants for gentamicin resistance in both *S. epidermidis* and *S. aureus* during one outbreak[3] cannot be taken as proof that the plasmid has spread from *S. epidermidis* to *S. aureus*. Transfer of plasmids between cultures in nature is most likely to have occurred where the frequencies of transfer in vitro are high. In the outbreaks where gentamicin resistance has been determined by plasmids in both *S. epidermidis* and *S. aureus*,[3] the frequency of transfer of the marker in vitro is about 10^{-8}. It is doubtful whether transfer of plasmids between cultures at this frequency in vivo would significantly contribute to resistance since plasmids tend to be lost at much higher frequencies than this during cell division (see below).

4 β-Lactam Resistance in *Staphylococcus Aureus*

Staphylococcal infections are commonly treated with β-lactam antibiotics. It is not surprising therefore that many types of β-lactam resistance have been described (Table II). By far the most common mechanism exhibited by the cell is the production of β-lactamase. This enzyme is usually inducible; after exposure to a sub-inhibitory concentration of a β-lactam agent a culture produces about 50–80 times more enzyme than when uninduced. There are at least four serological types of β-lactamase;[25,26] there is also much variation in the extent to which the enzyme diffuses outside the cell membrane to become extracellular. Each β-lactam antibiotic differs in ability to cause enzyme induction, in resistance to hydrolysis by β-lactamase, and in inactivation of the enzyme. However some of the antibiotics that have been thought to be resistant to β-lactamase, e.g. the isoxazolyl penicillins, may sometimes be vulnerable.[27] It is still not known to what extent this vulnerability anticipates therapeutic failure. Indeed, there is uncertainty whether the formation of small amounts of β-lactamase does cause therapeutic failure with the simple penicillins. This doubt stems from the possibility that such resistant cultures might have been selected by the 'accidental' exposure of commensals to low concentrations of penicillins in, for example, the nasal secretions. Because of the above variables, testing for sensitivity to the β-lactam agents should always include the particular compound used in the patient. The effect of hydrolysis of β-lactam antibiotic is readily demonstrated in disk testing with the use of heavy inocula or with actively growing cultures at the time of application of the disk.

Methicillin resistance is unique. Such cultures contain a

TABLE II. Mechanisms of resistance to β-lactam antibiotics in clinical isolates of *Staphylococcus aureus*

Mechanism	Comment
β-lactamase	Common; the enzyme rapidly hydrolyses simple penicillins, ampicillins and 'broad spectrum penicillins'. Has some lytic activity against isoxazolyl penicillins and some cephalosporins, e.g. cephaloridine
Methicillin resistance	Resistance to all β-lactam agents best demonstrated by growth at 30°C or in the presence of hypertonic media. Clinical significance not established
Penicillin tolerance	β-lactam antibiotics fail to destroy (although growth is inhibited) a proportion of certain cultures in vitro. Unlikely to be clinically important in most patients
Cephalosporin resistance	Rare: two cultures have been isolated that are defective in penicillin binding protein 3 after prolonged therapy with cephradine
L-forms	Staphylococci deficient in cell walls; extremely unlikely to be important clinically except in a few patients with renal infections

minority of cells that are resistant to all the β-lactam agents at 37°C or higher temperatures. In the presence of hypertonic media, or at low temperatures, the proportion of resistant cells increases so that, at 30°C, cultures are uniformly resistant to β-lactam antibiotics.

The genes coding for methicillin resistance are determined by a large chromosomal element that has no allelic equivalent in sensitive cells.[22] The instability of methicillin resistance in some aging cultures can be due to loss of all or part of this extra linkage group. Doubt has arisen concerning the clinical significance of methicillin resistance because (a) most of these cultures also produce high amounts of β-lactamase, (b) the resistant bacteria are slow-growing in the presence of the antibiotic and (c) the resistance is not expressed fully under physiological conditions. There have been reports of patients infected with methicillin-resistant staphylococci in whom β-lactam agents have failed.[28] These failures have been seen mainly in patients who were debilitated or immunosuppressed. The relative roles of methicillin resistance and other types of β-lactam resistance in causing therapeutic failure are uncertain. However, these methicillin-resistant cultures rarely produce primary staphylococcal sepsis in otherwise healthy people. The biochemical mechanism of the methicillin resistance of these strains is still largely unknown;[29] unfortunately, several workers have studied cultures which differ in properties in addition to methicillin resistance.

We have proposed that all methicillin-resistant cultures have evolved from a single clone.[30] Most cultures isolated recently still resemble the earlier strains and are probably derived from them.[2] If it is accepted that these cultures are all related, then once the mechanism and clinical significance of the resistance has been established in a few cultures, it may be reasonable to extend these findings generally.

Penicillin tolerance is seen in a minority of cultures of *S. aureus*.[31] These cultures contain a proportion of cells that resist the usual bactericidal concentrations of β-lactams and some other antibiotics, so the antibiotic appears bacteriostatic rather than bactericidal towards these cells. Penicillin-tolerant cultures have been isolated after therapeutic failure with β-lactam antibiotics. However, the exact role that penicillin tolerance plays in therapeutic failure is uncertain. Further information is needed before laboratories should be encouraged to seek penicillin tolerance routinely.

Another type of β-lactam resistance has been detected following prolonged cephalosporin therapy. Two cultures were selected that contained defective penicillin binding protein 3. These cultures had normal growth characteristic in vitro and were associated with morbidity in two patients. However, the occurrence of these mutants seems to be rare in vivo.[32]

Finally, L-forms of *S. aureus* might be encountered occasionally in renal infections.

5   Relationship of Antibiotic Resistance to Virulence in *Staphylococcus Aureus*

There is still uncertainty over the precise role of each of the 'virulence factors' of *S. aureus* in causing disease. Despite this, a few trends are apparent. First, recently isolated multi-resistant strains of *S. aureus* do not appear to produce primary sepsis in otherwise healthy people—certainly not to the same extent of the phage type 80/81 strains in the 1950s and 1960s. In parts of the world where multi-resistant staphylococci are currently producing outbreaks of infection, e.g. Greece, Australia, USA and the Republic of Ireland, the strains involved resemble those isolated from elsewhere, and the high incidence of nosocomial infection due to the strains in Australia has probably resulted from environmental and host factors rather than from enhanced virulence of the organism.[33] Experimental studies suggest that, in general, resistance is not likely to be associated with enhanced virulence—rather the reverse may happen.[34] Strains constructed in vitro to contain considerable amounts of extra DNA have reduced doubling times and some of the plasmids become unstable. However multi-resistance has been found by others to be associated with full virulence.[35] The multi-resistant strains have a similar capacity to survive in the environment compared to the sensitive strains. The properties of the organism associated with prolonged survival are production of pigment and resistance to unsaturated fatty acids. There is little evidence that resistant strains have abnormalities in either of these.

Multi-resistant *S. aureus* are less prevalent in the UK than a decade ago. The reason for this decline in the incidence of multi-resistant staphylococci is probably multifactoral, involving the better use of antibiotics (see below) and improved control of cross-infection. Many of the resistance determinants involved are unstable. Our own figures for the incidence of resistance in recently isolated strains of *S. aureus* are shown in Table III. It is notable that the incidences of resistant cultures from general practice and from hospital sources are very similar, although resistance to fusidic acid is now more common in general practice than in hospital cultures. We attribute these findings to the lavish use of topical fusidic acid in general practice and the careful control over its topical use within that particular hospital.

6   Macrolide Resistance in *Staphylococcus Aureus*

During the 1950s and early 1960s, hospital epidemics due to erythromycin resistant *S. aureus* were reported in the UK. This led to the restriction of the use of erythromycin on the grounds that it was particularly likely to select resistance. At that time the extent to which the high incidence of resistance was due to the epidemic spread of a few strains or indeed their plasmids, or was due to the

TABLE III. Incidence of antibiotic resistance* in *Staphylococcus aureus* isolated in the King's Lynn Health District Jan 1981–Jan 1983

Total number studied	No (%) resistant to:							
	Penicillin	Cephradine	Methicillin	Tetracycline	Erythromycin	Fusidic acid	Gentamicin	Neomycin
1075 (hospital)	866 (80.6)	4 (0.5)	0	93 (8.7)	58 (5.4)	20 (1.8)	1 (0.1)	12 (1.2)
1125 (general practice)	909 (80.8)	2 (0.2)	0	103 (9.2)	55 (4.9)	30 (2.7)	0	22 (1.9)

* Disk testing supplemented by MICs

TABLE IV. Genetic studies on 58 erythromycin-resistant cultures of *Staphylococcus aureus* isolated between January 1981 and January 1983 from hospital sources, King's Lynn Health District

Number in category	Nature of erythromycin resistance	Resistance to spectinomycin	Bacteriophage types (routine test dilution)	Loss of resistance on storage at room temperature for 2–6 months*	Doubling time of resistant cell relative to sensitive (%) mean of four experiments. Range (mean)	Transfer of erythromycin resistance in mixed cultures to *S. aureus* 6936†	Erythromycin resistance determined by plasmid genes‡ (size, approx. no. copies cell)	Unstable chromosomal resistance, probably transposon	Undetermined genetic basis of erythromycin resistance
26	Inducible§	Sensitive‖	NT¶ (14) 84 (5) 85 (2) 29/79/53/54 (2) 29 (2) 95 (1)	All: 0.7%–30.7% of cells sensitive (mean 7.8%)	89–119 (103)	7/26, frequency $\sim 10^{-6}$–10^{-8} per total bacteria	1.8×10^6 daltons, 2–3 copies/cell	–	–
7	Inducible	Sensitive	NT (3) 84 (2) 29 (2)	0	Not tested	0/7	1.8×10^6 daltons, 2–3 copies/cell	–	–
3	Inducible	Sensitive	Group I/III (3)	0.4%–6.0% (mean 2.9%)	95–112 (101)	0	3.0×10^6 daltons, 6–8 copies/cell	–	–
6	Inducible	Sensitive	Variable	0	Not tested	0	No plasmid DNA	–	6
5	Inducible	Resistant	Variable	0.26%–4.0% (1.3%)	88–116 (104)	0	No plasmid DNA	Probably, see text	–
2	Constitutive**	Resistant	NT (1) Group III (1)	0	Not tested	0	No plasmid DNA	–	2
9	Inducible	Resistant	Variable	0	Not tested	0	No plasmid DNA	–	9

* Detected by replica plating, careful identification of sensitive derivatives, including bacteriophage typing. Up to 4000 colonies screened after inoculation of stored culture to nutrient broth and plating after incubation at 37° 20h
† By method of Lacey (Reference 10)
‡ After first transduction/transfer in mixed cultures to plasmid-free culture 1030 plasmids isolated by ultracentrifuge and electrophoresis[1,16]
§ Inducible resistance to erythromycin only; erythromycin induces resistance to other macrolides, lincosamides, and streptogramin (MLS) antibiotics
‖ MIC <50 µg/ml
¶ NT = Non-typable at routine test dilution
** Constitutive resistance to all MLS antibiotics

evolution *de novo* of the resistance in a variety of strains, was not known. We have studied this problem over the years and come to the conclusion that the high incidence of erythromycin resistance is predominantly due to the epidemic spread of just one or a few clones[36]—i.e. the reported high incidence was essentially a result of bad cross-infection control. As a result of this we have not attempted to restrict the use of erythromycin specifically and despite the freer use of erythromycin in the King's Lynn Hospitals the number of resistant staphylococci has not increased (Table IV). In most of the erythromycin-resistant cultures isolated over the last two years the resistance is unstable in vitro (Table IV). This instability is most easily shown by storage at room temperature and identifying sensitive derivatives by replica plating. The great majority of the recently isolated erythromycin-resistant strains are inducibly resistant to erythromycin (dissociated resistance); resistance to spectinomycin in these cultures has become less common than previously (Table IV). The instability of the resistance is accounted for by two mechanisms: firstly, the spontaneous loss of a small plasmid (1.8×10^6 daltons) present in only 2–3 copies per cell, and secondly, the loss of chromosomal genes coding for erythromycin resistance. In five cultures, the resistance was not associated with plasmid DNA and transduction kinetics gave chromosomal features for the genes in question (see also reference 9). Yet on storage, the resistance was lost at high frequency. The precise mechanism of the loss is uncertain, although it is known that chromosomal genes determining erythromycin resistance can be transposed from plasmids to the chromosome in vitro. In these cultures, the reverse process may have occurred since three of the erythromycin-sensitive derivatives had lost penicillinase plasmids, and in all five of the cultures, it was possible to transpose the genes for erythromycin resistance from the chromosome to a penicillinase plasmid in the wild strain. Loss of resistance could be explained as excision of the transposon from the chromosome.

We conclude from these studies that resistance to erythromycin in *S. aureus* very closely follows the general pattern of antibiotic resistance where an equilibrium exists between the incidence of resistant and sensitive cells. Resistance is favoured by antibiotic use and bad cross-infection control. Sensitivity is favoured by the removal of selection pressure. In the King's Lynn hospitals, all clinical and representative 'environmental' isolates of *S. aureus* have been bacteriophage typed for seven years and only two trivial instances of cross-infection have been identified. This enables the role of cross-infection to be separated from selection of resistance by antibiotic use as an explanation for the amount of resistance. The incidence of erythromycin resistance has been consistently lower than that of penicillin and tetracycline, suggesting that the use of erythromycin is not specifically prone to select resistance—certainly not to the same extent as streptomycin, rifampicin, penicillin or ampicillin. During the last three years, the use of erythromycin in these hospitals has comprised about 10% (10000 g) of total antibiotics used.

7   Why Do So Many Staphylococci Produce Penicillinase?

Since the introduction of penicillin forty years ago, penicillin resistance appears to have increased inexorably in this organism, initially in hospital isolates, then in strains from general practice. Now at least 80% of staphylococci from developed countries produce β-lactamase. Some hospital cultures produce higher amounts of the enzyme than cultures from non-hospital sources. It is necessary to find explanations for this other than the use of simple penicillins (which are now rarely used for treating staphylococcal infections). Firstly, the frequent use (usually for non-staphylococcal infections) of ampicillin or amoxycillin might have selected cultures that produce β-lactamase. Secondly, the isoxazolyl penicillins, e.g. cloxacillin and flucloxacillin, may be vulnerable to β-lactamse, and their use might also select bacteria that produce these enzymes. Thirdly, it is possible that genes linked to β-lactamase determined by the 'penicillinase plasmid' might produce a selective advantage. Where mixtures of penicillin-resistant and sensitive bacteria are seen both in patients' noses and on their skin, there is a higher proportion of β-lactamase positive cultures on the skin than in the nose,[37] and Noble has found that β-lactamase-producing cultures survive better on murine skin than those that do not produce the enzyme.[38] However, Dyke and his co-workers have found that penicillinase can confer increased sensitivity to a fatty acid, linolenic acid, that may be important in removing *S. aureus* from the skin.[39]

Many dermatophyte fungi produce antibiotics, including penicillin, and their presence may also select for resistance in both *S. aureus* and *S. epidermidis* (W C Noble, personal communication). The latter is now notoriously resistant to antibiotics, and can be expected to produce increasing therapeutic problems in debilitated patients, and in patients with implants. Certainly, the possibility does exist that the production of β-lactamase by staphylococci is not simply selected by the use of penicillin. Moreover, many plasmids that determine β-lactamase also carry the genes coding for resistance to salts of cadmium, arsenic, mercury and other heavy metals and it is difficult to explain why these bacteria are resistant to these. That is, resistance to them may be fortuitous; if so, production of β-lactamase may also be! It is hoped that these ideas may encourage futher work with this problem.

8   Antibiotic Resistance in Streptococci

Some species of streptococci have acquired resistance to several antibiotics whereas others have remained uniformly sensitive to antibiotics such as the penicillins. The genetic basis of resistance in individual species varies. Thus, while all three 'classical' mechanisms of gene transfer—transformations, transduction and conjugation—can occur in vitro, any particular species had been manipulated by one, or two at the most, of these techniques. In particular, the only form of gene transfer that has been detected in group D streptococci is conjugation,[40,41] whilst transformation and transduction are characteristic of group A streptococci.[42] One interesting aspect of antibiotic resistance in various streptococci is the enormous variation of its incidence. For example, in group A streptococci isolated in Japan, the proportion of resistance to macrolide antibiotics may be greater than 50%[43] but this incidence of resistance is not seen elsewhere. It is also necessary to establish that the resistance detected is relevant clinically. The commonest resistances in group D streptococci are to tetracycline and macrolide antibiotics, but these agents are used rarely for treating infections due to group D streptococci, by far the commonest infection due to the group D streptococcus being urinary. Fortunately, β-lactamase production has never been described in streptococci and most streptococci are still treatable by simple penicillins or ampicillins.

9   Resistance Transfer in Group D Streptococci

Many group D streptococci from human and animals sources are resistant to tetracyclines, erythromycin, and aminoglycoside antibiotics. Many plasmids have been isolated that determine resistance.[41] However, resistance to both tetracyclines and to some aminoglycoside antibiotics can apparently be determined by chromosomal genes that are capable of transfer to recipients at relatively high frequencies ('conjugative transposons').[41,44] There are two types of conjugal transfer of plasmids in group D streptococci. One requires high cell-to-cell contact that can be achieved on the surface of solid agar or on filters, and the other occurs in broth cultures of density of 10^6–10^8 bacteria/ml.[41] There is little known about the mechanism of conjugation that requires high cell densities. However, where plasmids transfer between cells in dilute broth cultures, the recipient secretes a heat-stable peptide and this induces the donor cells to adhere to the recipients and it also promotes the subsequent transfer of plasmids from the donor to the recipient. This peptide is known as clumping inducing agent (CIA) and can be titred by dilution of the culture. Recipients may secrete several CIAs, each one having a specificity for different plasmids in a donor. Once a particular plasmid has transferred from a donor cell to the recipient, then that recipient now ceases to synthesize the corresponding CIA. Thus recipient cultures have the ability to signal to potential donors to cause aggregation with them, and then to direct transfer of DNA to them.[41,45] It is difficult to account for the evolution of such a system. This mechanism probably occurs widely in nature because about one third of clinical cultures of group D streptococci produce CIAs and are antibiotic resistant. In vitro, it is possible to transfer resistance from group D streptococci to group B and some other groups.[46] However, it is much less easy to transfer resistance from group D streptococci to group A or C (Engel *et al.*[47] and R W Lacey, unpublished observations). This is to be expected since the only known means of gene transfer in group D streptococci is conjugation, which does not apparently occur in group A or C strains. The suggestion that group D streptococci may provide a reservoir of antibiotic resistance plasmids that can be disseminated to other bacteria including group A streptococci or even staphylococci or gram-positive bacilli[41] is speculative.

10   Group A Streptococci

During the last thirty years, the incidence of macrolide resistance in group A streptococci has been approximately 0.1–1.0% and is often of a low level—MIC about 2–4 µg/ml. It is not known how often cultures with this low-level resistance are associated with therapeutic failure with the usual doses of erythromycin. However, some cultures have been found to be resistant to high levels of antibiotic and these should anticipate therapeutic failure. In the UK, resistance to erythromycin in streptococci has not increased recently. In Japan, the high incidence of streptococci resistant to erythromycin is due to the prevalence of a few types so that, as with *S. aureus*, the dissemination of one of a very few resistant clones has been responsible[43] rather than the frequent evolution of the resistance *de novo*. Apart from resistance to macrolide antibiotics, only resistance to tetracyclines is common. However, the incidence of this has declined during the last decade—presumably due to the diminishing use of tetracycline. In King's Lynn, about 4–5% of group A streptococci are now resistant to this antibiotic. There are apparently still very few group A streptococci resistant to penicillin or cephalosporins. The reason for this persistent sensitivity is not known but may be due to the inability of the cell to support the relevant DNA or, more likely, be due to the inability of the cell to synthesize β-lactamase.

11   Pneumococci

There have been several reports since 1978 of pneumococci resistant to penicillin and other antibiotics.[48] The resistance is relatively low level, but probably clinically important, and is not due to the synthesis of β-lactamase nor due to the presence of plasmids. However, plasmids have been detected in pneumococci and it is possible to transfer them between cultures in vitro by a mechanism that resembles conjugation in group D streptococci.[49] As with group A streptococci, it is still not known whether we can anticipate permanent absence of pneumococcal β-lactamase.

12   Origins of Antibiotic Resistance in Streptococci

Differing species of streptococci that are resistant to macrolides contain plasmids of $\sim 16 \times 10^6$ daltons. Some of the DNA sequences in these plasmids is similar to those in other gram-positive organisms that have been isolated from a variety of sources,[41,46,50–53] including the soil.[54] This raises the possibility that macrolide resistance in one bacterial species has spread to others. Since the use of macrolide antibiotics in both animals and man can select macrolide resistance, the use of macrolides such as tylosin in growth promotion in animals has been thought responsible for selecting macrolide resistance in human streptococci. However, a number of factors argue against this. Firstly, the nature of macrolide resistance in animal cultures (this includes both staphylococci and streptococci) is usually different to that in clinical cultures. Characteristically, animal organisms are constitutively resistant to all macrolides, lincosamines, and streptogramin B antibiotics although this may not be fully expressed.[47] In contrast, clinical strains of streptococci (and also staphylococci) show characteristic cross-resistance patterns including zonal resistance to lincomycin.[55] Secondly, it is difficult to transfer genes coding for macrolide resistance from streptococci and staphylococci from animal sources to human cultures. The only exception is resistance to macrolide antibiotics in animal group D streptococci that can transfer to human group D, but not A or C, streptococci. Thirdly, few streptococcal species produce disease in both man and animals. Fourthly, antibiotics are used to a greater extent in human medicine than in veterinary medicine and agriculture, at least in the UK, so the major selecting pressure for man must be the human use of these agents.

For further information on staphylococci the reader should consult the excellent reviews by Shanson[56] and Rosypal & Rosypalova,[57] and that by Clewell on streptococci.[42]

13   Conclusions

In both *Staphylococcus aureus* and *Streptococcus pyogenes*, acquired resistance has appeared erratically. There is uncertainty as to the clinical significance of a number of phenomona detected in vitro. There is scope to improve the relevance of laboratory sensitivity testing to the contexts of the patient. In general, the incidence of antibiotic resistance has correlated with total antibiotic consumption, but there are some exceptions to this: the proportion of staphylococci resistant to penicillin is higher than might be expected and that of *S. pyogenes* lower. The genetic basis of resistance in these gram-positive organisms are varied, and the actual appearance of resistance unpredictable. Once resistance strains have arisen, antibiotic use in man rather than animals is responsible for their selection. However, the incidence of multiple antibiotic resistance in *S. aureus* obtained from UK sources has declined over the last decade, and that of tetracycline resistance in group A streptococci has also become less. Antibiotic resistance is thus potentially reversible. Recent studies on erythromycin resistance show that both plasmid and chromosomally mediated resistance is unstable in vitro. The use of this antibiotic should not be specifically limited.

There is no evidence that resistance in these organisms is associated with enhanced virulence; it is possible that one factor responsible for the eclipse of the multi-resistant staphylococcus in the UK is its reduced viability compared to more sensitive strains.

However, the potential for gene reassortment in these organisms is immense, and epidemics due to highly virulent and multi-resistant strains might occur. Certainly, there are at present epidemics due to multi-resistant *S. aureus* in Dublin and throughout most of Australia. I believe (and hope) that the main reason for these is antibiotic abuse and bad cross-infection control, rather than enhanced virulence, but I may be wrong.

ACKNOWLEDGEMENTS

I thank Mrs V Lord and Mrs G Howson for technical assistance with some of the results reported here.

REFERENCES

1 Chopra I, Bennett P M, Lacey R W. A variety of staphylococcal plasmids present as multiple copies. J Gen Microbiol 1973; 79: 343–345

2 El Solh N, Fouace J M, Pillet J, Chabbert, Y A. Plasmid DNA content of multiresistant *Staphylococcus aureus* strains. Ann Microbiol 1981: 132B: 131–156

3 Jaffe H W, Sweeney H M, Weinstein R A. Structural and phenotypic varieties of gentamicin resistance plasmids in hospital strains of *Staphylococcus aureus* and coagulse-negative staphylococci. Antimicrob Agents Chemother 1982; 21: 773–779

4 El Solh N, Ehrlich S D. A small cadmium resistance plasmid isolated from *Staphylococcus aureus*. Plasmid 1982; 7: 77–84

5 Dunny G M, Christie P J, Adsit J C, Baron E S, Novick R P. Effects of antibiotics in animal feed on the antibiotic resistance of the Gram positive bacterial flora of animals and man. In: Levy S B, Clowes R C, Koenig E L, eds. Molecular biology, pathogenicity and ecology of bacterial plasmids. New York: Plenum Press, 1981; 557-565

6 Lacey R W. Properties of an unusual genetic element in *Staphylococcus aureus*. J Med Microbiol 1979; 12: 311–319

7 Novick R P. Penicillinase plasmids of *Staphylococcus aureus*. Fed Proc 1967; 26: 29–38

8 Lacey R W, Rosdahl V T. An unusual "penicillinase plasmid" in *Staphylococcus aureus*: evidence for its transfer under natural conditions. J Med Microbiol 1974; 7: 1–9

9 Novick R P. Analysis by transduction of mutations affecting penicillinase formation in *Staphylococcus aureus*. J Gen Microbiol 1963; 33: 121–136

10 Lacey R W. Evidence for two mechanisms of plasmid transfer in mixed cultures of *Staphylococcus aureus*. J Gen Microbiol 1980; 119: 423–435

11 Sjöström J-E, Löfdahl S, Philipson L. Transformation of *Staphylococcus aureus* by heterologous plasmids. Plasmid 1979; 2: 529–535

12 Cafferkey M T, Hone R, Falkiner R F, Keane C T, Pomeroy H. Gentamicin and methicillin resistant *Staphylococcus aureus* in Dublin hospitals: clinical and laboratory studies. J Med Microbiol; In press

13 Lyon B R, May J W, Marshall J H, Skurray R A. Plasmid-mediated antibiotic resistance in methicillin-resistant *Staphylococcus aureus*. Med J Aust 1981; 1: 468–469

14 Lacey R W, Chopra I. Genetic studies on a multi-resistant strain of *Staphylococcus aureus*. J Med Microbiol 1974; 7: 285–297

15 Novick R P, Edelman I, Schwesinger M D, Gruss A D, Swanson E C, Pattee P A. Genetic translocation in *Staphylococcus aureus*. Proc Natl Acad Sci USA 1979; 76: 400–404

16 Phillips S, Novick R P. Tn554—a site-specific repressor-controlled transposon in *Staphylococcus aureus*. Nature 1979; 278: 476–478

17 Khan S A, Novick R P. Terminal nucleotide sequences of Tn551, a transposon specifying erythromycin resistance in *Staphylococcus aureus*; homology with Tn3. Plasmid 1980; 4: 148–154

18 Murphy E, Novick R P. Site-specific recombination between plasmids of *Staphylococcus aureus*. J Bacteriol 1980; 141: 316–326

19 Novick R P, Iordanescu S, Surdeanu M, Edelman I. Transduction-related cointegrate formation between staphylococcal plasmids: a new type of site-specific recombination. Plasmid 1981; 6: 159–172

20 Novick R P, Murphy E, Gryczan T J, Baron E, Edelman I. Penicillinase plasmids of *Staphylococcus aureus*: Restriction-deletion maps. Plasmid 1979; 2: 109–129

21 Kühl S A, Pattee P A, Baldwin J N. Chromosomal map location of the methicillin resistance determinant in *Staphylococcus aureus*. J Bacteriol 1978; 135: 460–465

22 Stewart G C, Rosenblum E D. Genetic behavior of the methicillin resistance determinant in *Staphylococcus aureus*. J Bacteriol 1980; 144: 1200–1202

23 Murphy E, Novick R P. Physical mapping of *Staphylococcus aureus* penicillinase plasmid p1524: characterization of an invertible region. MGG 1979; 175: 19–30

24 Polak J, Novick R P. Closely related plasmids from *Staphylococcus aureus* and soil bacilli. Plasmid 1982; 7: 152–162

25 Richmond M H. Wild-type variants of exopenicillinase from *Staphylococcus aureus*. Biochem J 1965; 94: 584–593

26 Rosdahl V T. Naturally occurring constitutive β-lactamase of novel serotype in *Staphylococcus aureus*. J Gen Microbiol 1973; 77: 229–231

27 Lacey R W. Stability of the isoxazolyl penicillins to staphylococcal β-lactamase. J Antimicrob Chemother 1982; 9: 239–240

28 Giamarellou H, Papapetropoulou M, Daikos G K. 'Methicillin resistant' *Staphylococcus aureus* infections during 1978–1979: clinical and bacteriologic observations. J Antimicrob Chemother 1981; 7: 649–655

29 Smith P F, Wilkinson B J. Differential methicillin susceptibilities of peptidoglycan syntheses in methicillin-resistant *Staphylococcus aureus*. J Bacteriol 1981; 148: 610–617

30 Lacey R W, Grinsted J. Genetic analysis of methicillin-resistant strains of *Staphylococcus aureus*: evidence for their evolution from a single clone. J Med Microbiol 1973; 6: 511–526

31 Sabath L D, Wheeler N, Laverdiere M, Blazenic D, Wilkinson B J. A new type of penicillin resistance of *Staphylococcus aureus*. Lancet 1977; i: 443–445

32 Lacey R W, Lord V L. New type of β-lactam resistance in *Staphylococcus aureus*. Lancet 1981; i: 1049–1050

33 Gedney J, Lacey R W. Properties of methicillin-resistant staphylococci now endemic in Australia. Med J Aust 1982; i: 448–450

34 Lacey R W, Chopra I. Effect of plasmid carriage on the virulence of *Staphylococcus aureus*. J Med Microbiol 1975; 8: 137–147

35 Cutler R R. Relationship between antibiotic resistance, the production of "virulence factors", and virulence for experimental animals in *Staphylococcus aureus*. J Med Microbiol. 1979; 12: 55–62

36 Lacey R W. Do bacteria mutate to erythromycin resistance? Scot Med J 1977; 22: 367–374

37 Noble W C. Variation in the prevalence of antibiotic resistance of *Staphylococcus aureus* from human skin and nares. J Gen Microbiol 1977; 98: 125–132

38 Noble W C. Selection of penicillin resistant staphylococci on murine skin. Br J Exp Path (In press)

39 Butcher G W, King G, Dyke K G H. Sensitivity of *Staphylococcus aureus* to unsaturated fatty acids. J Gen Microbiol 1976; 94: 290–296

40 Jacob A E, Hobbs S J. Conjugal transfer of plasmid-borne multiple antibiotic resistance in *Streptococcus faecalis* var. *zymogenes*. J Bacteriol 1974; 117: 360–372

41 Clewell D B. Plasmids, drug resistance, and gene transfer in the genus *Streptococcus*. Microbiol Rev 1981; 45: 409–436

42 Malke H. Transduction in group A streptococci. In: Wannamaker L W, Matsen J M, eds. Streptococci and streptococcal disease. New York: Academic Press, 1972; 119–133

43 Miyamoto Y, Takizawa K, Matsushima A, Asai Y, Nakatsuka S. Antibiotic-resistance patterns among group-A streptococci isolated in Japan and their relation to serotype. In: Parker M T, ed. Pathogenic streptococci. Surrey: Reedbooks, 1978; 271–272

44 Franke A E, Clewell D B. Evidence for a chromosome-borne resistance transposon (Tn*916*) in *Streptococcus faecalis* that is capable of "conjugal" transfer in the absence of a conjugative plasmid. J Bacteriol 1981; 145: 494–502

45 Dunny G M, Craig R A, Carron R L, Clewell D B. Plasmid transfer in *Streptococcus faecalis*: Production of multiple sex pheromones by recipients. Plasmid 1979; 2: 454–465

46 Hershfield V. Plasmids mediating multiple drug resistance in group B streptococcus: transferability and molecular properties. Plasmid 1979; 2: 137–149

47 Engel H W B, Soedirman N, Rost J A, van Leeuwen W J, van Embden J D A. Transferabiity of macrolide, lincomycin and streptogramin resistances between group A, B and D streptococci, *streptococcus pneumoniae* and *Staphylococcus aureus*. J Bacteriol 1980; 142: 407–413

48 Jacobs M R, Koornhof H J, Robins-Browne R M. Emergence of multiply resistant pneumococci. New Eng J Med 1978; 299: 735–740

49 Buu-hoï A, Horodniceanu T. Conjugative transfer of multiple antibiotic resistance markers in Streptococcus pneumoniae. J Bacteriol 1980; 143: 313–320

50 Courvalin P M, Carlier C, Croissant O, Blangy D. Identification of two plasmids determining resistance to tetracycline and to erythromycin in group D streptococcus. MGG 1974; 132: 181–192

51 Horodniceanu T, Bouanchaud D H, Bieth G, Chabbert Y A. R plasmids in *Streptococcus agalactiae* Group B. Antimicrob Agents Chemother 1976; 10: 795–801

52 El-Solh N, Bouanchaud D H, Horodniceanu T, Roussel A, Chabbert Y A. Molecular studies and possible relatedness between R plasmids from groups B and D streptococci. Antimicrob Agents Chemother 1978; 14: 19–23

53 Weisblum B, Holder S B, Halling S M. Deoxyribonucleis acid sequence common to staphylococcal and streptococcal plasmids which specify erythromycin resistance. J Bacteriol 1979; 138: 990–998

54 Docherty A, Grandi G, Grandi R, Gryczan T J, Shivakumar A G, Dubnau D. Naturally occurring macrolide-lincosamide—streptogramin B resistance in *Bacillus licheniformis*. J Bacteriol 1981; 145: 129–137

55 Malke H, Reichardt W, Hartmann M, Walter F. Genetic study of plasmid-associated zonal resistance to lincomycin in *Streptococcus pyogenes*. Antimicrob Agents Chemother 1981; 19: 91–100

56 Shanson D C. Antibiotic-resistance *Staphylococcus aureus*. J Hosp Inf 1981; 2: 11–36

57 Rosypal S, Rosypalova A. Genetics of *Staphylococcus aureus*. Folia Facultatis Scientiarum Naturalium Universitatis Purkynianae Brunensis 1981; Tomus 23 Opus 6: 5–147

British Medical Bulletin (1984) Vol. 40, No. 1, pp. 84–90

DRUG RESISTANCE IN MYCOBACTERIA

D A MITCHISON MB FRCP FRCPath

MRC Unit for Laboratory Studies of Tuberculosis
Royal Postgraduate Medical School
London

1   Origins of drug resistance
2   Mutant structure and response to chemotherapy
3   Nomenclature
4   Factors influencing the emergence of resistance
    a Cross-resistance
    b Initial resistance
    c Drug potency
    d Numbers of viable bacilli
5   Prognostic importance of resistance
6   Uses for sensitivity testing in tuberculosis
    a Epidemiological
    b Failure and relapse
7   The prevalence of drug-resistant strains
    References

The treatment of tuberculosis has been revolutionized over the past 25 years by the advent of potent antibacterial drugs. Although, worldwide, about 10 million persons still contract the disease and at least 3 million die each year, modern chemotherapy is almost always capable of achieving longlasting quiescent disease, or in other words a cure, if the disease is recognized sufficiently early and effective drug regimens are prescribed and taken for sufficiently long. The success of this treatment has been due to the prevention of the emergence of drug-resistant tubercle bacilli by the use of combined chemotherapy, in which more than one drug is given to the patient, at least in the initial months of the regimen. Efficient, available chemotherapy is essential for the success of a case-finding and treatment programme, now recognized as the most effective measure for controlling tuberculosis.

In the second most important mycobacterial disease, leprosy, the necessity of using combined chemotherapy has only been recognized in recent years. Because dapsone is so effective and so cheap, it has unfortunately been given in monotherapy on a world-wide scale and, despite evidence of the increasing frequency of infections due to dapsone-resistant strains, it continues to be used in this way in many countries. The alternative policy of combined treatment, including substantially more expensive antibacterial drugs, is only being introduced gradually at present.

1   Origins of Drug Resistance

Drug resistance can emerge to all of the antibacterial drugs used in the treatment of mycobacterial disease. It occurs most commonly when a single drug is given alone and when the viable bacterial population in the lesions is large. In tuberculosis, it first appears after an interval of at least 2 weeks and more usually 1–4 months after the start of chemotherapy. In leprosy, dapsone resistance was first recognized in patients with multibacillary (lepromatous) disease some 20 years after the introduction of the drug.[1] The occurrence of drug resistance is widely thought to be due to the overgrowth of sensitive organisms by mutant resistant bacilli present in wild strains before they were ever in contact with the drug concerned. Performance of the fluctuation test of Luria and Delbrück indicated mutation rates in *Mycobacterium tuberculosis* of about 2×10^{-8} for resistance to isoniazid and streptomycin, 2×10^{-10} for rifampicin and 1×10^{-7} for ethambutol.[2] The proportion of resistant mutants is variable from one culture to another and, for most drugs, is much greater for mutants with low minimal inhibitory concentrations (MICs) than for those with higher MICs.[3,4] In very approximate terms, the ratio of mutants able to grow during treatment to sensitive organisms in wild strains is about $1:10^6$ for isoniazid and streptomycin and $1:10^7$ for rifampicin.[2,3]

Mutation to drug resistance is usually thought to occur in bacterial chromosomes. The isolation of plasmids from opportunist or saprophytic mycobacteria has been described[5,6,7] (though not from *M. tuberculosis*, *M. bovis* or *M. leprae*). Although it has been claimed that these plasmids are associated with aminoglycoside resistance, the issue is still uncertain. It seems reasonable to assume that resistance to isoniazid, rifampicin, pyrazinamide, dapsone and other non-aminoglycoside drugs is always chromosomal and that resistance to streptomycin and other aminoglycosides in tubercle bacilli is probably also chromosomal. In the treatment of tuberculosis, the pattern of the emergence of resistance suggests little linkage between unrelated drugs, even among the aminoglycosides, though there are several well-established patterns of cross-resistance between closely related drugs. The species of mycobacteria that are well adapted to a parasitic role in man, *M. tuberculosis*, *M. africanum*, *M. bovis* and *M. leprae*, all exist within closed lesions in human or animal hosts and do not come into contact with other bacteria, including other strains of mycobacteria, which might transmit plasmids to them. Thus a plasmid-mediated resistance system could not readily be exploited by them to increase their genetic variability.

2   Mutant Structure and Response to Chemotherapy

The relationship between mutant structure, drug dosage and the response of newly diagnosed patients with pulmonary tuberculosis to treatment with isoniazid was thoroughly explored during the period when this drug was being used alone in clinical studies.[8,9,10] The rate at which isoniazid is acetylated to microbiologically inactive acetylisoniazid in man is genetically controlled by a single gene, about 40% of most populations (including Indians) being virtually indistinguishable homozygous or heterozygous rapid inactivators and the remainder slow inactivators. In a comparison of the plasma isoniazid concentration time curves for rapid and slow inactivators, rapid inactivators had only a slightly lower peak concentration than slow inactivators, but had much smaller areas under the curve (exposure) and much shorter durations of coverage during which a bacteriostatic concentration is maintained. Table I shows that there was a good association between response and peak concentration but little with exposure or coverage. According to the mechanism suggested to explain the association, isoniazid-resistant mutants with increasingly high degrees of resistance were inhibited by the concentrations reached near the peak as the size of the dose of isoniazid was raised.[11] It is of interest that the improvement in response with increasing dose size appeared to flatten off at about 8.7 mg/kg body weight in slow inactivators, when the peak concentration was about 6 mg/l. Canetti & Grosset[3] found that mutants capable of growth on 5 mg/l or more in vitro were all highly

TABLE I. Response to treatment with isoniazid alone related to peak serum concentrations of isoniazid

Dosage of isoniazid (mg/kg)	No. of doses per day	Inactivator status	Patients		Peak concentration (mg/l)	Coverage after 1 day's dose (h)	Exposure per day*
			Total	Favourable (%)			
2.2[8]	2	rapid	36	44	0.7	4—12	4.5
		slow	46	48	1.2	26+	10.8
4.4[8]	2	rapid	27	56	1.9	26+	8.7
		slow	39	59	2.6	26+	20.9
8.7[8]	1	rapid	32	66	4.2	14	8.7
		slow	36	72	6.6	26+	20.9
13.9[9,10]	1	rapid	62	66	8.4	15	13.9
		slow	81	69	9.2	26+	33.4

* The dose size of isoniazid in mg/kg body weight multiplied by 1.0 for rapid inactivators and by 2.4 for slow inactivators, i.e. a value proportional to the area under the serum concentration–time curve

resistant, so that one would expect no increase in the numbers of mutants inhibited in the lesions when patients were treated with doses higher than about 8.7 mg/kg.

A similar relationship between dose size, mutant structure and response has been postulated in recommending the dose of dapsone to be used in the treatment of leprosy. There is indirect evidence, derived from the stepwise pattern of the evolution of resistance to *M. leprae*[12,13] and from biochemical genetic studies on the mechanism of sulphonamide and dapsone resistance in *Streptococcus pneumoniae*,[14] that a mutant structure exists consisting of numerous mutants with low levels of resistance and much rarer mutants with higher degrees of resistance. If this is true, then dosage with as little as 1 mg dapsone daily, though capable of inhibiting sensitive *M. leprae* as effectively as does higher conventional dosage,[15,16] would allow the numerous, low resistance mutants to grow. Thus, the conventional dose size of 100 mg daily continues to be recommended to reduce the mutants selected to those that have high degrees of resistance and occur relatively rarely.

3 Nomenclature

A specialized nomenclature is used to describe the isolation of resistant organisms from patients in relation to their history of previous chemotherapy. Primary resistance is the term used when the strains of mycobacteria are either naturally resistant to the drug, for instance the universal pyrazinamide-resistance of *M. bovis*, or have acquired resistance in another person as a result of ineffective chemotherapy. Initial resistance is the isolation of a resistant strain from a patient who claims never to have had chemotherapy; it includes primary resistance and also undisclosed acquired resistance—undisclosed either because the patient is unaware that he has received chemotherapy previously—e.g., isoniazid in a simple cough medicine—or because there is insufficient trust between him and his new medical advisers. Finally, a patient may give a frank history of previous unsuccessful chemotherapy and is then said to have disclosed acquired resistance.

4 Factors Influencing the Emergence of Resistance

In theory, giving two drugs together should eliminate the emergence of resistant organisms since one drug should prevent the growth of mutants resistant to the other drug. As mutants comprise about $1:10^6$ of the bacterial population in tuberculosis, a doubly resistant mutant should only occur once if the total population were about 10^{12}, perhaps 100 times higher than the occurrence rate even in extensive pulmonary tuberculosis. In multibacillary leprosy, the bacterial population may well exceed that found in tuberculosis. However, peak serum and tissue

dapsone concentrations exceed its minimal inhibitory concentration by about 500 times,[17] so that the proportion of resistant mutants capable of growth while a patient is receiving a full dose of 100 mg daily is likely to be very low[18] and double-drug therapy should be effective. There are several reasons why the ideal of total protection by two-drug therapy might not be achieved.

a *Cross-Resistance*

There may be cross-resistance between the two drugs, so that inhibition of one or both sets of mutants is absent or incomplete. Examples in *M. tuberculosis* are partial cross-resistance between thiacetazone and ethionamide[19] and between capreomycin, viomycin and kanamycin,[20,21] while complete cross-resistance occurs between kanamycin and amikacin.[22] In practice, cross-resistance is a rare cause of the emergence of resistance.

b *Initial Resistance*

A patient may be started on treatment with two drugs, but have initial resistance to one of them, so that there is little or no inhibition of the mutants resistant to the other drug. However, it should be noted that 10 of 20 patients with severe pulmonary tuberculosis and primary isoniazid resistance showed a definite initial bacteriological response to treatment with isoniazid alone or isoniazid and *para*-aminosalicylic acid (PAS),[23] and 4 of 10 patients with strains initially resistant to PAS, streptomycin and isoniazid nevertheless attained quiescent disease when treated with these three drugs.[24]

c *Drug Potency*

Drugs vary in their ability to suppress the emergence of resistance to another drug. A highly potent drug is able to prevent the growth of—and usually kills—all the organisms in the lesion, and continue to do so despite minor irregularity in drug taking by the patient. This implies that drug concentrations considerably higher than the MIC are present for some of the time, that drug action is not reduced by pH or other environmental factors, and that exposure to the drug is followed by a period of several days (in tuberculosis) or several weeks (in leprosy) in which the organisms do not begin to grow again.[25] Examples of less potent drugs are: streptomycin, because it does not act on bacilli in an acid environment, as may occur inside macrophages or extracellularly in areas of acute inflammation; pyrazinamide because it only acts on bacilli at pH values of less than about 5.6; thiacetazone because it is only bacteriostatic and bacilli will start to grow again if a dose is missed. Other drugs, such as ethambutol, kanamycin and ethionamide can only be given in suboptimal dosages because of the risks of toxicity.

While we can hope to explain the efficacy of a drug in preventing the emergence of resistance from its in-vitro characteristics and its pharmacology, the ultimate evaluation depends upon its behaviour

TABLE II. Relative activity of antibacterial drugs in preventing the emergence of resistance to isoniazid or rifampicin

Study	Drug combination		No. of patients	Failures of treatment	
	Primary	Secondary		No.	%
E. Africa	isoniazid	rifampicin	183	1	0.5
	isoniazid	streptomycin	96	2	2
Madras	isoniazid	ethambutol*	105	4	4
	isoniazid	PAS	309	37	12
E. Africa	isoniazid	thiacetazone	423	68	16
Hong Kong**	rifampicin	ethambutol	57	10	18

* With an initial supplement of streptomycin daily for 2 weeks
** Reserve regimen for failure patients

in clinical studies. Table II sets out the efficacy of several drugs (the secondary drug) in preventing the emergence of resistance to isoniazid or rifampicin (the primary drug), when given with this drug in double-drug chemotherapy for severe pulmonary tuberculosis.[26,27] The same methods have been used throughout these studies for measuring the emergence of isoniazid resistance. In the studies with isoniazid as the primary drug, all patients were newly diagnosed. However, in the study with rifampicin and ethambutol, the patients were being re-treated after failure with a first-line regimen. It is evident that rifampicin was highly effective in preventing the emergence of isoniazid resistance in almost all patients. Streptomycin and ethambutol were less effective, allowing failure with emergence of ioniazid resistance to occur in 2–4% of patients, while thiacetazone and PAS were much less effective, with 12–16% of failures. The finding (Table II) that ethambutol failed to prevent rifampicin resistance emerging in 18% of patients while failure occurred in only 4% of patients treated with ethambutol and isoniazid, suggests that rifampicin is less potent than isoniazid. This conclusion is in keeping with evidence that the usual dosage of rifampicin (10mg/kg body weight/day) may not be optimal, whereas no advantage has ever been found to result from increasing the usual dose size of isoniazid (300mg/day).[28] In practice, it is usual for the treatment of pulmonary tuberculosis to be started with three drugs, partly because even the most effective pair (isoniazid and rifampicin) does not always prevent the emergence of resistance and partly to guard against the possibility that the occurrence of initial isoniazid resistance might lead in effect to giving monotherapy.

d *Numbers of Viable Bacilli*

The probability of resistance emerging is clearly greatly influenced by the number of viable bacilli in the lesions at the time that chemotherapy is started or a regimen changed. In tuberculosis, the risk is greatest in cavitated, pulmonary lesions with bacillary populations of perhaps 10^8–10^9 colony forming units

(c.f.u.) which are usually treated with three drugs initially. However, the risk is so small in closed tuberculomata, with populations usually of less than 100c.f.u., that monotherapy is justified. Lesions with fairly small bacterial populations, such as bone and joint tuberculosis and tuberculosis meningitis, could probably be safely treated with a two-drug regimen of isoniazid and rifampicin, since even if there was initial resistance to isoniazid, the probability of there being sufficient organisms to allow rifampicin resistance to emerge would be small. Again, monotherapy with isoniazid or, on an experimental basis, with rifampicin is to be recommended for chemoprophylaxis in contacts or patients with minimal inactive lesions. While chemotherapy for pulmonary lesions is usually started with two or three drugs given together for the first 2–3 months, the continuation can safely be with isoniazid alone because the numbers of viable bacilli at risk from which mutants might grow has by then been reduced to a very low level.[29]

Ellard[18] has outlined the rationale behind the current recommended treatment for multibacillary leprosy, which is daily dapsone and clofazimine supplemented by supervised once-monthly doses of rifampicin and clofazimine. Studies are required to assess the benefits of adding a fourth drug, ethionamide or prothionamide. This regimen of three (or four) drugs is designed to provide effective therapy even if initial dapsone resistance is present. A further recommendation is that paucibacillary (tuberculoid) leprosy patients should be treated with daily dapsone supplemented with once-monthly doses of rifampicin for six months, on the grounds that even if initial dapsone resistance is present, rifampicin should be sufficiently effective on its own.

5 Prognostic Importance of Resistance

Data on the prognostic influence of initial drug resistance in tuberculosis have been drawn entirely from studies carried out under the auspices of the Medical Research Council, since it is only in these studies that treatment was continued without alteration despite a finding of initial resistance, and the methods of sensitivity testing were also the same. The influence of primary or initial drug resistance on the results of the chemotherapy of newly diagnosed, severe, pulmonary tuberculosis with isoniazid alone or isoniazid and a weak second drug such as PAS or thiacetazone are summarized in Table III. The prognostic effect was considerable. Thus, in the pooled results of four controlled clinical trials carried out at the Tuberculosis Chemotherapy Centre, Madras, 15 (71%) of 21 patients with primary isoniazid resistance had an unfavourable response with bacteriologically active disease at the end of treatment, as compared with only 14% of patients with sensitive organisms on admission to the study. Similar results were obtained in four co-operative studies in East African centres in which patients were treated either with isoniazid and PAS or with

TABLE III. Response of patients with primary or initial resistance to isoniazid to chemotherapy with isoniazid alone or to isoniazid plus PAS or thiacetazone

Study and reference	Resistant organisms					Sensitive organisms		
	Type of resistance	Chemotherapy given	No. of patients	Unfavourable		No. of patients	Unfavourable	
				No.	%		No.	%
Madras: 1 study[23]	primary	H	6	5	83	216	93	43
Madras: 4 studies[41]	primary	PH	21	15	71	389	53	14
E. Africa: 4 studies[45]	initial	PH	21	10	48	176	30	17
		TH	39	24	62	304	84	28

Abbreviations: H: isoniazid; PH: PAS plus isoniazid; TH: thiacetazone plus isoniazid

isoniazid and thiacetazone. These results were obtained in the 1960s when there was little alternative to PAS or thiacetazone as companion drugs to be given to prevent the emergence of resistance to isoniazid, particularly in developing countries.

The position has, however, completely changed as the result of the introduction of newer and more potent drugs and the development during the last decade of short-course regimens which greatly reduce the period of treatment necessary to obtain a bacteriologically quiescent status.[30] The most important of these drugs, whose action has been reviewed elsewhere,[31] is rifampicin, excellent both as a sterilizing drug which kills the last few semi-dormant organisms in the lesion (and thereby reduces the duration of therapy) and also, as we have seen, in preventing growth of organisms throughout the lesions and therefore the emergence of resistance to a companion drug. Pyrazinamide is almost as good as a sterilizing drug, but is much less effective than rifampicin in preventing the emergence of resistance. Ethambutol appears to be of no value as a sterilizing drug, but is moderately effective in preventing resistance. The prognostic influence of initial resistance to isoniazid alone or to isoniazid and streptomycin in the pooled results from a series of studies of short-course regimens including these drugs[32] is set out in Table IV. The results obtained in patients with initially sensitive organisms are not included since they are, with very few exceptions, uniformly favourable, irrespective of the regimen. Results in patients with initial resistance to streptomycin only are also omitted, since this resistance did not appear to influence the response to treatment. The first two lines of the table describe regimens in which four drugs, including rifampicin, were given for one or two months in an initial intensive phase and were followed by a continuation regimen of thiacetazone and isoniazid or twice-weekly streptomycin, isoniazid and pyrazinamide lasting 6–8 months in all. These regimens are particularly useful for developing countries who wish to minimize the high cost of rifampicin and who also wish to confine its prescription to patients being treated initially in hospital and thereby avoid wider-scale uncontrolled use for other diseases in the community. Although the regimen with a one-month initial intensive phase was highly successful, at least under clinical trial conditions, in patients with initially sensitive organisms, 20% of those with initial resistance to isoniazid only and 100% of those with double resistance to isoniazid and streptomycin failed, with the emergence of positive bacteriology during chemotherapy. As might be expected, the proportions of failures were lower when the initial intensive phase lasted two months. It is of interest that of the 20 patients in the regimens with initial intensive phases of one or two months who failed, additional

resistance emerged in only seven (four to rifampicin and three to streptomycin), so that a failure usually did not compromise further treatment of the patient. When the duration of the treatment with rifampicin was extended to 4–6 months, much better results were obtained in those with initial resistance. Addition of streptomycin to the basic regimen of rifampicin and isoniazid prevented failures in those with initial resistance to isoniazid only, but, as might be expected, not in those with double resistance. However, if pyrazinamide was added, only 2 of 51 patients with initial resistance failed and if the regimen included ethambutol as well, there were no failures among the 50 patients with initial resistance who were then treated for six months. The reason for these excellent results is clear enough. Initial resistance to rifampicin, pyrazinamide and ethambutol is still very rare in previously untreated patients. Even at the start of treatment, when high viable bacterial populations were present, the emergence of resistance was prevented by rifampicin together with ethambutol and pyrazinamide; in the later phases, the populations were sufficiently small to prevent resistance emerging to rifampicin given in effect alone, or even to other weaker drugs. The duration of the treatment with rifampicin was, however, the dominant factor determining the result. Cultures from all of the 14 patients whose treatment for four or more months with rifampicin failed, had developed additional resistance to rifampicin.

An aspect of these findings of practical value in the UK and other technically advanced countries, is that the occurrence of initial drug resistance to isoniazid or to isoniazid and streptomycin is not a reason for changing chemotherapy with the current three-drug regimens of isoniazid, rifampicin and ethambutol introduced by the British Thoracic Association.[33] The same argument applies with even greater force when the regimen, under current study, of isoniazid, rifampicin, pyrazinamide and ethambutol[34] is widely used. No change is necessary because the results will be so good in any case.

There is as yet no evidence from clinical studies that regimens with three or four drugs will be capable of curing multibacillary leprosy in the presence of initial dapsone resistance. However, the rationale is similar to that underlying short-course chemotherapy of tuberculosis and the analogies suggest that it will be just as successful.

6   Uses for Sensitivity Testing in Tuberculosis

There are two circumstances under which tests for sensitivity of strains of *M. tuberculosis* to antibacterial drugs are recommended.

TABLE IV. Response of patients with initial resistance to short-course chemotherapy with regimens containing rifampicin

Duration of rifampicin administration (months)	Drugs in addition to HR	Regimen	Resistance to H only			Resistance to SH		
			No. of patients	Unfavourable		No. of patients	Unfavourable	
				No.	%		No.	%
1	SZ	1SHRZ/TH or SHZ(2)*	20	4	20	5	5	100
2	SZ	2SHRZ/TH or SHZ(2)	39	3	8	19	8	42
4–6	–	HR	9	1	11	8	3	12
	S	SHR	32	0	0	22	8	36
	SZ	2SHRZ/HRZ or HR, SHRZ(3), 4SHRZ(3)/SHZ(2)	33	0	0	18	2	11
	EZ, ESZ	HRZE, HRZE(3), HRSZE(3)	22	0	0	28	0	0

Abbreviations: H: isoniazid; S: streptomycin; R: rifampicin; Z: pyrazinamide; T: thiacetazone; E: ethambutol
* A number at the start of the drug list describing the regimen indicates the duration in months of an initial intensive phase of chemotherapy. A number in parentheses after the drug list indicates the number of drug doses given in a week. The absence of a number in parentheses indicates daily dosage

TABLE V. Prevalence of primary or initial drug resistance of *M. tuberculosis* in selected national surveys

Country	Date	Type of resistance	Total patients	Per cent prevalence of resistance to:				
				Any	H	S	SH	SHR
UK[46]	1955–6	primary	976	3.1	0.5	2.0	0.2	–
England & Wales[47]	1960	primary	1338	3.4	0.5	1.6	0.4	–
UK[48]	1963	primary	896	4.1	0.7	2.0	0.8	–
England & Wales[35]	1978–9	primary	1038	3.0	1.1	1.1	0.7	0.1
UK[49]	1960–1	acquired	410	81.7	17.8	7.3	55.9	–
Hong Kong[50]	1962	initial	302	20.0	8.0	4.0	6.3	–
	1962	acquired	262	61.8	24.0	6.9	30.2	–
Kenya[51,52]	1964	initial	632	14.7	8.9	0.8	1.4	–
	1974	initial	702	10.1	7.3	1.4	1.4	–
Tanzania[53]	1969–70	initial	636	9.3	4.9	4.4	1.4	–
India[54]	1964–5	initial	1838	20.4	8.2	5.8	6.5	–

Abbreviations: H: isoniazid; S: streptomycin; R: rifampicin

a *Epidemiological*

Surveys have been done to estimate the prevalence of drug resistance in newly diagnosed patients, and, more rarely, in patients with a history of previous treatment to obtain information about the pool of drug-resistant strains within the community. Surveys may also monitor other aspects of the national tuberculosis service, such as the types of disease being encountered, the chemotherapy given and its results. Such surveys are of great value in guiding policy decisions for the service, highlighting weaknesses in its practice and establishing its success in diagnosing and treating the disease. Estimates of initial drug resistance are fairly easy to obtain but it is much more difficult to establish data for primary resistance, particularly in developing countries. Unless circumstances are exceptional, surveys carried out in developing countries on patients claiming not to have had previous treatment usually estimate initial resistance, whose incidence may be at least twice that of primary resistance. In technically advanced countries, patients have fewer reasons for hiding a history of previous treatment and usually know more about its details, so that an estimate of true primary resistance can often be obtained.

Several surveys of the prevalence of drug resistance have been done in UK (Table V) and other technically advanced countries. In general, they demonstrate that the prevalence of primary resistance is low, occurring in about 3–4% of patients, and has not altered appreciably over the past 25 years. In fact, in the UK 1978–9 survey,[35] the prevalence among white patients had fallen to 1.6% and was only maintained at the overall 3.0% level by a much higher rate (7.5%) in those of Indian subcontinent extraction. An important reason for continuing to do these surveys is to see whether primary resistance to rifampicin, pyrazinamide and ethambutol is appearing. In the UK 1978–9 survey, 1 of 1070 strains with sensitivity tests was resistant to rifampicin as well as to isoniazid and streptomycin.

Surveys in developing countries (Table V) serve more directly useful purposes. Initial resistance reflects not only the level of primary resistance but also such matters as the degree of co-operation between patients and the tuberculosis service, the availability of sufficient drug for the administration of effective chemotherapy and the mishandling of treatment by general practitioners before the patients reach the government services. Thus a high prevalence of resistance usually means inefficient arrangements for treatment (as viewed in all of its aspects). The prevalence of resistance is also a good indicator of the type of chemotherapy that should be used in a community. Thus a prevalence of initial isoniazid-resistant strains of over 15% might be taken to indicate that regimens which are capable of giving highly successful results in patients with pretreatment resistance should be used, if they can be afforded, for the routine treatment of newly diagnosed cases. Such regimens would start with an initial phase of four drugs, and would include rifampicin for at least four months. On the other hand, simpler and cheaper regimens would be acceptable if a prevalence of 10% or less were found.

Occasional surveys have been carried out on patients known to have received previous chemotherapy (Table V). A high proportion (62–82%) of their strains had acquired resistance, often to both isoniazid and streptomycin. These patients constitute a reservoir which acts as a source of primary resistance. When possible, public health authorities should attempt to estimate the size of the problem and take steps, principally by improving the standards of primary chemotherapy, to reduce the size of the reservoir.

b *Failure or Relapse*

If a patient with pulmonary tuberculosis converts from positive to negative smears or cultures of sputum during chemotherapy and then reverts to having several positive results again, the fall and rise phenomenon has occurred. Alternatively, occasional patients may show no apparent changes in serial bacteriological examinations despite several months of chemotherapy. In either circumstance, a failure is said to have occurred if the positive bacteriology has taken place during chemotherapy and a relapse if it has happened after the end of chemotherapy. A failure, when it occurs during chemotherapy including isoniazid, is always accompanied by the emergence of resistance to isoniazid and often to the other drugs being used in treatment.[36] On the other hand, the organisms obtained at relapse, as after completion of regimens of short-course chemotherapy, are usually still sensitive and the patient responds well to repetition of treatment with the drugs used previously.[37] While these conclusions are useful in guiding the choice of further treatment, the situation is seldom so simple. A failure may occur because the patient is not in fact taking drugs or is taking them very irregularly, despite regular attendance at a clinic, and the organisms may then remain sensitive. Alternatively, grossly irregular drug-taking may lead to the emergence of resistance only evident when a bacteriological relapse occurs after the end of the prescribed period of treatment. These uncertainties point to the necessity of doing sensitivity tests on cultures obtained at failure or relapse to decide to which drugs the organisms are still sensitive and so determine the most effective further chemotherapy.

In summary, the collection of epidemiological data on the prevalence of primary or initial drug resistance and the sensitivity testing of cultures from patients whose treatment has failed or have had a relapse are of considerable importance both in technically advanced and in developing countries. The sensitivity test service should be confined to a small number of laboratories, to ensure a continuing interest in the specialized techniques that are used. In developing countries, the service, if available at all, may only be provided by a single central laboratory usually in the capital city. If so, it would be advantageous for other less specialized laboratories to undertake the culture of specimens and then to send the cultures to the central laboratory for sensitivity testing.

7 The Prevalence of Drug-Resistant Strains

As far as is known from tests of dubious accuracy on limited numbers of strains, all isolates of *M. tuberculosis* had similar degrees of sensitivity to each of the antibacterial drugs when these were first introduced for chemotherapy. This suggests that the mutation rate to resistance is balanced by a tendency for resistant strains to revert to sensitivity or by a failure of the resistant mutants to grow as successfully as the sensitive organisms. The occurrence of reversion from isoniazid resistance to sensitivity was shown by Schmidt et al.,[38] who first passaged a resistant strain several times in isoniazid-containing medium to remove any residual sensitive bacilli, then infected monkeys by the tracheal route to allow multiplication within the tissues and finally injected lesional material into guinea pigs. Highly isoniazid-resistant, catalase-negative, organisms are of low virulence in the guinea pig, which therefore acted as selective agents for sensitive organisms.[39, 40] The organs of 50 of the 62 guinea pigs infected with monkey tissue yielded cultures that were isoniazid sensitive or had mixtures of sensitive and resistant organisms. There is some evidence that highly isoniazid-resistant *M. tuberculosis* are also of slightly reduced pathogenicity in man. Thus, resistant strains from patients with primary resistance have been found to have a lower degree of resistance and therefore a higher catalase activity and guinea-pig virulence than strains from patients with acquired resistance.[41] This finding suggests selection of the more virulent organisms during establishment of an active lesion in the contact of a patient with acquired resistance. Further evidence is provided by a study of the infectivity of groups of patients who were treated with different regimens of isoniazid alone or isoniazid plus PAS and therefore excreted widely different numbers of resistant organisms in their sputum. Over a five-year period, the risk of their family contacts developing tuberculosis, or indeed disease due to isoniazid resistant strains, was not related to the degree of exposure to the resistant organisms.[42] Similar data is not available for resistance to other drugs, though in-vitro studies have shown that strains of *Escherichia coli* with low degrees of resistance to streptomycin are rapidly overgrown in mixtures by their sensitive parents.[43]

We have already seen that in UK and probably other technically advanced countries, the balance between creation of resistance and reversion to sensitivity tends towards the slow elimination of resistance. In developing coutnries, standards of chemotherapy are far less satisfactory and the selection pressure in favour of resistance much greater. Estimates of initial resistance, usually the

TABLE VI. Prevalence of primary drug-resistance at the Tuberculosis Chemotherapy Centre, Madras, 1957–1974

(data from SP Tripathy, personal communication)

Year	No. of patients	Per cent prevalence of resistance to:		
		H	S	SH
1957	211–229	4	4	1
1958	263–269	6	3	1
1961	248–249	5	3	1
1962	204	6	8	2
1963	127	6	10	4
1964	194–196	5	5	2
1965	255	6	7	2
1967	238–242	7	7	4
1968	192–195	9	7	3
1969	191	9	4	1
1970	176	8	10	3
1971	264	9	9	5
1972	265	10	9	5
1973	255–256	11	13	5
1974	206	7	15	4

Abbreviations: H: isoniazid; S: streptomycin

only data available, are of little value in measuring the trend, but the Tuberculosis Chemotherapy Centre, Madras has been sufficiently effective in eliciting true histories of previous treatment in newly diagnosed patients to estimate approximate rates of primary resistance. The rates found in successive chemotherapy studies from 1957–1974 are set out in Table VI. There is probably an increase in the proportions found resistant to isoniazid, streptomycin and both drugs, though the prevalence is still only moderate at the end of the period. Furthermore, some of the apparent increase might be an artifact due to less successful questioning of patients and the inclusion of some with undisclosed acquired resistance. In summary, the accumulation of resistance in the community does not pose a serious threat to the control programme for tuberculosis, partly because it is small and slow, even in developing countries, and partly because of the introduction of short-course regimens which are effective in the presence of initial resistance. However, this happy state could easily be changed if initial rifampicin resistance were to become more common, as may well be occurring,[44] and every attempt should be made to prevent this happening, if necessary by confining the use of the drug to hospitals and the government health services in developing countries.

In contrast to the findings in tuberculosis there has been a striking increase in the prevalence of dapsone resistance in leprosy, due to the heavy selection pressure of monotherapy with this drug over a 30-year period. Ellard[18] estimates that there has been a 100-fold increase in the past 20 years, so that 10% of newly diagnosed patients in some centres may have resistant strains. This is a serious threat to the success of the leprosy control programme and is a very strong reason for learning the lesson provided by tuberculosis and rapidly introducing combined chemotherapy, even though it may increase the drug costs appreciably.

References

1 Pettit JHS, Rees RJW. Sulphone resistance in leprosy. An experimental and clinical study. Lancet 1964; 2: 673–674

2 David HL. Probability distribution of drug-resistant mutants in unselected populations of *Mycobacterium tuberculosis*. Appl Microbiol 1970; 20: 810–84

3 Canetti G, Grosset, J. Teneur des souches sauvages de *Mycobacterium tuberculosis* en variants résistants a l'isoniazide et en variants résistants a la streptomycine sur milieu de Loewenstein–Jensen. Ann Inst Pasteur 1961; 101: 28–46

4 Mitchison DA. The segregation of streptomycin-resistant variants of *Mycobacterium tuberculosis* into groups with characteristic levels of resistance. J Gen Microbiol 1951; 5: 596–604

5 Jones WD, David HL. Preliminary observations on the occurrence of a streptomycin R-factor in *Mycobacterium smegmatis* ATCC 607. Tubercle 1972; 53: 35–42

6 Crawford JT, Bates JH. Isolation of plasmids from mycobacteria. Infect Immun 1979; 24: 979–981

7 Mizuguchi Y, Fukunga M, Taniguchi H. Plasmid deoxyribonucleic acid and translucent-to-opaque variation in *Mycobacterium intracellulare* 103. J Bacteriol 1981; 146: 656–659

8 Tuberculosis Chemotherapy Centre, Madras. A concurrent comparison of isoniazid plus PAS with three regimens of isoniazid alone in the domiciliary treatment of pulmonary tuberculosis in South India. Bull WHO 1960; 23: 535–585

9 Mitchison DA. Plasma concentrations of isoniazid in the treatment of tuberculosis. In: Davies DS, Pritchard BNC, eds. Biological effects of drugs in relation to their plasma concentrations. London: Macmillan, 1973; 169–182

10 Tuberculosis Chemotherapy Centre, Madras. The prevention and treatment of isoniazid toxicity in the therapy of pulmonary tuberculosis. 2. An assessment of the prophylactic effect of pyridoxine in low dosage. Bull WHO 1963; 29: 457–481

11 Selkon JB, Devadatta S, Kulkarni KG et al. The emergence of isoniazid-resistant cultures in patients with pulmonary tuberculosis during treatment with isoniazid alone or isoniazid plus PAS. Bull WHO 1964; 31: 273–294

12 Rees RJW. Drug resistance of *Mycobacterium leprae* particularly to DDS. Int J Lepr 1967; 35: 625–638

13 Shepard CC, Levy L, Fasal P. The sensitivity to dapsone (DDS) of *Mycobacterium leprae* from patients with and without previous treatment. Am J Trop Med Hyg 1969; 18: 258–263

14 Hotchkiss RD, Evans AH. Fine structure of a genetically modified enzyme as revealed by relative affinities for modified substrate. Fed Proc 1960; 19: 912–925

15 Waters MFR, Rees RJW, Ellard GA. Experimental and clinical studies on the minimal inhibitory concentration (MIC) of dapsone (DDS) in leprosy [Abstract]. Int J Lepr 1968; 36: 651

16 Ellard GA, Gammon PT, Rees RJW, Waters MFR. Studies on the determination of the minimal inhibitory concentration of 4,4′-diamino-diphenyl-sulphone (Dapsone, DDS) against *Mycobacterium leprae*. Lepr Rev 1971; 42: 101–117

17 Colston MJ, Ellard GA, Gammon PT. Drugs for combined therapy: experimental studies on the antileprosy activity of ethionamide and prothionamide, and a general review. Lepr Rev 1978; 49: 115–126

18 Ellard G. Rationale of the multi-drug regimens recommended by a World Health Organisation study group on chemotherapy of leprosy. Int J Lepr 1983; In press

19 Bartmann K. Kreutzresistenz zwischen d-'A'thylthioisonicotinamid (1314 Th) und Thiosemicarbazon (Conteben). Tuberkulosearzt 1960; 14: 525–529

20 Tsukamura M, Mizuno S. Cross-resistance relationships among the aminoglucoside antibiotics in *Mycobacterium tuberculosis*. J Gen Microbiol 1975; 88: 269–274

21 McClatchy JK, Kanes W, Davidson PT, Moulding TS. Cross-resistance in *M. tuberculosis* to kanamycin, capreomycin and viomycin. Tubercle 1977; 58: 29–34

22 Allen BW, Mitchison DA, Chan YC, Yew WW, Allen WGL, Girling DJ. Amikacin in the treatment of tuberculosis. Tubercle 1983; 64: 111–118

23 Devadatta S, Bhatia AL, Andrews RH et al. Response of patients infected with isoniazid-resistant tubercle bacilli to treatment with isoniazid plus PAS or isoniazid alone. Bull WHO 1961; 25: 807–829

24 Hong Kong Tuberculosis Treatment Services/British Medical Research Council. A study in Hong Kong to evaluate the role of pretreatment susceptibility tests in the selection of regimens of chemotherapy for pulmonary tuberculosis. Am Rev Respir Dis 1972; 16: 1–22

25 Dickinson JM, Aber VR, Mitchison DA. Studies on the treatment of experimental tuberculosis of the guinea pig with intermittent doses of isoniazid. Tubercle 1973; 54: 211–224

26 Mitchison DA. Treatment of tuberculosis. The Mitchell Lecture 1979. J R Coll Physicians Lond 1980; 14: 91–99

27 Hong Kong Tuberculosis Treatment Services/Brompton Hospital/British Medical Research Council. A controlled trial of daily and intermittent rifampicin plus ethambutol in the retreatment of patients with pulmonary tuberculosis: Results up to 30 months. Tubercle 1975; 56: 179–189

28 Jindani A, Aber VR, Edwards EA, Mitchison DA. The early bactericidal activity of drugs in patients with pulmonary tuberculosis. Am Rev Respir Dis 1980; 121: 939–949

29 East and Central African and British Medical Research Council 5th Collaborative Study. Controlled trial of 5 short-course regimens of chemotherapy (three 6-month and one 8-month) for pulmonary tuberculosis. Tubercle 1983; 64: 53–66

30 Fox W. Whither short-course chemotherapy? Br J Dis Chest 1981; 75: 331–357

31 Mitchison DA. Basic mechanisms of chemotherapy. Chest 1979; 76S: 771–781S

32 Mitchison DA. Effect of initial drug resistance on short-course chemotherapy of pulmonary tuberculosis. In: Periti P, Grassi GG, eds. Current chemotherapy and immunotherapy. Proceedings of the 12th international congress of chemotherapy, Florence, Italy, 19th–24th July, 1981. Washington: American Society for Microbiology, 1982; 1004–1005

33 British Thoracic Association. Short-course chemotherapy in pulmonary tuberculosis. Lancet 1980; 1: 1182–1183

34 British Thoracic Association. A controlled trial of 6 months chemotherapy in pulmonary tuberculosis. Second report: results during the 24 months after the end of chemotherapy. Am Rev Respir Dis 1982; 126: 460–462

35 Medical Research Council Tuberculosis and Chest Diseases Unit. National survey of tuberculosis notifications in England and Wales 1978–9. Br Med J 1980; 281: 895–898

36 Tuberculosis Chemotherapy Centre, Madras. A controlled comparison of a twice-weekly and three once-weekly regimens in the initial treatment of pulmonary tuberculosis. Bull WHO 1970; 43: 143–206

37 Hong Kong Tuberculosis Treatment Services and East African and British Medical Research Councils. First-line chemotherapy in the retreatment of bacteriological relapses of pulmonary tuberculosis following a short-course regimen. Lancet 1976; 1: 162–163

38 Schmidt LH, Grover AA, Hoffmann R, Rehm J, Sullivan R. The emergence of isoniazid-sensitive bacilli in monkeys inoculated with isoniazid-resistant strains. In: Transactions 17th conference on the chemotherapy of tuberculosis, Washington DC. Veterans Administration Department of Medicine and Surgery, 1958; 264–269

39 Barnett M, Bushby SRM, Mitchison DA. Tubercle bacilli resistant to isoniazid: virulence and response to treatment with isoniazid in guinea-pigs and mice. Br J Exp Pathol 1953; 34: 568–581

40 Cohn ML, Kovitz C, Oda U, Middlebrook G. Studies on isoniazid and tubercle bacilli. II. The growth requirements, catalase activities, and pathogenic properties of isoniazid-resistant mutants. Am Rev Tuberc 1954; 70: 641–664

41 Tripathy SP, Menon NK, Mitchison DA et al. Response to treatment with isoniazid plus PAS of tuberculous patients with primary isoniazid resistance. Tubercle 1969; 50: 257–268

42 Devadatta S, Dawson JJY, Fox W et al. Attack rate of tuberculosis in a 5-year period among close family contacts of tuberculous patients under domiciliary treatment with isoniazid plus PAS or isoniazid alone. Bull WHO 1970; 42: 337–351

43 Mitchison DA. The occurrence of independent mutations to different types of streptomycin resistance in *Bacterium coli*. J Gen Microbiol 1953; 8: 168–185

44 Hong Kong Chest Service and British Medical Research Council. Controlled trial of 4 three-times-weekly regimens and a daily regimen all given for 6 months for pulmonary tuberculosis. Second report: the results up to 24 months. Tubercle 1982; 63: 89–98

45 East African and British Medical Research Councils. Influence of pretreatment bacterial resistance to isoniazid, thiacetazone or PAS on the response to chemotherapy of African patients with pulmonary tuberculosis. Tubercle 1963; 44: 393–416

46 Fox W, Wiener A, Mitchison DA, Selkon JB, Sutherland I. The prevalence of drug-resistant tubercle bacilli in untreated patients with pulmonary tuberculosis: a national survey, 1955–56. Tubercle 1957; 38: 71–84

47 Public Health Laboratory Service. Drug resistance in untreated pulmonary tuberculosis in England and Wales during 1960. Tubercle 1961; 42: 308–313

48 Miller AB, Tall R, Fox W, Lefford MJ, Mitchison DA. Primary drug resistance in Great Britain: second national survey, 1963. Tubercle 1966; 47: 92–108

49 British Tuberculosis Association. Acquired drug resistance in patients with pulmonary tuberculosis in Great Britain—a national survey, 1960–61. Tubercle 1963; 44: 1–26

50 Hong Kong Government Tuberculosis Service and British Medical Research Council. Drug-resistance in patients with pulmonary tuberculosis presenting at chest clinics in Hong Kong. Tubercle 1964; 45: 77–95

51 East African and British Medical Research Councils. Tuberculosis in Kenya: a national sampling survey of drug resistance and other factors. Tubercle 1968; 49: 136–169

52 East African and British Medical Research Councils. Tuberculosis in Kenya: a second national sampling survey of drug resistance and other factors, and a comparison with the prevalence data from the first national sampling survey. Tubercle 1978; 59: 155–177

53 East African and British Medical Research Council. Tuberculosis in Tanzania: a national sampling survey of drug resistance and other factors. Tubercle 1975; 56: 269–294

54 Indian Council of Medical Research. Prevalence of drug resistance in patients with pulmonary tuberculosis presenting for the first time with symptoms at chest clinics in India. Part I. Findings in urban clinics among patients giving no history of previous chemotherapy. Indian J Med Res 1968; 56: 1617–1630

British Medical Bulletin (1984) Vol. 40, No. 1, pp. 91–95

ANTIBIOTIC-RESISTANT BACTERIA IN ANIMAL HUSBANDRY

A H LINTON PhD DSc FRCPath

Department of Microbiology
University of Bristol

1   Acquired resistance in animal pathogens
2   Acquired antibiotic resistance in non-pathogenic bacteria
    associated with animals
3   The importance of antibiotic-resistant bacteria
    a   For animals
    b   For man
    References

The problem of antibiotic-resistant bacteria in animals parallels very closely that experienced in man. It arises by the same mechanisms under the selective pressure imposed by the use of antibiotics; the incidence of resistant bacteria is directly related to the intensity of antibiotic usage. Beside being used therapeutically, antibiotics are used widely in animals for prophylaxis, often on a herd basis.[1] They are also added in low concentrations to animal feeds to promote growth.

The amounts of antibiotics used for these purposes varies from country to country. Following the implementation in 1971 of the Swann recommendations,[2] the legal use of veterinary antibiotics in the UK was restricted to antibiotics issued on prescription but there have been many breaches of the legislation, largely helped by the availability of black-market antibiotics.[3] Many EEC countries have adopted similar control. It is difficult to obtain accurate information on the amounts of antibiotics used in animals in the UK, but in the USA, where antibiotics as feed additives are not restricted, approximately half of all antibiotics available are used for this purpose (Fig. 1).[4] In most Third World countries, antibiotics are as freely available for use in animals as in man.

In the light of these differences, it is not surprising that the incidence of antibiotic resistance varies from country to country. Other factors also influence this incidence; for instance, the heavier the stocking rate, especially in intensive systems of animal husbandry, the higher the incidence of infectious disease and, correspondingly, the greater the therapeutic use of antibiotics. Antibiotics are frequently administered prophylactically to counter the risks of infection in animals liable to stress during transportation.

Whether or not the route by which an antibiotic is administered has a greater or lesser influence on the indigenous microflora depends, at least in part, on the pharmokinetics of the antibiotic. For instance, chloramphenicol when given by injection can attain sufficient levels in the gut to exert an influence on the gut flora. In general, however, oral administration of antibiotics influences the indigenous flora of the alimentary tract more profoundly than administration by other routes.[5] This is highly relevant in the animal use of antibiotics since they are often mixed with animal feeds for therapy and growth promotion.

Antibiotic resistance arises both in pathogenic and non-pathogenic species of bacteria and the resistance may be

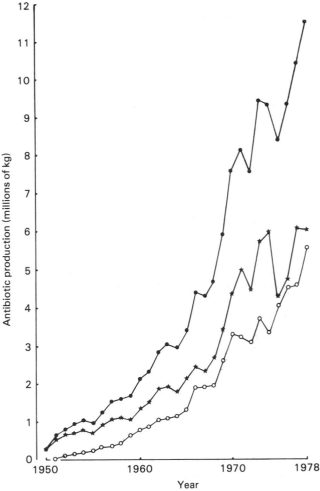

FIG. 1. Data on the quantities and uses of antibiotics produced in the USA from 1950–1978[4]

● total antibiotic produced; ★ quantities used medicinally in man and animals; ○ quantities incorporated in animal feeds as feed additives

transferred between them. Each will be considered separately and their potential interaction and importance for animals and man discussed.

1   Acquired Resistance in Animal Pathogens

Many groups of animal pathogens have not demonstrated acquired resistance even after many years of antibiotic usage. The streptococci causing mastitis in cows, for instance, are still as sensitive to benzyl penicillin as when they were first used. Rather, this one-time commonest cause of mastitis has fallen in incidence and has been superceded by infections with naturally penicillin-insusceptible bacteria e.g. *Escherichia coli*[6] and penicillin-resistant staphylococci.

In animals, acquired antibiotic resistance occurs mainly in two groups of organisms: *Staphylococcus aureus* and gram-negative rods, particularly the enteric organisms. Shortly after intramammary penicillin was introduced, strains of penicillin-resistant *S. aureus* began to appear. By 1961, 70% of all isolates were

TABLE I. The percentage of all salmonella isolates, submitted to the Central Veterinary Laboratory, resistant to individual drugs

(Data from Sojka & Wray, 1980[9] and personal communication)

	Su	Sm	Te	Cm	Ne	Ap	Fz	Tp
1971	55*	81	1	<1	<1	4	2	0
1972	39	91	3	1	4	1	<1	0
1973	66	76	5	<1	1	<1	1	0
1974	64	48	5	<1	1	<1	<1	0
1975	77	39	3	<1	1	<1	1	<1
1976	75	65	5	<1	1	1	1	<1
1977	49	46	9	6	1	1	1	<1
1978	66	54	18	12	6	7	1	1
1979	56	54	16	11	7	8	2	5
1980	54	35	15	7	4	4	1	8
1981	77	42	22	5	4	5	1	7

Abbreviations:
Su Sulphonamide (50 µg), Sm Streptomycin (10 µg), Te tetracycline (10 µg), Cm Chloramphenicol (10 µg), Ne Neomycin (10 µg), Ap Ampicillin (10 µg), Fz Furazolidone (15 µg), Tp Trimethoprim/sulphamethoxazole (25 µg).
* Data 1% and above rounded up to the nearest %.

Table II. Percentage of salmonella isolates from animals and their environment resistant to five important antibacterials

(after WJ Sojka and C Wray, personal communication)

	Te			Cm			Ne			Ap			Tp		
	A	B	C	A	B	C	A	B	C	A	B	C	A	B	C
1971	3	<1	1	<1	<1	0	1	<1	0	5	3	2	0	0	0
1972	3	<1	6	3	0	<1	9	<1	<1	<1	0	<1	0	0	0
1973	6	<1	7	<1	0	<1	3	0	<1	1	0	<1	0	0	0
1974	8	<1	3	<1	0	<1	2	0	<1	2	0	<1	0	0	0
1975	5	<1	2	<1	<1	<1	2	<1	<1	1	0	<1	<1	0	<1
1976	7	<1	4	1	0	<1	2	0	<1	1	1	1	1	<1	<1
1977	23	2	3	16	1	1	2	1	1	2	<1	11	<1	<1	<1
1978	38	2	4	28	2	1	14	1	<1	14	2	2	3	0	<1
1979	35	5	3	24	5	1	16	<1	<1	17	5	<1	11	<1	1
1980	33	1	4	17	<1	<1	8	1	<1	1	<1	<1	18	0	2
1981	48	1	5	12	<1	<1	12	0	<1	12	0	<1	14	0	2

A: *S. typhimurium*   B: *S. dublin*   C: Other serotypes
Abbreviations as for Table I.

penicillin-resistant,[7] mainly because they had acquired R plasmids coding for the production of the penicillin-destroying enzyme, β-lactamase; this percentage has been maintained to date.

Among the gram-negative pathogens, the presence of antibiotic resistance has been confined chiefly to the salmonella. The incidence of antibiotic resistance in these organisms differs markedly from that in the gram-negative members of the indigenous gut flora (see below). It varies also from one country to another but, in general, is not a serious therapeutic problem in most salmonella infections arising in animals. Oral antibiotics have been used extensively in animal husbandry and veterinary medicine over the last 30 years and, throughout this period, many outbreaks of salmonellosis in animals have occurred involving a wide range of serotypes.[3]

Despite the ongoing antibiotic selective pressure, relatively few outbreaks with multiple antibiotic-resistant strains have occurred in the UK.[3,8-13] An analysis of isolates of all salmonella serotypes submitted to the Central Veterinary Laboratory in the UK over the last 20 years demonstrated that resistance to only a few antibacterial agents has been encountered. For instance, resistance to sulphonamides and streptomycin has been found in over 50% of all isolates and, up to 1976, 1–5% of all isolates were resistant to tetracyclines. None of these antibiotics, however, are indicated in the treatment of animal salmonellosis. Resistance to the broad-spectrum antibiotics (ampicillin, chloramphenicol etc.) which are useful in treatment remained ≤1% up till 1976 (Table I).

Serious problems of multiple antibiotic resistance in animal salmonella in the UK have occurred in one serotype only: *S. typhimurium* (Table II). In the 1960s, an increasing range of R determinants was experienced in *S. typhimurium* phage type 29.[14] Initially, this endemic phage type in calves was sensitive to the majority of therapeutic antibiotics available. However, it progressively demonstrated an ever-widening range of R determinants in parallel with the range of antibiotics administered, mainly prophylactically. The outbreak suddenly came to an end in 1968–69 and *S. typhimurium* was superceded in prevalence by a fully sensitive *S. dublin* despite no obvious change in antibiotic usage.

More recently, a series of phage types of *S. typhimurium* (types 204, 193, 204c etc.), derived from a parent phage type 49 by R plasmid colonization, has caused a series of outbreaks in calves that spread to man.[15-22] These strains carried from four to seven determinants. In 1975 and 1979, approximately 70% of all animal isolates of *S. typhimurium* were from cattle and, of these, 46% and 57% were of phage types 193 and 204 respectively.[23]

Since epidemics in the UK caused by multiple-resistant strains have been relatively few, it must be inferred that the genetic events whereby R plasmids are transferred to salmonella from other bacteria, or the conditions which predispose to them, rarely occur in vivo. However, the situation in other countries indicates that local factors may increase the potential for R-plasmid transfer to occur. In the Netherlands, there has been a considerable build-up in veal calves of multiple-resistant *S. dublin* since 1975 and, since

1972, of *S. typhimurium*; these strains appeared to be highly virulent.[24] The plasmids carried by the *S. dublin* were shown to be different from those carried by the *S. typhimurium* strains, indicating no direct plasmid relationship between the two serotypes.

Mutiple-resistant strains of *S. gallinarum* (carrying nine R determinants) have been reported in poultry in Greece following treatment by a combination of antibiotics and coccidiostats.[25] In Germany, multiple-resistant strains of salmonella, including resistance to gentamicin, have been described in poultry. This is attributed to the highly questionable practice of using this antibiotic for egg-dipping as a protection against mycoplasma infections in newly hatched chicks.[26]

Antibiotic resistance has been encountered in other pathogens, namely in isolates of *Pasteurella multocida* and *P. haemolytica* from cattle and pigs, and multiple resistance to penicillin, tetracycline, streptomycin and chloramphenicol has been reported.[27] Some R determinants in pasteurellae have been shown to be located on R plasmids.[28]

2 Acquired Antibiotic Resistance in Non-Pathogenic Bacteria Associated with Animals

In contrast to the unequal distribution of antibiotic resistance among animal pathogens, the oral administration of antibiotics in animals over many years and often for long periods has selected a predominantly antibiotic-resistant flora in the oral cavity and alimentary tract of many meat animals.[29-31] The microbial composition of the normal animal's gut flora is not only highly complex but varies between species and with age in the same species. It is not surprising, therefore, that the incidence of antibiotic resistance in these indigenous bacteria varies between animal species and the bacterial species which make up their complex flora. In addition to *E. coli*, antibiotic resistance—often plasmid-mediated—has been demonstrated in many bacterial species associated with the animal and its environment. These include *Proteus* spp., *Pseudomonas* spp., *Acinetobacter* spp., *Providence* spp. and *Klebsiella pneumoniae* (unpublished data). The most definitive work has been done on *E. coli* from meat animals and this will be reviewed here.

In the non-ruminant meat animal, the numbers of *E. coli* in rectal contents are similar to those in man (approx. 10^6/g), but in older ruminants, especially cattle, they are fewer; of the order of 10^3/g or even undetectable.[32] Cattle and sheep kept at pasture receive comparatively few antibiotics and little antibiotic resistance is found among their *E. coli*.[30] Housed animals, in contrast, especially those managed intensively, frequently receive antibiotics and carry large numbers of antibiotic-resistant *E. coli* in their dominant flora. Consequently calves, pigs and poultry are commonly colonized by large numbers of multiple-resistant strains, often carrying seven to eight R determinants (Table III).[33]

In non-hospitalized man, antibiotic resistant *E. coli* may constitute 0.02% of all *E. coli* in the gut,[34] whereas in calves, pigs and poultry, the proportion of resistant strains is regularly 60% or higher, whether or not the individual animal is on antibiotics.[30] No doubt this is due to the extensive oral use of antibiotics in housed meat animals over many years which has selected a mainly resistant flora. These strains have now become established as the stable components of the animals' gut flora and persist even in the absence of antibiotic pressure. Persisting in the animals' environment, these antibiotic-resistant strains are ingested and colonize the gut where they are able to compete on equal terms with sensitive ones for colonization. Carriage of R plasmids has been shown by some workers[34] to discourage colonization but others[35] have demonstrated a link between R plasmid carriage (H2 plasmid) and persistence in the gut.

Antibiotic-resistant strains of *E. coli* from the gut of meat animals regularly contaminate the carcass of the animal from which the *E. coli* were derived and by cross-contamination, other carcasses on the same slaughter line.[36-38] They pass along the food chain and have been shown to colonize the alimentary tract of man for at least 10 days.[39]

Furthermore, the range of O-serogroups of *E. coli* commonly isolated from meat animals is very similar to that found regularly in the human gut.[40]

3 The Importance of Antibiotic-Resistant Bacteria

a For Animals

Antibiotic-resistant, pathogenic bacteria inevitably present a greater therapeutic problem for the veterinarian than sensitive ones. This is particularly important in animal salmonellosis which, in contrast to the disease in man, frequently takes a septicaemic form. Where infection is by a multiple-resistant strain of *S. typhimurium*, very few useful antibiotics remain available to the veterinarian. The importance of antibiotic resistance in *E. coli* infections is less clear. Coliform mastitis in cows is most certainly an endogenous infection by strains originating in the cow's gut[41] and, as stated earlier, most of these are fully sensitive to the regularly available antibiotics. In a recent study, only 10% of isolates from bovine mastitis carried one or two R determinants.[6] Little data is available on the resistance patterns of enteropathogenic *E. coli*.[33] Penicillin-resistant *Staphylococcus aureus* from bovine mastitis can be successfully treated using an intramammary preparation of newer β-lactam antibiotics.

The high incidence of antibiotic resistance in indigenous *E. coli*

TABLE III. The percentages of *Escherichia coli* resistance to each of six antibacterial agents on eleven sampling occasions from calves reared intensively for veal[33]

Antibacterial agent	Days of sampling											% of all isolates
	1	2	6	9	13	15	21	23	27	30	34	
Ampicillin	38.5*	24	72.5	46.5	48	32	43	42	32.5	30.5	26.5	39.5
Chloramphenicol	15	3	49.5	45.5	70	75	58	57	52.5	59	57.5	49.0
Kanamycin	42.5	17	66.5	88	100	98	99	96	100	96.5	97.5	81.5
Streptomycin	60	48	90.5	100	100	96	100	95	99	99	100	89.0
Sulphonamide	78	72	92.5	100	100	100	100	100	99	100	100	94.0
Tetracycline	45.5	18	96	96.5	100	100	100	98	97	93	100	82.5
No. of strains of *E. coli* examined	99	100	95	90	100	100	100	100	99	85	87	1055

* Numbers to nearest 0.5%.

must be viewed as a rich source of R plasmids. Transfer of R plasmids between strains of *E. coli* has been regularly demonstrated. Even H2 plasmids which are thermosensitive for transfer have been shown to be transferred outside the calf in the cooler environment and later colonize the calf by the oral route.[35]

Using agarose gel electrophoresis the plasmid profiles of strains of *E. coli* of the different O-serogroups, isolated from the same ecological niche, have been studied. Within the same O-serogroup the plasmid profiles were found frequently to be very similar, whilst the profiles of strains of other serogroups were often very different. But certain strains of *E. coli* and *S. typhimurium* phage type 193, isolated from the same batch of calf slurry, demonstrated some similarities in plasmid profiles (unpublished data). These observations give added weight to the theory that the H2 plasmids in the present outbreak of salmonellosis in calves were derived from *E. coli* or some other common bacterial component of the calf's environment.

b *For Man*

S. aureus causing bovine mastitis are of different phage types to those causing infection in man. Antibiotic-resistant strains from udder infection in cows are therefore unlikely to cause staphylococcal infections in man.

The zoonotic nature of salmonella food poisoning in man is well established and meat is the commonest vehicle. Should infection occur with an antibiotic-resistant strain, chemotherapy, if neces-sary, would be complicated. Fortunately, salmonellosis in man rarely requires antibiotic therapy which, indeed, is contra-indicated. There is some evidence that multiple-resistant strains may be more virulent than sensitive ones.[24,35]

The risk of human infections by multiple-resistant strains may be affected by different eating habits. In the UK, poultry meat is responsible for 80% of human salmonella food poisoning but rarely are resistant strains encountered in poultry. Beef is the main meat consumed in the USA and, because resistant strains are more commonly encountered in cattle, the chances of human infections arising with these strains is greater.

The significance to man of antibiotic-resistant animal *E. coli* is less clear. It has been shown that animal strains reach man via the food chain but there is no evidence that they cause human infections (such as urinary tract infection). However, during their temporary colonization of the human gut they have the potential to transfer their R plasmids to the indigenous flora of the gut. It must be stressed that, under normal conditions, transfer of plasmids in vivo is a rare event. However, if the right conditions are created in the gut, especially as a consequence of antibiotic selection pressure with its resultant change in bacterial population dynamics, transfer of R plasmids will occur and the recipient bacteria will multiply rapidly to become dominant in the microflora. These, in turn, may transfer their R plasmids to human pathogens. R plasmids common to *E. coli* have been demonstrated not only in other Enterobacteriaceae but also in *Haemophilus influenzae* and *Neisseria gonorrhoea*.[42,43]

REFERENCES

1 Council for Agricultural Science and Technology. Report: Antibiotics in animal feeds. Ames, IA, USA: 1981: 79

2 Joint Committee on the use of Antibiotics in Animal Husbandry and Veterinary Medicine. Report. London: HMSO 1969: 83

3 Linton AH. Has Swann failed? Vet Rec 1981; 108: 328–331

4 Report. The effects of human health of subtherapeutic use of antimicrobials in animal feeds. Washington DC: National Academy Science 1980: 8

5 Stabler SL, Fagerberg DJ, Quarles CL. Effects of oral and injectable tetracyclines on bacterial drug resistance in feedlot cattle. Am J Vet Res 1982; 30: 1763–1766

6 Linton AH, Robinson TC. Studies on the association of *Escherichia coli* with bovine mastitis. Br Vet J 1983; In press

7 Pearson JKL. Intramammary therapy: its achievements and limitations. In: Woodbine M, ed. Antibiotics and antibiosis in agriculture. London: Butterworths, 1977; 217–228

8 Sojka WJ, Hudson EB. A survey of drug resistance in Salmonella isolated from animals in England and Wales during 1972. Br Vet J 1976; 132: 95–104

9 Sojka WJ, Wray C. A survey of drug resistance in salmonellae isolated from animals in England and Wales 1975 to 1978. Br Vet J 1980; 136: 463–477

10 Sojka WJ, Hudson EB, Slavin G. A survey of drug resistance in *Salmonella* isolated from animals in England and Wales during 1971. Br Vet J 1974; 130: 128–138

11 Sojka WJ, Wray C, Hudson EB. A survey of drug resistance in salmonellae isolated from animals in England and Wales 1973 and 1974. Br Vet J 1977; 133: 292–311

12 Sojka WJ, Slavin G, Brand TF, Davies G. A survey of drug resistance in salmonellae isolated from animals in England and Wales. Br Vet J 1972; 128: 189–198

13 Linton AH. The Swann Report and its impact. In: Stuart-Harris CH, Harris DM, eds. The control of antibiotic-resistant bacteria. London: Academic Press, 1982; 183–200

14 Anderson ES. Drug resistance in *Salmonella typhimurium* and its implications. Br Med J 1968; 3: 333–339

15 Davies G. Chloramphenicol-resistant *S. typhimurium*. Vet Rec 1979; 104: 128

16 Threlfall EJ. Multiresistant epidemic strains of *Salmonella typhimurium* in Britain. In: Pohl P, Leunen J, eds. Resistance and pathogenic plasmids. CEC Seminar. Brussels: National Institute for Veterinary Research, 1982; 103–114

17 Threlfall EJ, Hall MLM, Rowe B. Plasmid-mediated antimicrobial drug resistance in *Salmonella dublin* in food animals. Vet Rec 1979; 105: 20–21

18 Threlfall EJ, Ward LR, Ashley AS, Rowe B. Plasmid-encoded trimethoprim resistance in multiresistant epidemic *Salmonella typhimurium* phage types 204 and 193 in Britain. Br Med J 1980; 280: 1210–1211

19 Threlfall EJ, Ward LR, Rowe B. Spread of multi resistant strains of *Salmonella typhimurium* phage types 204 and 193 in Britain. Br Med J 1978; 2: 997

20 Threlfall EJ, Ward LR, Rowe B. Epidemic spread of a chloramphenicol-resistant strain of *Salmonella typhimurium* phage type 204 in bovine animals in Britain. Vet Rec 1978; 103: 438–440

21 Threlfall EJ, Ward LR, Rowe B. Chloramphenicol-resistant *Salmonella typhimurium*. Vet Rec 1979; 104: 60–61

22 Rowe, B, Threlfall EJ, Ward LR, Ashley AS. International spread of multiresistant strains of *Salmonella typhimurium* phage types 204 and 193 from Britain to Europe. Vet Rec 1979; 105: 468–469

23 Anonymous. Increase in antibiotic resistance. Vet Rec 1980; 106: 472

24 van Leeuwen WJ, Voogd CE, Guinée PAM. Antibiotic resistance in Salmonella in the Netherlands. In: Pohl P, Leunen J, eds. Resistance and pathogenic plasmids. CEC Seminar. Brussels: National Institute for Veterinary Research, 1982; 115–127

25 Kontomichalou P, Paraskevopoulu P, Karapentelaki I *et al*. Trimethoprim resistance plasmids, from Enterobacteriaceae causing nosocomial infections and from human and animal salmonella isolated in Greece. In: Pohl P, Leunen J, eds. Resistance and pathogenic plasmids. CEC Seminar. Brussels: National Institute for Veterinary Research, 1982; 131–152

26 Helmeuth R, Pietzsch O, Stephen R, Chakraborty T, Bulling E. Gentamicin resistant Sallmonellae in turkey rearing. In: Woodbine M, ed. Antibiotics and antibiosis in agriculture. London: Butterworth, 1984; In press

27 Chang WH, Carter GR. Multiple drug resistance in *Pasteurella multocida* and *Pasteurella haemolytica* from cattle and swine. J Am Vet Med Assoc 1976; 169: 710–712

28 Zimmerman ML, Hirsch DC. Demonstration of an R-plasmid in a strain of *Pasteurella haemolytica* isolated from feedlot cattle. Am J Vet Res 1980; 41: 166–169

29 Jackson G. A survey of antibiotic resistance of *Escherichia coli* isolated from farm animals in Great Britain from 1971 to 1977. Vet Rec 1981; 108: 325–328

30 Linton AH. Antibiotic resistance: the present situation reviewed. Vet Rec 1977; 100: 354–360

31 Linton AH, Howe K, Osborne AD. The effects of feeding tetracycline, nitrovin and quindoxin on the drug-resistance of coli-aerogenes bacteria from calves and pigs. J Appl Bacteriol 1975; 38: 255–275

32 Howe K, Linton AH, Osborne AD. A longitudinal study of *Escherichia coli* in cows and calves with special reference to the distribution of O-antigen types and antibiotic resistance. J Appl Bacteriol 1976; 40: 331–340

33 Linton AH, Timoney JF, Hinton M. The ecology of chloramphenicol-resistance in *Salmonella typhimurium* and *Escherichia coli* in calves with endemic salmonella infection. J Appl Bacteriol 1981; 50: 115–129

34 Hartley CL, Howe K, Linton AH, Linton KB, Richmond MH. Distribution of R plasmids among the O-antigen types of *Escherichia coli* isolated from human and animal sources. Antimicrob Agents Chemother 1975; 8: 122–131

35 Timoney JF, Linton AH. Experimental ecological studies on H2 plasmids in the intestine and and faeces of the calf. J Appl Bacteriol 1982; 52: 417–424

36 Howe K, Linton AH, Osborne AD. An investigation of calf carcass contamination by *Escherichia coli* from the gut contents at slaughter. J. Appl Bacteriol 1976; 41: 37–45

37 Linton AH, Handley B, Osborne AD, Shaw BG, Roberts TA, Hudson WR. Contamination of pig carcasses at two abattoirs by *Escherichia coli* with special reference to O-serotypes and antibiotic resistance. J Appl Bacteriol 1977; 42: 89–110

38 Linton AH, Howe K, Hartley CL, Clements HM, Richmond MH, Osborne AD. Antibiotic resistance among *Escherichia coli* O-serotypes from the gut and carcasses of commercially slaughtered broiler chickens: a potential public health hazard. J Appl Bacteriol 1977; 42: 365–378

39 Linton AH, Howe K, Bennett PM, Richmond MH, Whiteside EJ. The colonization of the human gut by antibiotic resistant *Escherichia coli* from chickens. J Appl Bacteriol 1977; 43: 465–469

40 Linton AH. Animal to man transmission of Enterobacteriaceae. R Soc Health J 1977; 97: 115–118

41 Linton AH, Howe K, Sojka WJ, Wray C. A note on the range of *Escherichia coli* O-serotypes causing clinical bovine mastitis and their antibiotic resistance spectra. J. Appl Bacteriol 1979; 46: 585–590

42 Elwell LP, Roberts M, Mayer LW, Falkow S. Plasmid-mediated beta-lactamase production in *Neisseria gonorrhoeae*. Antimicrob Agents Chemother 1977; 11: 528–533

43 Saunders JR, Elwell LP, Falkow S. β-lactamases an R-plasmids of *Haemophilus influenzae*. Scand J Infect Dis 1978; 13 (suppl): 16–122

British Medical Bulletin (1984) Vol. 40, No. 1, pp. 96–101

COUNTERACTING ANTIBIOTIC RESISTANCE: NEW DRUGS

R B SYKES PhD

D P BONNER PhD

*The Squibb Institute for Medical Research
Princeton, New Jersey*

1 β-Lactam antibiotics
   a Enzyme inhibitors
   b Chemical modification
   c Novel β-lactams from nature
2 Aminoglycosides
3 Chloramphenicol
4 Tetracyclines
5 Pyridone carboxylic acids
6 Rifamycins
7 Discussion
   References

The emergence of microbial resistance to antibiotics has stimulated research and development in the antibiotic field over the past 40 years. From knowledge gained over this period, we can point to five basic mechanisms by which bacteria develop resistance to antibiotics: interference with antibiotic transport into the cell by reduced antibiotic uptake or increased energy dependent efflux; the antibacterial target may be altered or overproduced to mitigate the drug effect; the antibiotic may be modified or inactivated by bacterial enzymes; the bacterial requirement for a metabolite to which the antibiotic is targeted may be reduced; the cells may synthesize a new enzyme which allows a new metabolic pathway to overcome a previously blocked reaction.

A knowledge of these resistance mechanisms has proved essential for the rational development of new antimicrobial agents in extending or supplementing the activity spectra of existing compounds. A number of strategies have been used in new drug development with specific reference to overcoming resistance mechanisms. These approaches fall within three major categories, encompassing the search for natural products, semi-synthesis and total synthesis.

Sulphonamides and penicillins, the first antimicrobial families to be used successfully in the treatment of bacterial diseases, provide a striking comparison in terms of resistance and drug development. Although resistance to sulphonamides was recognized soon after their introduction, the mechanisms of resistance to this group of drugs were to remain a mystery for many years. In contrast, penicillin-inactivating enzymes had already been identified before penicillin became generally available.

Following the discovery of sulphanilamide and its mechanism of action, large numbers of sulphonamides were synthesized on an empirical basis in the search for compounds with increased antibacterial 'power'. Additionally, analogues of other essential metabolites were prepared in abundance. In terms of successfully competing against the problem of resistance development to sulphonamides, trimethoprim, a 2:4 diaminopyrimidine, was the only useful compound to emerge from these studies. Thus, sulphonamide resistance was overcome to some degree by a novel, rather than a traditional approach, i.e. the discovery of a new class of antimicrobial agents which could be used in combination with the sulphonamides, as opposed to chemically modifying the existing molecule. Co-trimoxazole, a combination of sulphamethoxazole and trimethoprim was introduced in 1969, more than 30 years after the discovery of sulphonamides.

The euphoria which developed over the discovery, development and successful use of penicillin in the treatment of bacterial diseases, waned with the appearance of penicillin-resistant strains of *Staphylococcus aureus*. The compound which had, to some degree, supplanted the sulphonamides was now itself a victim of resistance. The 1950s provided the staging point for the largest and most successful of all antibiotic programmes, the development of β-lactam antibiotics. These compounds will be used as a framework on which to build the story of how the pharmaceutical industry approaches the science of antibiotic development, with specific reference to drug resistance.

1 β-Lactam Antibiotics

The continuing development of β-lactam antibiotics, of which penicillin is the progenitor, can be directly attributed to the constant fight against resistance. The serious resistance problems confronting penicillin in the early 1950s led to intensified efforts in all areas of antibacterial research. Knowledge that resistance was the result of a penicillin-inactivating enzyme, penicillinase, stimulated the development of new concepts in antibiotic research. Approaches taken to overcome the resistance problem included modification of the penicillin molecule and the search for penicillinase inhibitors. It took ten years of intensive research from the realization of the problem to a resulting solution.

Work on penicillinase inhibitors during this initial period met with little success and was superseded by the development of penicillinase-stable, semi-synthetic penicillins and the discovery of cephalosporin C.

Modification of the penicillin molecule from a biosynthetic or chemical approach produced no breakthroughs before the isolation of the penicillin nucleus, 6-aminopenicillanic acid (6-APA) in 1959.[1] The identification of 6-APA in penicillin fermentation broths opened the door to one of the most successful approaches in the development of antibiotics: chemical modification of an existing antibiotic molecule. Preparation of the semi-synthetic, β-lactamase-stable penicillins, such as methicillin and cloxacillin, offered relief against penicillinase-producing staphylococci. In addition, these compounds provided an important example of antibiotic development directed toward overcoming a specific resistance problem.

The concept of searching for novel agents with stability to the penicillin-hydrolysing enzyme had started to yield results by the mid-1950s. About this time, Newton & Abraham[2] reported on the isolation of cephalosporin C. The antibacterial activity of this novel agent was not impressive but the apparent relationship of the substance to penicillin, coupled with its resistance to staphylococcal penicillinase, was of immediate clinical interest. Consequently, an enormous effort was devoted to the development of cephalosporin C by a number of pharmaceutical companies. However, due to manufacturing difficulties, cephalosporin C failed to reach the clinic before the introduction of the semi-synthetic penicillins and so it became redundant. It did, however, provide a second β-lactam nucleus, 7-aminocephalosporanic acid (7-ACA), which formed a basis for chemical modification.

By the mid-1960s, broad-spectrum penicillins and cephalosporins had made their appearance in the clinical setting to counteract the growing prevalence of gram-negative pathogens. It was during this period that penicillin- and cephalosporin-inactivating enzymes (β-lactamases) produced by gram-negative bacteria were recognized as clinically important (see Fig. 1).

Before 1960, penicillin-resistant staphylococci invariably produced a penicillinase responsible for the resistant phenotype. Once the penicillinase problem had been controlled, staphylococci once again succumbed to the action of β-lactam antibiotics. In contrast to staphylococci, gram-negative bacteria produce a plethora of β-lactamases which are equally diverse in their β-lactam hydrolysing abilities as these pathogens are in their taxonomic distribution.[3,4] The open-knit peptidoglycan-teichoic acid structure of the gram-positive cell wall is generally believed to present no effective barrier to the entry of β-lactam antibiotics. In contrast, the outer membrane of gram-negative organisms can undoubtedly impede the access of penicillins and cephalosporins to their killing sites on the inner cell membrane.[5] Factors such as these add additional levels of complexity to the killing of gram-negative bacteria by antibiotics.

During the 1970s, penicillin-sensitive enzymes or penicillin-binding proteins (PBPs) were identified as the possible targets of penicillin action.[6] Firm evidence has now accumulated that mutation in certain PBPs is responsible for penicillin resistance in strains of pneumococci[7] and methicillin-resistant staphylococci.[8]

These additional challenges have driven β-lactam research to new heights over the last decade and the success has been impressive. Progress has resulted from three distinct approaches, each having its own philosophy but all three being closely intertwined. The first is the search for enzyme inhibitors, with the concept of developing compounds capable of inactivating β-lactamases and to be used in conjunction with β-lactamase-susceptible compounds. The second approach has been to modify existing structures chemically, (e.g., penicillins and cephalosporins) to produce highly potent non-substrate antibiotics. The search for novel β-lactam-containing molecules from nature constitutes the third approach.

a Enzyme Inhibitors

Narrow-spectrum penicillins, such as cloxacillin and methicillin, exclusively active against gram-positive organisms, show a high degree of stability to a wide range of β-lactamases. However, broad-spectrum penicillins, including such compounds as amoxycillin and carbenicillin and the ureidopenicillins, azlocillin, mezlocillin and piperacillin, are readily inactivated by plasmid-mediated β-lactamases from gram-positive and gram-negative bacteria.[9] β-Lactamase-stable, broad spectrum penicillins are futuristic curiosities, a fact that has led to the development of β-lactamase inhibitors.

Although many examples of semi-synthetic β-lactam antibiotics which act as competitive inhibitors of β-lactamase are known,[10] none show the desired effect of protecting β-lactamase-susceptible β-lactams against enzyme attack. In an attempt to find potentially novel β-lactamase inhibitors, several laboratories turned their attention to the screening of soil micro-organisms. Specific testing procedures were developed to detect β-lactamase inhibitory activity. A well-documented screen is that developed by the Beecham workers,[11] which became known as the 'KAG' assay. In this test system, an assay plate is prepared from agar seeded with a β-lactamase-producing strain of *Klebsiella aerogenes* and containing penicillin G at a concentration well below the inhibitory concentration for the test organism. Samples of broth filtrates are placed on plates, either on filter paper disks or in wells, and the plates incubated overnight. A clear zone of inhibition around the well indicates the presence of a presumptive β-lactamase inhibitor. A duplicate plate, prepared as described above but lacking penicillin G, acts as a control to eliminate samples containing antibiotic rather than enzyme inhibitory activity. The naturally occurring β-lactamase inhibitors clavulanic acid,[12] olivanic acids,[13] izumenolide[14] and panosialin[15] were the products of such screening systems.

The isolation of clavulanic acid from a strain of *Streptomyces clavuligerus* by workers at Beecham in the mid-1970s provided the first known example of a β-lactamase inactivator. Although exhibiting weak antibacterial activity against gram-positive and gram-negative bacteria, clavulanic acid is a potent inhibitor of a wide range of clinically important β-lactamases.[16] Augmentin, a combination of clavulanic acid and amoxycillin, shows a high degree of activity against β-lactamase-producing strains of *S. aureus*, *Bacteroides fragilis*, *Neisseria gonorrhoeae*, *Haemophilus influenzae*, and TEM-producing strains of *Escherichia coli*.[17]

Following the isolation and development of clavulanic acid the field of β-lactamase inhibitors blossomed forth, with such compounds as the semi-synthetic penicillanic acid sulphones[18] and halo-penicillanic acids.[19] In addition to protecting β-lactamase-susceptible penicillins, β-lactamase inhibitors are also being developed for use with enzyme-susceptible cephalosporins such as cefoperazone.[20]

The present crop of β-lactamase inhibitors are referred to mechanistically as suicide inactivators. Characteristically, these compounds interact with the enzyme to form the inactivating species.[21]

b Chemical Modification

i Penicillins

Development of new penicillins over the past decade has been restricted to modification of the 6 β-side chain on the β-lactam nucleus. New penicillins having broad spectrum activity, including significant activity against *Pseudomonas aeruginosa*, are all related chemically and referred to as ureidopenicillins. Included in this group are piperacillin, azlocillin and mezlocillin. Although active against a broader range of gram-negative bacteria than earlier penicillins, these compounds are unstable to plasmid-mediated β-lactamases produced by gram-positive and gram-negative bacteria, making them prime candidates for combination with β-lactamase inhibitors.

FIG. 1. Interaction of penicillins and cephalosporins with β-lactamases

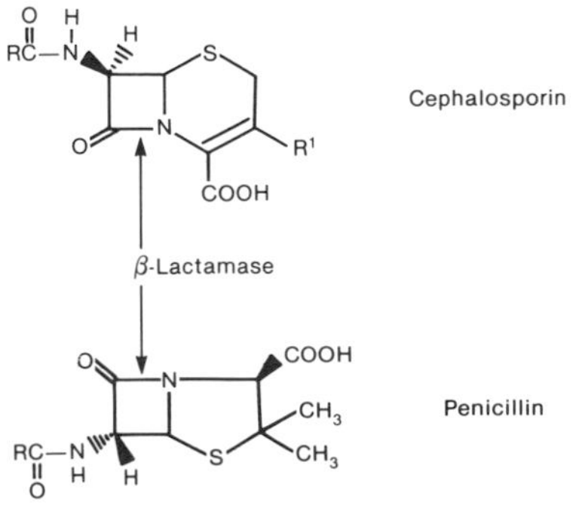

A novel series of amidinopenicillins, exemplified by mecillinam, was discovered by workers in Denmark.[22] Potently active against gram-negative organisms, these compounds bind preferentially to a target PBP not previously observed in binding studies with penicillins and cephalosporins.[23] Although scientifically of great interest, this knowledge has not at this time led to the development of significant applications.

ii *Cephalosporins*

Derivatization of the cephalosporin molecule led independently to the development of oxime cephalosporins by workers at Glaxo and Fujisawa. These broad-spectrum cephalosporins show a greater degree of stability to hydrolysis by gram-negative β-lactamases than previous compounds of this class. Cefuroxime[24] is a product of early oxime research. A further breakthrough came in 1975 with the development of aminothiazole oxime cephalosporins at a number of pharmaceutical companies throughout the world. Addition of the aminothiazole moiety to the oxime side chain of certain cephalosporins results in compounds having a high degree of activity against aerobic gram-negative bacteria, including β-lactamase-producing strains. Since the mid-70s, aminothiazole oximes have dominated cephalosporin research, leading to such compounds as ceftizoxime,[25] ceftriaxone,[26] and ceftazidime.[27] In addition to its high activity against the Enterobacteriaceae, ceftazidime is equally active to aminoglycoside antibiotics against strains of *P. aeruginosa*.

c *Novel β-Lactams from Nature*

Until 1970, penicillins and cephalosporins were the sole representatives of the naturally occurring β-lactam antibiotics. However, with a greater commitment to selective screening and major advances in isolation technology, a variety of novel β-lactam-containing molecules have made their appearance over the last decade. In all cases, the discovery of novel molecular types has been the focus for chemical modification programmes aimed at producing superior β-lactam antibiotics.

During the 1970s, molecules represented by the cephamycins,[28] nocardicins[29] and carbapenems[30] were described. In contrast to the fungal-produced penicillins and cephalosporins, these novel molecules are produced by members of the actinomycetes.

The finding that a 7-α-methoxyl group on the cephalosporin nucleus gave the molecule exceptional stability to a wide range of β-lactamases led to the development of the semi-synthetic cephamycins, cefoxitin,[31] cefmetazole[32] and cefotetan.[33] The 7α-methoxy oxacephem, Latamoxef (Moxalactam),[34] was also modelled from the cephamycins. All these molecules exhibit broad spectrum antibiotic activity including activity against anaerobic pathogens such as *Bacteroides fragilis*. In addition, they exhibit exceptional stability to hydrolysis by β-lactamases.

The carbapenems, ubiquitous products of streptomycetes, combine the properties of high intrinsic activity against a wide range of bacteria and stability to β-lactamases.[35] The carbapenem *N*-formimidoyl thienamycin[36] is presently under study as one of the most powerful broad-spectrum antibacterial agents being developed.

The discovery of bacterially-produced monocyclic β-lactam antibiotics by workers at Squibb and Takeda has led to a flurry of excitement in yet another area of β-lactam research. Unlike the bicyclic molecules produced by streptomycetes and fungi, the monobactams[37] lend themselves to total synthesis. Azthreonam,[38] a synthetic monobactam highly potent against aerobic gram-negative bacteria and stable to β-lactamases, is presently under development.

2. Aminoglycosides

The first aminoglycoside, streptomycin, was available for clinical use in 1945. This was soon to be followed by a range of other naturally occurring molecules of the same class. One of the most frequently observed and better understood mechanisms of resistance to these drugs, is associated with the presence of drug-inactivating enzymes. The three classes of enzymes involved, *N*-acetyltransferases, *O*-adenylyltransferases and *O*-phosphotransferases, catalyse the reaction of antibiotics with ATP or acetyl-CoA (Fig. 2). Catalysis is mediated via two structural sites binding to adenosine and aminoglycoside antibiotics containing 2-deoxy-streptamine or streptidine. As with the β-lactams two strategies have been employed to prevent inactivation. The more successful approach has been to generate non-substrate derivatives. Synthesis of 3′,4′-dideoxykanamycin (dibekacin) by Umezawa and co-workers[39] provided a compound resistant to 3′-*O*-phosphotransferase. Netilmicin, the 1-*N* ethyl derivative of sissomicin, has been prepared and is unable to serve as a substrate for 2″-*O*-modifying and many 3-*N*-acetylating enzymes.[40] Amikacin, the 1-*N*-aminohydroxybutyryl derivative of kanamycin A, has proven to be a non-substrate for most aminoglycoside-inactivating enzymes and consequently has found an increasing role in treating infections caused by gentamicin and tobramycin-resistant bacteria.[41]

Strategies toward enzyme inhibition, on the other hand, while not as far advanced as those with the β-lactamase inhibitors, are certainly under study. Recently, workers at Lilly isolated 7-hydroxytropolone from a strain of *Streptomyces neyagawaensis* which proved to be an inhibitor of the 2″-*O*-adenylyltransferase-inactivating enzyme.[42] Formycins A and B have also been reported to inhibit aminoglycoside phosphotransferases.[43] In these situations, and in contrast to the case with β-lactamase inhibitors, we appear to be dealing with co-substrate (ATP) inhibition. While 7-hydroxytropolone does show in-vitro synergism with gentamicin and tobramycin against resistant bacteria,[44] the future role of such inhibitors is unclear. The potential for toxicity must be seriously considered when involving a competitor for a primary metabolite such as ATP.

In addition to enzyme modification, it is now believed that other factors play an important role in aminoglycoside resistance. These include reduced target binding and decreased intracellular accumulation. In the case of spectinomycin, resistance to the drug can be the result of one of three unrelated mechanisms. These are: enzyme modification, altered binding on the 30S ribosomal subunit, or a change in permeability. Werner *et al.*,[45] have recently synthesized 4(*R*)amino spectinomycin derivatives which show activity against a range of spectinomycin-resistant strains. This increased activity appears to be a function of binding to a different site, resistance to enzymatic modification and increased uptake of the drug.

FIG. 2. Enzymatic modification of aminoglycosides

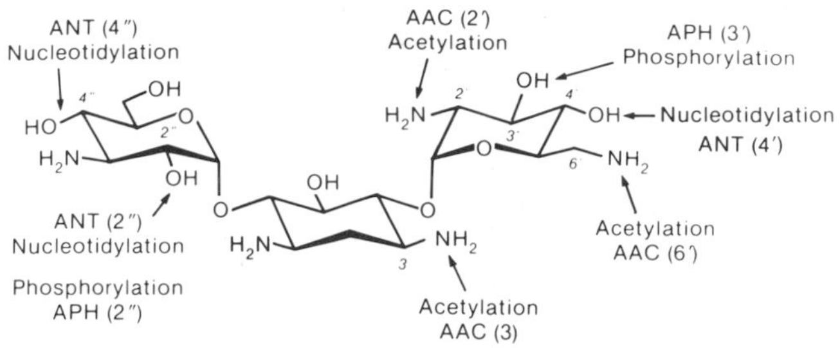

3 Chloramphenicol

The majority of bacterial isolates resistant to chloramphenicol can convert this antibiotic successively to its 3-acetyl and then its 1,3-diacetyl ester, both of which lack inhibitory activity. The modifying enzyme is chloramphenicol acetyl transferase (Fig. 3). Acetylation of the chloramphenicol molecule at position 3 is followed by chemical rearrangement, resulting in the transfer of the acetyl group to position 1, thus allowing further enzymatic acetylation at position 3 to give the diacetate. Both the monoacetate and diacetate are inactive. A less common enzyme-mediated inactivation is observed in some strains of *Flavobacterium* where hydrolysis of the amide bond liberates dichloroacetate, resulting in a loss of antibiotic activity.

Screening for inhibitors of chloramphenicol acetyl transferase has been reported and recently a streptomycete product capable of inhibiting this enzyme has been described.[46] However, high levels of inhibitor were required to potentiate the action of chloramphenicol against resistant bacteria and the effects were marginal.

Chemical modification of the chloramphenicol structure in search for nonsubstrate derivatives has been carried out. Substitution of a fluorine on the 3' carbon position for the normally present hydroxyl results in a compound refractory to hydrolysis by chloramphenicol acetyl transferase and active against resistant strains harbouring the enzyme.[47]

4 Tetracyclines

Resistance to tetracycline is commonly found among different bacterial species but no mechanism for destroying or modifying the drug has been discovered. Resistance appears to result from decreased accumulation of the drug secondary to an energy dependent efflux.

FIG. 3. Interaction of chloramphenicol with chloramphenicol acetyl transferase

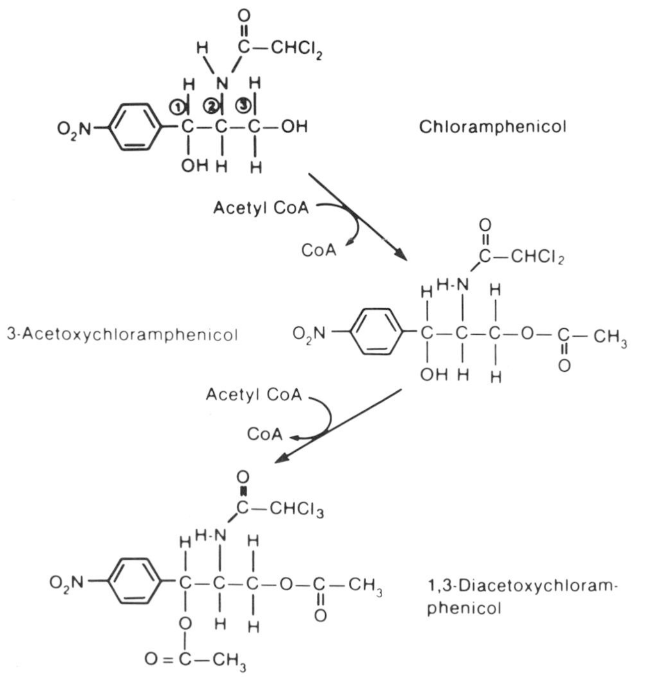

While newer analogues of the tetracyclines, including minocycline and doxycycline, have been synthesized, gains in overcoming bacterial resistance have been small. This is particularly true among the Enterobacteriaceae, where tetracycline resistance is plasmid-mediated. These organisms are cross-resistant to minocycline and doxycycline. A recent advance in this area has been the synthesis of a new thiotetracycline derivative active against tetracycline-resistant organisms.[48] While the exact mechanism by which thiotetracycline overcomes resistance is unclear, it is interesting to note that this new analogue is bactericidal to gram-negative rods where the older tetracyclines are bacteriostatic.[49]

5 Pyridone Carboxylic Acids

DNA gyrase is the enzyme responsible for DNA supercoiling in bacteria. The enzyme from *E. coli* is made up of two different subunits, A and B, each of which is the target for antibiotic action. Pyridone carboxylic acids, including such compounds as nalidixic acid and oxolinic acid, inhibit the A subunit. Resistance to this group of compounds develops due to a change in the A subunit structure.

As with other classes of antimicrobials, programmes have been directed to synthesize congeners of nalidixic acid active against resistant strains. Existence in some organisms of a possible dual mode of resistance initially hampered efforts. Early studies on pipemidic acid demonstrated that this derivative was active to some extent against a subgroup of nalidixic acid resistant organisms. Investigation of this subgroup revealed baseline changes in the DNA synthesizing system, conferring decreased sensitivity to both nalidixic and pipemidic acids and altered permeability further restricting the activity of nalidixic acid but not impeding the influx of pipemidic acid.[50] More recently, new derivatives such as norfloxacin[51] and AT-2266[52] have appeared and show activity against a variety of nalidixic-acid-resistant organisms. Studies have not yet been reported detailing how these new compounds overcome resistance but it is interesting to note that norfloxacin is a fluorinated derivative of pipemidic acid which had already nullified the permeability aspect of resistance. It will be of interest to see what effect the presence of a fluorine has on the interaction with the DNA synthesizing system.

6 Rifamycins

Rifamycins owe their activity to the inhibition of bacterial RNA polymerase by forming a very stable complex with the enzyme. Rifampicin, a semi-synthetic derivative of the rifamycins, is used mainly for the treatment of tuberculosis and gram-positive infections. Mutations to rifampicin resistance are readily obtained and resistant organisms exhibit a great variety of phenotypes. In search of rifamycins which would affect rifampicin-resistant bacteria, a large number of semi-synthetic derivatives have been prepared. Many of these are capable of inhibiting the RNA polymerase of rifampicin-resistant *E. coli* mutants.[53] However, the mechanism of action of these compounds against rifampicin-resistant RNA polymerase differs from the mechanism of rifampicin on this enzyme.[54] In addition, a number of rifamycins which inhibit rifampicin-resistant RNA polymerase by a mechanism similar to the action of rifampicin on a sensitive RNA polymerase have recently been reported.[55]

7 Discussion

In the microbial world today, resistance mechanisms exist to all classes of antibiotics currently in clinical use. In many cases, the incidence of resistance is related to antibiotic usage; however, this general explanation may be overly simplistic. For antibiotics like penicillin G which has been used extensively for almost 40 years, the resistance patterns are rather remarkable. The majority of staphylococci are resistant to the action of penicillin whereas the majority of streptococci remain susceptible. In contrast, resistance mechanisms are already in existence for antibiotics which have yet to make their appearance in the clinic.

Following the introduction of the penicillinase-resistant penicillins, staphylococci were relatively well controlled. Within the last decade we have seen the emergence of what appear to be a new breed of antibiotic-resistant strains of staphylococci. Many of these are multi-resistant and only susceptible to vancomycin, an antibiotic introduced in the 1950s. The mechanisms by which these organisms resist the action of β-lactam antibiotics are not presently fully understood. Considering the virulent nature of staphylococci and their widespread role in infectious disease, elucidation of these resistance mechanisms is certainly a priority for the future. Certain strains of streptococci also exhibit high resistance to antibiotic action through mechanisms that are not fully understood. Consequently, developing drugs specifically directed against groups of antibiotic resistant gram-positive organisms is assuming a new importance.

Gram-negative organisms, which play an ever increasing role in infectious disease, present a formidable resistance problem to antibiotic therapy. Organisms such as *Neisseria gonorrhoeae* and *Haemophilus influenzae*, which have acquired resistance against traditional penicillin therapy, are now more reliably treated with newer and more powerful drugs. Similarly, pathogens such as *Pseudomonas*, *Enterobacter* and *Acinetobacter*, not readily killed by older antibiotics, are being covered to some extent by newly developed compounds. Even so, these organisms continue to pose a serious threat to immunocompromised patients. Development of more potent antibiotics to treat such infections also becomes a priority for the foreseeable future.

There is little doubt that bacteria have enormous potential to overcome the deluge of antibiotics with which they are bombarded. In this regard, we can anticipate a continued battle between antibiotics and bacteria.

REFERENCES

1 Batchelor FR, Doyle FP, Nayler JHC, Rollinson GN. Synthesis of penicillin: 6-aminopenicillanic acid in penicillin fermentations. Nature 1959; 183: 257–258

2 Newton GGF, Abraham EP. Isolation of cephalosporin C, a penicillin-like antibiotic containing D-α-aminoadipic acid. Biochem J 1956; 62: 651–658

3 Richmond MH, Sykes, RB. The β-lactamases of gram-negative bacteria and their possible physiological role. In: Rose AH, Tempest DW, eds. Advances in microbial physiology 9. New York: Academic Press, 1973; 31–88

4 Sykes RB, Matthew M. The β-lactamases of gram-negative bacteria and their role in resistance to β-lactam antibiotics. J Antimicrob Chemother 1976; 2: 115–157

5 Sykes RB, Georgopapadakou NH. Bacterial resistance to β-lactam antibiotics: an overview. In: Salton MRJ, Shockman GD, eds, β-Lactam antibiotics. Mode of action, new developments and future prospects. New York: Academic Press, 1981; 199–214

6 Spratt BG. The mechanism of action of penicillin. Sci Prog 1978; 65: 101–128

7 Williamson R, Zighilboim S, Tomasz A. Penicillin-binding proteins of penicillin-resistant and penicillin-tolerant *Streptococcus pneumonia*. In: Salton M, Shockman GD, eds, β-Lactam antibiotics. Mode of action, new developments and future prospects. New York: Academic Press, 1981; 215–225

8 Hayes MV, Curtis NAC, Wyke AW, Ward BJ. Decreased affinity of a penicillin-binding protein for β-lactam antibiotics in a clinical isolate of *Staphylococcus aureus* resistant to methicillin. Fems Micro Lett 1981; 10: 119–122

9 Nev HC. Structure–activity relations of new β-lactam compounds and in-vitro activity against common bacteria. Rev Infect Dis 1983; 5 (Suppl 2) S319–337

10 Cole M. Inhibition of β-lactamases. In: Hamilton-Miller JMT, Smith JT, eds. Beta-lactamases. New York: Academic Press, 1979; 205–289

11 Brown AG, Butterworth D, Cole M et al. Naturally-occurring β-lactamase inhibitors with antibacterial activity. J Antibiot 1976; 29: 668–669

12 Howarth TT, Brown AG, King TJ. Clavulanic acid, a novel β-lactam isolated from *Streptomyces calvuligerus*; X-ray crystal structure analysis. J Chem Soc Chem Commun 1977; 523–525

13 Brown AG, Corbett DF, Eglington AJ, Howarth TT. Structures of olivanic acid derivatives MM4550 and MM13902; two new fused β-lactams isolated from *Streptomyces olivaceous*. J Chem Soc Chem Commun 1977; 15: 523–525

14 Liu W-C, Astle G, Wells JS Jr et al. Izumenolide—a novel β-lactamase inhibitor produced by *Micromonospora I*. Detection, isolation and characterization. J Antibiot 1980; 1256–1261

15 Bush K, Freudenberger J, Sykes RB. Inhibition of *Escherichia coli* Tem-2 β-lactamase by the sulfated compounds izumenolide, panosialin and sodiumdodecyl sulfate. J Antibiot 1980; 33: 1560–1562

16 Reading C, Cole M. Clavulinic acid: a beta-lactamase-inhibiting beta-lactam from *Streptomyces clavuligerus*. Antimicrob Agents Chemother 1977; 11: 852–857

17 Hunter PA, Colman K, Fisher J, Taylor D. *In vitro* synergistic properties of clavulanic acid, with ampicillin, amoxicillin and ticarcillin. J Antimicrob Chemother 1980; 6: 455–470

18 English AR, Retsema JA, Girard AE, Lynch JE, Barth WE. CP-45,899 a beta-lactamase inhibitor that extends the antibacterial spectrum of beta-lactamases: initial bacteriological characterization. Antimicrob Agents Chemother 1978; 14: 414–419

19 Pratt RF, Loosemore MJ, 6-β-bromopenicillanic acid, a potent β-lactamase inhibitor. Proc Natl Acad Sci USA 1978; 75: 4145–4149

20 Foulds G, Stankewich JP, Marshall DC et al. Pharmacokinetics of sulbactam in humans. Antimicrob Agents Chemother 1983; 23: 692–699

21 Charnas RL, Fisher J, Knowles JR. Chemical studies on the inactivation of *Escherichia coli* RTEM β-lactamase by clavulanic acid. Biochem 1978; 17: 2185–2189

22 Lund F, Tybring L. 6 β-amidinopenicillanic acids—a new group of antibiotics. Nature (New Biol) 1972; 135–137

23 Spratt BG. Distinct penicillin binding proteins involved in the division, elongation, and shape of *Escherichia coli* K12. Proc Natl Acad Sci USA 1975; 72: 2999–3003

24 O'Callaghan CH, Sykes RB, Ryan DM, Foord RD, Muggleton PW. Cefuroxime—a new cephalosporin antibiotic. J Antibiot 1976; 29: 29–37

25 Kamimura T, Matsumoto Y, Okada N et al. Ceftizoxime (FK 749), a new parenteral cephalosporin: in vitro and in vivo antibacterial activities. Antimicrob Agents Chemother 1979; 16: 540–548

26 Angehrn P, Probst PJ, Reiner R, Then RL. R013-9904, a long-acting broad-spectrum cephalosporin: in vitro and in vivo studies. Antimicrob Agents Chemother 1980; 18: 913–921

27 O'Callaghan CH, Acred P, Harper, PB et al. GR 20263, a new broad-spectrum cephalosporin with anti-pseudomonal activity. Antimicrob Agents Chemother 1980; 17: 876–883

28 Nagarajan R, Boeck LD, Gorman M et al. β-lactam antibiotics from *Streptomyces*. J Am Chem Soc 1971; 93: 2308–2310

29 Aoki H, Sakai H, Kohsaka M et al. Nocardicin A, a new monocyclic β-lactam antibiotic. I. Discovery, isolation and characterization. J Antibiot 1976; 29: 492–500

30 Ratcliffe RW, Albers-Schönberg G. Nontraditional β-lactam antibiotics. In: Morin RB, Gorman M, eds. Chemistry and biology of β-lactam antibiotics. Vol 2. New York: Academic Press, 1982; 227

31 Birnbaum J, Stapley EO, Miller AK, Wallick H, Hendlin D, Woodruff HB. Cefoxitin, a semi-synthetic cephamycin: a microbiological overview. J Antimicrob Agents Chemother 1978; 4(SB): 15–32

32 Nakao H, Yanagisawa H, Ishihara S et al. Semisynthetic cephamycins II. Structure–activity studies related to cefmetazole (CS-1170). J Antibiot 1979 1979; 32: 320–329

33 Wise R, Andrews JM, Hancox J. In vitro activity of cefotetan, a new cephamycin derivative compared with that of other β-lactam compounds. Antimicrob Agents Chemother 1982; 21: 486–491

34 Yoshida T, Matsuura S, Mayama M, Kameda Y, Kuwahara S. Moxalactam (6059-S), a novel 1-oxa-β-lactam with an expanded antibacterial spectrum: laboratory evaluation. Antimicrob Agents Chemother 1980; 17: 302–312

35 Sykes RB, Bush K. Physiology, biochemistry and inactivation of β-lactamases. In: Morin RB, Gorman M, eds. Chemistry and biology of β-lactam antibiotics. Vol 3. New York: Academic Press, 1982; 155–207

36 Kropp H, Sundelof JG, Kahan JS, Kahan FM, Birnbaum J. MK0787 (N-formimidoylthienamycin: evaluation of in vitro and in vivo activities. Antimicrob Agents Chemother 1980; 17: 993–1000

37 Sykes RB, Cimarusti CM, Bonner DP et al. Monocyclic β-lactam antibiotics produced by bacteria. Nature 1981; 291: 482–491

38 Sykes RB, Bonner DP, Bush K, Georgopapadakou NH. Azthreonam (SQ 26,776), a synthetic monobactam specifically active against aerobic gram-negative bacteria. Antimicrob Agents Chemother 1982; 85–92

39 Umezawa H, Umezawa S, Tsuchiya T, Okazaki Y. 3′,4′-dideoxy-kanamycin B active against kanamycin-resistant *Escherichia coli* and *Pseudonomas aeruginosa*. J Antibiot 1971; 24: 485–487

40 Wright JJ. Synthesis of I-N-ethylsisomicin: a broad-spectrum semi-synthetic animoglycoside antibiotic. J Chem Soc Chem Commun 1976; 6: 206–208

41 Kawaguchi H, Naito T, Nakagawa S, Fujisawa K. BB-K8, a new semisynthetic aminoglycoside antibiotic. J Antibiot 1972; 25: 695–708

42 Allen NE, Alborn WE Jr, Hobbs JN Jr, Kirst HA. 7-hydroxytropolone: an inhibitor of aminoglycoside-2″-O-adenyltransferase. Antimicrob Agents Chemother 1982; 22: 824–831

43 Doi O, Kondo S, Tanaka N, Umezawa H. Purification and properties of kanamycin–phosphorylating enzyme from *Pseudomonas aeruginosa*. J Antibiot 1969; 22: 273–282

44 Kirst HA, Marconi GG, Counter FT et al. Synthesis and characterization of a novel inhibitor of an aminoglycoside-inactivating enzyme. J Antibiot 1982; 35: 1651–1657

45 Werner RG, Lechner UL, Goeth H. Derivatives of 4-dihydro-deoxy-4(R)-aminospectinomycin and their activity against susceptible and resistant *Escherichia coli* strains. Antimicrob Agents Chemother 1982; 21: 101–106

46 Miyamura S, Koizuma K, Nakagawa Y. An inhibitor of chloramphenicol acetyltransferase produced by *Streptomyces*. J Antibiot 1979; 1217–1218

47 Syriopoulou VP, Harding AL, Goldman DA, Smith AL. In vitro antibacterial activity of fluorinated analogs of chloramphenicol and thiamphenicol. Antimicrob Agents Chemother 1981; 19: 294–297

48 Russell AD, Ahonkhai I. Antibacterial activity of a new thiatetracycline antibiotic, thiacycline, in comparison with tetracycline, doxycycline and minocycline. J Antimicrob Chemother 1982; 9: 445–449

49 Bakhtiar M, Selwyn S. Antibacterial activity of a new thiatetracycline. J Antimicrob Chemother 1983; 11: 291

50 Inoue S, Ohue T, Yamagishi J, Nakamura S, Shimizu M. Mode of incomplete cross-resistance among pipemidic, piromidic and nalidixic acids. Antimicrob Agents Chemother 1978; 14: 240–245

51 Ito A, Harai K, Inoue M et al. In vitro antibacterial activity of AM-715, a new nalidixic acid analog. Antimicrob Agents Chemother 1980, 17: 103–108

52 Shimizu M, Takase Y, Nakamura S et al. AT-2266, a new oral antipseudomonal agent. In: Nelson JD, Grassi C, eds. Current chemotherapy and infectious disease. Washington DC: American Society of Microbiology, 1980; 451–454

53 Riva S, Fietta A, Silvestri AG. Mechanism and action of a rifamycin derivative (AF/013) which is active on the nucleic acid polymerases insensitive to rifamycin. Biophys Res Commun 1972; 49: 1263–1271

54 Meilhac M, Tysper Z, Chambon P. Animal DNA-dependent RNA polymerases. 4. Studies on inhibition by rifamycin derivatives. Eur J Biochem 1972; 28: 291–300

55 Nikiforov VG, Trapkova AA, Gragerov AI, Maslin DN. A derivative of rifimycin SV inhibiting rifampicin-resistant RNA polymerase of *Escherichia coli*. FEBS Lett 1982; 150: 416–418

British Medical Bulletin (1984) Vol. 40, No. 1, pp. 102–106

IMPACT OF BACTERIAL RESISTANCE TO ANTIBIOTICS ON THERAPY

H P LAMBERT MD FRCP FFCM

Communicable Diseases Unit
St George's Hospital
London

1 Meningitis
2 Respiratory infections
3 Gastrointestinal infections
4 Sexually transmitted diseases
5 Hospital infections
6 Control of antibiotic-resistant bacterial infection
   a Control of antibiotics
   b Control of hospital infection
References

The emergence and spread of antibiotic resistance to bacteria of medical importance has exercised a profound effect on clinical practice, imposing serious constraints on the options available for the treatment of many infections. The problems resulting from increasing drug resistance affect infections acquired in the community as well as those acquired in hospital[1] and are relevant to a wide variety of infections important by virtue of their severity, or frequency, or both.

1 Meningitis

Meningitis presenting after the neonatal period and affecting previously normal patients is most commonly caused by one of three organisms, *Neisseria meningitidis*, *Haemophilus influenzae* and *Streptococcus pneumoniae*. Problems of drug resistance have become important in all three forms of infection.

The value of sulphonamides in the treatment of meningococcal septicaemia and meningitis was firmly established soon after their introduction in the late 1930s. They remained the treatment of first choice until 1963, when sulphonamide resistance emerged into clinical significance. By 1969, 70% of meningococcal strains in the USA were sulphonamide resistant.[2] Although the prevalence of resistance among invasive strains has remained low in the UK, their existence means that this group of drugs cannot now be employed in the initial treatment of this serious and often rapidly progressive infection. Benzyl penicillin by high-dose intravenous injection is now used initially, although sulphonamides are permissible as continuation treatment when the blood or cerebro-spinal fluid (CSF) isolate has been shown to be susceptible to sulphonamide and when the patient's condition allows a change to oral therapy. A hint that penicillin treatment of meningococcal meningitis might itself be threatened is given by the identification of a strain of *N. meningitidis* with penicillinase-producing and transfer plasmids probably acquired from a strain of *Neisseria gonorrhoeae*.[3]

Several successful forms of chemotherapy have been authenticated for meningitis caused by *H. influenzae*. Chloramphenicol as the sole drug was widely used but the slight risk of marrow aplasia associated with its use remained a cause of concern. For this reason, when the efficacy of high-dose ampicillin by intravenous injection had been established, this regimen came to be widely used in the USA and, to a lesser extent, in the UK. Transferable drug resistance associated with β-lactamase production, and thus with resistance to ampicillin emerged in 1974,[4] and its frequency is now too great to permit ampicillin as initial choice of therapy. A recent multicentre study showed that 9 of 79 capsulated strains (11%) were β-lactamase producers.[5]

Chloramphenicol resistance has also been identified in *H. influenzae*[6] but such strains are so far rare. Chloramphenicol has, for the moment, resumed its role as first-choice treatment for haemophilus meningitis, although many physicians follow the recommendation of the American Academy of Pediatrics in employing both chloramphenicol and ampicillin. These policies too may have to be abandoned, since invasive infections caused by *H. influenzae* resistant both to chloramphenicol and to ampicillin have been identified in several countries.[7,8] The correct choice of treatment for invasive haemophilus infections caused by such resistant strains is not yet established. Fortunately, although the earlier cephalosporins were relatively ineffective in the treatment of bacterial meningitis, some of the newer compounds, with their high intrinsic activity and high degree of β-lactamase resistance, are proving much more successful. A controlled trial using cefuroxime gave favourable results in the common forms of meningitis,[9] and information is rapidly accumulating on the relevant pharmacokinetic properties and clinical effectiveness of several of the extended spectrum compounds.[10]

Most strains of *Streptococcus pneumoniae* are fully susceptible to penicillin, which remains the preferred drug for this serious form of meningitis. Penicillin resistance in pneumococci has, however, emerged in two forms and its possible increase needs careful surveillance. The penicillin-insensitive pneumococci first identified in Papua New Guinea and in Australia in the late 1960s are inhibited by penicillin concentrations of 0·1–2·0 mg/l (in comparison with a minimum inhibitory concentration (MIC) for sensitive pneumococci of <0·02 mg/l). Plasma levels adequate for the treatment of pneumonia and other non-meningitic infections are therefore easily attainable. The low CSF levels achieved, even after high doses of benzyl penicillin given intravenously, make it possible that penicillin may be inadequate for the treatment of meningitis caused by these strains. Hansman[11] adduces evidence of this in Papua New Guinea, where penicillin-insensitive strains were isolated from 19 of 57 patients with severe pneumococcal infections.

Pneumococci with multiple drug resistance which included a high degree of penicillin resistance was first described in South Africa in 1977.[12] The two main agents available for pneumococcal meningitis, penicillin and chloramphenicol, are ineffective in infection caused by these resistant strains. Pneumococci with multiple drug resistance have been identified rarely, but in a wide range of countries including the UK[13] and one report[14] describes an epidemic in a day care centre for children, some of whom developed meningitis.

2 Respiratory Infections

i *Sore Throat*

The only common bacterial cause of acute sore throat is *Streptococcus pyogenes*, which has fortunately remained susceptible to penicillin. Resistance to sulphonamides emerged soon after their introduction, and tetracycline resistance in this species became prevalent in the 1960s. The frequency varies a good deal in different areas, in one large survey accounting for 36% of strains isolated in the UK.[15]

Resistance to macrolide antibiotics among haemolytic streptococci has also been commonly observed, arising in apparently unrelated foci[16] and emerging rapidly in the course of treatment in individual patients.[17] The use of tetracycline is therefore inappropriate as an agent of first choice for acute streptococcal infections. The prevalence of erythromycin resistance in haemolytic streptococci needs to be measured by repeated surveillance, since it is widely used as the agent of first choice for a variety of infections, and is often needed for penicillin-allergic patients.

ii *Other Upper Respiratory Tract Infections*

Acute otitis media and acute sinusitis often require antibiotic treatment. Here, too, the spread of antibiotic resistance has substantially diminished the available options. Recent studies have shown a variety of causal pathogens in both conditions, of which *S. pneumoniae*, *H. influenzae* and *S. pyogenes* are the most important. Several types of resistance affecting the use of these drugs have already been discussed. In addition, tetracycline and macrolide resistance are well documented in pneumococci as well as in β-haemolytic streptococci; erythromycin resistance, however, remains fairly uncommon in pneumococci. The multi-resistant strains isolated in South Africa and elsewhere showed resistance to this drug, as well as to penicillin, chloramphenicol, co-trimoxazole, clindamycin and tetracycline.

The problems posed in the treatment of haemophilus meningitis by changes in antibiotic resistance are also relevant to the management of acute epiglotitis, another life-threatening infection caused by capsulated strains of *H. influenzae*.

iii *Pneumonia*

S. pneumoniae remains the most common identified cause of pneumonia acquired in the community; the problems of antibiotic resistance in this species have already been discussed. It is evident that benzyl penicillin by injection, or a suitable oral penicillin in less seriously ill patients, remains the agent of first choice; any increase in the prevalence of penicillin resistance would present serious problems of drug choice and cost, especially since pneumococcal pneumonia shows its highest prevalence and severity in the poorer countries of the world.

Mycoplasma pneumoniae infections can best be treated by erythromycin or by tetracycline. Resistance is easily induced in vitro but appears rarely during treatment,[18] most re-isolates retaining their original antibiotic susceptibility.

Haemophilus influenzae must also be considered in relation to lower respiratory tract infections. Non-capsulated strains have long been recognized as an important component of the flora of bronchial secretions in patients with chronic bronchitis. The wider use of transtracheal aspiration in the diagnosis of acute pneumonia has shown this organism as a significant cause of acute pneumonia. The causal strains may be capsulated or non-capsulated.[19]

Pneumonia acquired by patients in hospital presents a somewhat different spectrum of causes. The pneumococcus is important in both hospital and community contexts, but the hospital patient is at risk from a wide variety of pathogens of no great significance to him previously as a healthy subject. Especially relevant in relation to antibiotic resistance are the so-called 'gram-negative pneumonias', that is, those caused by Enterobacteriaceae or pseudomonads, and pneumonia caused by *S. aureus*. Drug resistance as it affects the management of these hospital-acquired pneumonias will be discussed in a subsequent section.

3 Gastrointestinal Infections

Transferable drug resistance was first demonstrated in intestinal bacteria. The widespread presence of plasmids and transposons mediating resistance in normal and potentially pathogenic bacteria, and the emerging evidence of in-vivo transfer makes it easy to understand why important changes in the antibiotic sensitivity pattern of bowel pathogens have occurred so readily, and with such a detrimental effect on the options available for treatment.

S. typhi is easily inhibited in vitro by a variety of antimicrobial agents, but some of them are ineffective in treatment, and only two agents, chloramphenicol and co-trimoxazole, are widely used. Amoxycillin, mecillinam and trimethoprim alone are also effective. Drug resistance in *S. typhi* first became important in 1972, when a large outbreak of typhoid in Mexico was caused by a strain resistant to chloramphenicol, streptomycin, sulphonamide and tetracycline.[20] Since then, chloramphenicol-resistant strains have been isolated in many countries, although they are still uncommon enough in the UK to allow chloramphenicol (or co-trimoxazole) to be the treatment of first choice while the results of sensitivity testing are awaited. The in-vivo acquisition of drug resistance in typhoid was proved in 1981 by Datta *et al.*[21] in a patient with an initially drug-sensitive strain who was treated with chloramphenicol and then co-trimoxazole. The subsequent isolate of *S. typhi* was resistant to all three drugs, chloramphenicol and sulphonamide resistance being determined by one plasmid, and trimethoprim resistance by a transposon located on a different plasmid.

Drug resistance is also extremely common in non-typhoid salmonella, and the resistance patterns in human infections are generally similar to those found in the animal sources from which most human salmonella infections ultimately originate. This process, first thoroughly analysed in the 1960s in relation to *S. typhimurium* type 29 infections,[22] has been shown in relation to many salmonella species and many antibiotics. Most recently, a steady increase in trimethoprim resistance in human infections by *S. typhimurium* has been shown;[23] none were encountered until 1974, but by 1981, 6·7% of human strains were resistant. This trend followed a somewhat larger increase in trimethoprim resistance among cattle salmonellae, in which 14·0% had become resistant by 1981. Since most of the strains from human sources were of phage types associated with cattle, this increase in resistance was thought to have resulted from attempts to control bovine salmonellosis by trimethoprim. These extensive changes in the drug resistance of non-typhoid salmonella infection have no direct effect on the management of acute gastroenteritis, the most common clinical manifestation of salmonellosis, since antimicrobials have little or no place in its treatment. In invasive salmonellosis, however, the presence of drug resistance exercises a severe limitation and no effective therapy may be available in systemic infection caused by multi-resistant strains. Outbreaks of this type have been described in several developing countries, especially in paediatric wards,[24] and have been associated with human-to-human infection rather than directly from animal sources.

Human shigellosis exhibits a wide range of severity, from subclinical infection to severe dysentery accompanied by serious systemic illness and leading to a high rate of mortality. The efficacy of antimicrobial therapy in the more serious forms of bacillary dysentery has been fully established but the rapid spread of drug resistance in this genus has, in many areas, nullified its value. Ampicillin resistance became common in shigella infections soon after the drug was introduced so that by the late 1960s most strains of *S. sonnei* in London were resistant to ampicillin as well as to sulphamides. Transferable drug resistance was discovered in multi-resistant shigella isolates in Japan, and outbreaks caused by similar strains have been seen in many countries. The huge epidemic of *Shigella dysenteriae* type 1 infection in Central America in 1969 and 1970 was caused by a strain mostly resistant to sulphamides, streptomycin, tetracycline and chloramphenicol,[25] while in a later outbreak, an additional plasmid conferring ampicillin resistance was identified.[26] At present many shigella strains are susceptible to trimethoprim but the rapid increase in resistance of enterobacteriaceae to this agent suggests that this advantage may soon be lost.

Cholera is treated mainly by oral or intravenous fluid replacement but the use of antimicrobials to reduce the fluid requirement, and to lessen the likelihood of spread to contacts, are both well documented. Here, too, a useful form of therapy and chemoprophylaxis are easily vitiated by the spread of drug resistance. Mhalu *et al.*[27] describe an epidemic in Tanzania in which the strains were initially tetracycline-susceptible. After five months 76% had become resistant. An outbreak caused by a strain of *Vibrio cholerae* with a plasmid coding for resistance to tetracycline, ampicillin, kanamycin, streptomycin and co-trimoxazole has recently been described from Bangladesh.[28]

4 Sexually Transmitted Diseases

The main effects of changes in antibiotic resistance have been seen in the treatment of gonorrhoea. The initial success of sulphonamide was soon lost by the emergence of resistant strains. By 1958 treatment failures were being reported following penicillin treatment and these isolates were shown to have an increase in the MIC for penicillin which, although moderate (up to 1 g/l), was well correlated with treatment failure. The problem was partly solved by increasing the dose of penicillin or by the use of alternative drug regimens, although this form of penicillin resistance was often linked to tetracycline resistance. The huge variations in the speed with which drug resistance may arise is best shown in the gonococcus, for it was not until 1976 that penicillinase-producing organisms, with a high degree of resistance and causing infection untreatable by penicillin at any dose, appeared almost simultaneously in the UK[29] and the USA.[30] Two types bearing different plasmids were identified, one originating in East Asia and the other in West Africa. These strains have now spread all over the world. In the period of 18 months up to June 1982, 3177 cases of gonorrhoea caused by β-lactamase-producing strains were identified in 11 European countries.[31] The emergence of penicillinase-producing gonococci has serious consequences for the public health services. An increase in treatment failures leads to longer periods of infectivity, gonococci isolated from treatment failures must be tested for penicillinase production, and alternative therapies, some imposing an expensive additional item in health budgets, must be available. Isolates which produce β-lactamase and also resistant to spectinomycin, an important alternative drug, are now being reported.

5 Hospital Infections

Hospitals have long been recognized as important foci for the emergence and dissemination of drug-resistant bacteria. The dominant role of hospital staphylococcal infection in the 1950s and 1960s has now been supplanted to some extent by the problems of nosocomial infection caused by aerobic gram-negative bacteria. The extent of this change, the reasons which underlie it and the complex epidemiology of these infections are discussed elsewhere.[32] The principal factors underlying this modern epidemic appear to be the high frequency of impairment of resistance caused by disease or its treatment; the extensive use of antibiotics leading to selective pressure favouring the emergence of resistant strains, and the opportunities for cross-infection afforded by the hospital environment. The importance of plasmids and transposons in mediating these forms of resistance is well established, although some resistance factors in enteric bacteria are chromosomal. The relative importance of various sources of infection—bowel, skin, respiratory and urinary tract—and of different modes of cross-infection are still being evaluated; recent work in this field has been usefully reviewed by Casewell.[32]

Nearly one in ten of the patients admitted to an acute care hospital in the UK acquires an infection during his stay. Such infections vary from the trivial to fatal and many of them require antibiotic treatment. These drugs are often also mistakenly given to patients who are colonized but not apparently infected with hospital organisms. Overall, antibiotics are administered to about 20% of hospital in-patients. Thus antibiotic administration, some of it necessitated by hospital-acquired infection, contributes to the vicious circle by which such infections acquire drug resistance. The infections of clinical importance resulting from this process well show the significance of this special environment as many of them are rare outside hospital. The most serious are gram-negative septicaemias which account for the largest proportion of patients with bacterial shock syndrome in hospital, gram-negative pneumonias, especially severe in immune-suppressed patients, and hospital-acquired urinary tract infections. These forms of infection may occur anywhere in the hospital but are especially common in intensive care units and special care baby units.

Ampicillin resistance soon emerged in hospital-acquired gram-negative bacterial infections, and the most recent changes have concerned the development of resistance to the aminoglycosides and to trimethoprim. Gentamicin resistance, often associated with multiple resistance, emerged in many hospitals throughout the world after the drug had been used for several years as the mainstay in treating infections caused by Enterobacteriaceae and by pseudomonads. Infection caused by these gentamicin-resistant strains are endemic in many hospitals, although the distribution is patchy, and a large number of outbreaks of multi-resistant coliform infection has now been documented. Drug resistance factors may be so numerous as to abrogate all available antibiotic treatments; of the gentamicin-resistant klebsiellae in one study, for example, 89% were resistant to at least 10 antibiotics.[32] At present the antibiotic management of gentamicin-resistant infection relies on the use of amikacin, resistant to most of the aminoglycoside-destroying enzymes, and on a variety of newly introduced β-lactamase agents, some of them of very broad activity and others of specific value in pseudomonas infections. Several cephalosporins have a suitably high intrinsic activity and high degree of β-lactamase stability for use in coliform infections, of which cefotaxime, moxolactam, ceftazidime and the combination of amoxycillin with clavulinic acid have been most extensively evaluated. Azlocillin, piperacillin and ceftazidime are especially relevant in the treatment of pseudomonas infection.

Although infections of this type may be confined to hospitals, there is increasing evidence of the spread of resistance between hospital, nursing home and community. For example, Weinstein *et al.*[33] showed that one in four of the aminoglycoside-resistant

TABLE I. Valuable treatments under threat or no longer available

Type of infection	Treatments under threat	Treatments no longer available
Meningococcal meningitis and septicaemia		Sulphonamides (for initial treatment)
H. influenzae infections	Chloramphenicol	Ampicillin (for initial treatment)
Urinary infections	Ampicillin, trimethoprim	
Gonorrhoea	'High-dose' penicillin	'Low-dose' penicillin
Pneumococcal infections	Penicillin	
Salmonella infection	Chloramphenicol, co-trimoxazole, amoxycillin	
Methicillin-resistant staphylococcal infection	Many antibiotics	
Hospital coliform infection	Many antibiotics	Ampicillin
Shigellosis		Sulphonamides, ampicillin

strains they identified were present in admission specimens; of these, some were found in patients transferred from nursing homes or other hospitals and others in patients previously admitted to their own hospital.

Aminoglycosides, as relatively toxic agents given parenterally, are almost confined to institutional use but trimethoprim, at first in combination with sulphamethoxazole and now increasingly as a single agent, has been used widely in hospitals and in general practice. Surveys of the incidence of resistance have recorded widely variable results, but in nearly all the frequency of trimethoprim resistance has shown substantial increases. Datta et al.[34] showed that resistant isolates had increased to comprise 15% of the coliforms and both this study and that of Towner et al.[35] showed that the proportion of strains with transferable resistance has greatly increased.

Drug-resistant bacteria important in hospital infection are often distributed very erratically, presenting serious problems in some hospitals and scarcely occurring in others. This is a notable feature in the outbreaks of methicillin-resistant staphylococcal infection which have plagued hospitals in many countries and have spread from them to nursing homes and to the surrounding communities. Kayser[36] has reviewed this problem up to 1975 and the more recent epidemiology is discussed by Wenzel.[37] It is evident that these organisms can cause life-threating infection, and their resistance pattern imposes serious constraints upon the available antibiotic choices. Vancomycin, a relatively toxic drug requiring intravenous administration and regular monitoring in the laboratory, is often the only effective agent. It is, of course, unsuitable for use except in hospital. Many strains are additionally susceptible only to rifampicin, fusidic acid, and co-trimoxazole.

It is evident that the development of drug resistance has made unavailable a number of previously valuable treatments, and that in many other infections treatment is made more difficult, or more expensive, by the presence of drug-resistant bacteria. Examples of these consequences for therapy are given in Table I. Drug resistance in mycobacteria is discussed elsewhere in this Bulletin (pp. 84–90).

6 Control of Antibiotic-Resistant Bacterial Infection

a *Control of Antibiotics*

The widespread use of antibiotics and the ample evidence which relates their use to the emergence of drug resistance has stimulated a large volume of work aimed at analysing the ways in which these drugs are prescribed, and at attempting to limit their use. Most studies have shown substantial errors in the manner in which antibiotics are used. The most frequent concern optimal choice for bacterial infections, excessive use of topical preparations and,

especially, excessive prescribing, both in number and duration of courses, for surgical prophylaxis. The rational use of antibiotics in surgical prophylaxis is especially important since many valid indications for its use are now well established. Shapiro et al.[38] found that 10% of patients in acute care hospitals received antibiotics for surgical prophylaxis, but that this high usage accounted for 30% of total antibiotic consumption.

Methods used in attempting to limit antibiotic usage must clearly be adapted to the particular problems of individual countries and institutions. In general, the most fruitful have combined restrictive and educational methods. The latter include clinical and laboratory consultation, education of undergraduates and postgraduates, guidelines in the forms of bulletins and booklets, and various forms of monitoring and audit. Restrictive methods operate mainly through the pharmacy and the laboratory. For example, a restricted list of drugs may be stocked or consultation may be required if particular drugs are to be used, or the duration of a prescribed course may be limited unless a specific new order is given. The laboratory attempts to limit its reporting of bacterial isolates to those judged clinically significant and often reports on a limited number of antibiotic susceptibilities for these isolates.

Measuring the value of antibiotic control programmes has proved extremely difficult. Several well-documented examples have shown successful control of antibiotic use and the resultant control of antibiotic resistance, for example, in a burns unit[39] and in surgical prophylaxis.[40] On the other hand, some educational initiatives have had little influence on the quality of antibiotic prescribing.[41]

The limited success of antibiotic control programmes makes it especially important that vigorous efforts should be made to control cross-infection in hospital, a potent element in the spread of antibiotic resistant bacteria.

b *Control of Hospital Infection*

Established control methods used to limit the spread of hospital infection are as appropriate for the newer multiply resistant hospital pathogens as they were for the more traditional pathogens for which they were developed. Unfortunately, many of the most vulnerable hospital patients are inevitably exposed to many contacts and subjected to many procedures which may be followed by infection, and there is an inevitable conflict between the demands of barrier nursing and those of diagnosis and treatment. Furthermore, although many modern hospitals contain an ample supply of single rooms, barrier nursing in a single room which is part of a general ward area is often less efficiently maintained than in an isolation unit, in which the techniques of barrier nursing are an essential and routine component of the ward procedures. Despite these difficulties, patients harbouring resistant organisms should be barrier-nursed. The US Department of Health Education and Welfare has published an excellent system,[42] which has been adapted for use in general hospitals in the UK.[43] A simplified version of the latter system is in use at St George's Hospital, London and many hospitals have made their own adaptations. These procedures can be used whether or not the hospital possesses specific ventilation systems, and enteric cross-infection can be controlled even in old and unsuitable buildings if simple measures are vigorously implemented.[44]

Since the modes by which antibiotic-resistant bacteria emerge, flourish and spread within and outside the hospital vary so much from one organism to another, and since so much still remains unknown about their detailed ecology, it seems essential that attempts to control these organisms should include both of the main methods, an antibiotic control policy and an efficient system of cross-infection control.

REFERENCES

1 Finland M. Emergence of antibiotic resistance in hospitals 1935–1975. Rev Infect Dis 1979; 1: 4–21

2 Artenstein MS. Chemoprophylaxis of meningococcal carriers. N Engl J Med 1969; 281: 678

3 Dillon JR, Pauzé M, Yeung K-H. Spread of penicillinase-producing and transfer plasmids from the gonococcus to *Neisseria meningitidis*. Lancet 1983; 1: 779–781

4 Smith AL. Antibiotics and invasive *Haemophilus influenzae*. N Engl J Med 1976; 294: 1329–1331

5 Philpott-Howard J, Williams JD. Increase in antibiotic resistance in *Haemophilus influenzae* in the United Kingdom since 1977. Br Med J 1982; 2: 1597–1599

6 Kinmonth A-L, Storrs CN, Mitchell RG. Meningitis due to chloramphenicol-resistant *Haemophilus influenzae* type b. Br Med J 1978; 1: 694

7 Uchiyama N, Greene GR, Kitts DB, Thrupp LD. Meningitis due to *Haemophilus influenzae* type B resistant to ampicillin and chloramphenicol. J Pediatr 1980; 97: 421–424

8 Simasathien S, Duangmani C, Echeverria P. Haemophilus influenzae type B resistant to ampicillin and chloramphenicol in an orphanage in Thailand. Lancet 1980; 2: 1214–1217

9 Swedish Study Group. Cefuroxime versus ampicillin and chloramphenicol for the treatment of bacterial meningitis. Lancet 1982; 1: 295–298

10 Lambert HP. Treatment of bacterial meningitis. Br Med J 1983; 286: 741–742

11 Gratten M, Naraqi S, Hansman D. High prevalence of penicillin-insensitive pneumococci in Port Moresby, Papua New Guinea. Lancet 1980; 2: 192–195

12 Appelbaum PC, Bhamjee A, Scragg JN, Hallett AF, Bowen AJ, Cooper RC. Streptococcus pneumoniae resistant to penicillin and chloramphenicol. Lancet 1977; 2: 995–997

13 Williams EW, Watts JA, Potten MR. Streptococcus pneumoniae resistant to penicillin and chloramphenicol in the UK. Lancet 1981; 2: 699

14 Radetsky MS, Istre GR, Johansen TL *et al*. Multiply resistant pneumococcus causing meningitis: its epidemiology within a day-care centre. Lancet 1981; 2: 771–773

15 Tetracycline resistance in pneumococci and group A streptococci. Report of an ad-hoc study group on antibiotic resistance. Br Med J 1977; 1: 131–133

16 Dixon JMS, Lipinski AE. Infections with β-hemolytic *Streptococcus* resistant to lincomycin and erythromycin and observations on zonal-pattern resistance to lincomycin. J Infect Dis 1974; 130: 351–356

17 Sprunt K, Leidy G, Redman W. Cross resistance between lincomycin and erythromycin in viridans streptococci. Pediatrics 1970; 46: 84–88

18 Niitu Y, Hasegawa S, Suetake T, Kubota H, Komatsu S, Horikawa M. Resistance of *Mycoplasma pneumoniae* to erythromycin and other antibiotics. *J Pediatr* 1970; 76: 438–443

19 Wallace RJ Jr, Musher DM, Martin RR. *Haemophilus influenzae* pneumonia in adults. Am J Med 1978; 64: 87–93

20 Anderson ES. The problem and implications of chloramphenicol resistance in the typhoid bacillus. J Hyg 1975; 74: 289–299

21 Datta N, Richards H, Datta C. Salmonella typhi in vivo acquires resistance to both chloramphenicol and co-trimoxazole. Lancet 1981; 1: 1181–1183

22 Anderson ES. The ecology of transferable drug resistance in the enterobacteria. Annu Rev Microbiol 1968; 22: 131–180

23 Ward LR, Rowe B, Threlfall EJ. Incidence of trimethoprim resistance in salmonellae isolated in Britain: a twelve year study. Lancet 1982; 2: 705–706

24 Leading Article. Drug resistance in Salmonellae. Lancet 1982; 1: 1391–1392

25 Farrar WE Jr, Eidson M. R factors in strains of *Shigella dysenteriae* type 1 isolated in the Western hemisphere during 1969–70. J Infect Dis 1971; 124: 327–329

26 Crosa JH, Olarte J, Mata LJ, Luttropp LK, Peñaranda ME. Characterisation of an R-plasmid associated with ampicillin resistance in *Sigella dysenteriae* type 1 isolated from epidemics. Antimicrob Agents Chemother 1977; 11: 553–558

27 Mhalu FS, Mmari PW, Ijumba J. Rapid emergence of El Tor *Vibrio cholerae* resistant to antimicrobial agents during first six months of fourth cholera epidemic in Tanzania. Lancet 1979; 1: 345–347

28 Glass RI, Huq MI, Lee JV *et al*. Plasmid-borne multiple drug resistance in *Vibrio cholerae* serogroup O1, biotype El Tor: evidence for a point-source outbreak in Bangladesh. J Inf Dis 1983; 147: 204–209

29 Percival A, Rowlands J, Corkill JE *et al*. Penicillinase-producing gonococci in Liverpool. Lancet 1976; 2: 1379–1382

30 Ashford WA, Golash RG, Hemming VG. Penicillinase-producing *Neisseria gonorrhoeae*. Lancet 1976; 2: 657–658

31 World Health Organization. Surveillance of β-lactamase-producing *N. Gonorrhoeae* (PPNG). Weekly Epidemiological Record. 1983; 58: 5–8

32 Casewell MW. The role of multiply resistant coliforms in hospital-acquired infection. In: Reeves DS, Geddes AM, eds. Recent advances in infection 2. Edinburgh: Churchill Livingstone, 1982; 31–50

33 Weinstein RA, Nathan C, Gruensfelder R, Kabins SA. Endemic aminoglycoside resistance in gram-negative bacilli. Epidemiology and mechanisms. J Infect Dis 1980; 141: 338–345

34 Datta N, Dacey S, Hughes V *et al*. Distribution of genes for trimethoprim and gentamicin resistance in bacteria and their plasmids in a general hospital. J Gen Microbiol 1980; 118: 495–508

35 Towner KJ, Pearson NJ, Pinn PA, O'Grady F. Increasing importance of plasmid-mediated trimethoprim resistance in enterobacteria; two six-month clinical surveys. Br Med J 1980; 280: 517–519

36 Kayser FH. Methicillin-resistant staphylococci 1965–75. Lancet 1975; 2: 650–652

37 Wenzel RP. The emergence of methicillin-resistant *Staphylococcus aureus*. Ann Intern Med 1982; 97: 440–442

38 Shapiro M, Townsend TR, Rosner B, Kass EH. Use of antimicrobial drugs in general hospitals. II Analysis of patterns of use. J Infect Dis 1979; 139: 698–706

39 Lowbury EJL, Babb JR, Roe E. Clearance from a hospital of Gram-negative bacilli that transfer carbenicillin-resistance to *Pseudomonas aeruginosa*. Lancet 1972; 2: 941–945

40 Roberts NJ Jr, Douglas RD Jr. Gentamicin use and *Pseudomonas* and *Serratia* resistance; effect of a surgical prophylaxis regimen. Antimicrob Agents Chemother 1978; 13: 214–220

41 Swindell PJ, Reeves DS, Bullock DW, Davies AJ, Spence CE. Audits of antibiotic prescribing in a Bristol hospital. Br Med J 1983; 286: 118–122

42 National Communicable Disease Center. Isolation techniques for use in hospitals. Public Health Service Publication No 2054. Washington 1970: US Department of Health, Education and Welfare

43 Control of Infection Group, Northwick Park Hospital and Clinical Research Centre. Isolation system for general hospitals. Br Med J 1974; 2: 41–44

44 Taylor MRH, Keane CT, Kerrison IM, Stronge JL. Simple and effective measures for control of enteric cross-infection in a children's hospital. Lancet 1979; 1: 865–867

Notes on Contributors

DR S G B AMYES is a lecturer in bacteriology in the Medical School of the University of Edinburgh. He graduated in biochemistry at University College London and went on to receive an MSc degree in virology from the University of Reading. He obtained his PhD degree in microbiology in the Department of Pharmaceutics, School of Pharmacy, University of London. In 1974 he was appointed as a teaching Fellow at the School of Pharmacy and in 1977 he moved to his present position in Edinburgh. He has been involved in research into antimicrobial drug action and the mechanism of drug resistance employed by bacteria to overcome these agents. His publications include: with J T Smith, 'R-factor trimethoprim resistance mechanism: an insusceptible target site' (*Biochem Biophys Res Commun* 1974; 58: 412–418); 'Bacterial activity of trimethoprim alone and in combination with sulphamethoxazole on susceptible and resistant bacteria' (*Antimicrob Agents Chemother* 21: 288–293); and, with H Young, 'Trimethoprim resistance: An epidemic caused by two related transposons' (*13th International Congress of Chemotherapy*, Vienna).

DR D P BONNER is Assistant Department Director—Medical Microbiology in the Department of Microbiology at the Squibb Institute for Medical Research, Princeton NJ, where he has been since 1978. He received his MS and PhD from the Waksman Institute of Microbiology at Rutgers University, New Brunswick NJ, being the recipient of a Public Health Service Predoctoral Fellowship and later a Busch Postdoctoral Fellowship. His work until 1978 centred on the biological properties of the polyene macrolide antifungal antibiotics. More recently he has studied properties of the monobactams—monocyclic β-lactam antibiotics isolated from bacteria. Publications include: with R P Tewari, M Solotorovsky, W Mechlinski & C P Schaffner, 'Comparative chemotherapeutic activity of amphotericin B and amphotericin B methyl ester' (*Antimicrob Agents Chemother* 1975; 7: 724–729); and, with R B Sykes, K Bush & N Georgopapadakou, 'Aztreonam (SQ 26,776), a synthetic monobactam specifically active against aerobic gram-negative bacteria' (*Antimicrob Agents Chemother* 1982; 21: 85–92).

DR I CHOPRA is a lecturer in microbiology at the University of Bristol. He received his first degree in bacteriology at Trinity College, Dublin, and his PhD degree in the Department of Microbiology, University of Bristol, in Professor M H Richmond's laboratory. His research interests concern the mechanisms by which antibiotics are transported into bacteria and how the process can sometimes be prevented by plasmid-encoded products. His publications (some 40 papers) reflect these interests, the three most important being: with P R Ball & S W Shales, 'Plasmid-mediated tetracycline resistance involves increased efflux of the antibiotic' (*Biochem Biophys Res Commun* 1980; 93: 74–81); with P R Ball, 'Transport of antibiotics into bacteria' (*Adv Microb Physiol* 1982; 23: 183–240); and, with T J Foster *et al.* 'Analysis of tetracycline resistance encoded by transposon Tn10: deletion mapping of tetracycline-sensitive point mutations and identification of two structural genes' (*J Bacteriol* 1983; 153: 921–929). Dr Chopra's work has been supported by grants from the Medical Research Council, the Nuffield Foundation and various pharmaceutical companies in both the UK and USA. He is currently engaged in molecular studies on bacterial cell envelope composition in organisms cultured in the presence of low antibiotic levels.

DR E CUNDLIFFE, now Reader in Biochemistry at the University of Leicester, was formerly a Research Fellow of Churchill College, Cambridge, and a Beit Fellow. He graduated in biochemistry at Cambridge and received his PhD degree there in 1967. His long-term interests have been in ribosomal structure and function and also in antibiotic action and resistance. More recently, he has become interested in actinomycetes and the manner in which antibiotic-producing strains tolerate their products. He moved to Leicester from Cambridge in 1976, having also worked at Tufts University Medical School, Boston MA, and the University of Wisconsin in Madison. In addition to being co-author of a textbook (*The molecular basis of antibiotic action* 2nd ed. London: Wiley 1981) his publications include: with M Cannon & J E Davies, 'Mechanism of inhibition of eukaryotic protein sythesis by trichothecene fungal toxins' (*Proc Natl Acad Sci USA* 1974; 71: 30–34); with J Thompson & F Schmidt, 'Site of action of a ribosomal RNA methylase conferring resistance to thiostrepton' (*J Biol Chem* 1982; 257: 7915–7917); and, with C J Thompson, R H Skinner, J Thompson, J M Ward & D A Hopwood, 'Biochemical characterization of resistance determinants cloned from antibiotic-producing streptomycetes' (*J Bacteriol* 1982; 151: 678–685).

NAOMI DATTA is Professor of Microbial Genetics in the University of London. After qualifying in medicine she joined the Public Health Laboratory service for post-graduate training in microbiology and in 1957 joined the Department of Bacteriology, Royal Postgraduate Medical School, where she still works. Her professorial title relates to her work on the genetics of antibiotic resistance in bacteria, especially on resistance plasmids. She has studied various aspects of the latter including plasmid conjugation and its control, β-lactamases in enterobacteria, trimethoprim and gentamicin resistances and transposons that carry them. With colleagues supported by grants from the Medical Research Council, she has classified plasmids into incompatibility (Inc) groups, using this method for epidemiological studies. Her current research is on conjugative plasmids with no drug resistance genes in a collection of bacteria isolated before the medical use of antibiotics. Some of her publications are: 'Transmissible drug-resistance in an epidemic strain of *Salmonella typhimurium*' (*J Hyg Camb* 1962; 60: 301); 'Classification of plasmids as an aid to understanding their epidemiology and evolution' (*J Antimicrob Chemother* 1977; 3 (Suppl C): 19); and, with V M Hughes, 'Plasmids of the same Inc groups in enterobacteria before and after the medical use of antibiotics' (Nature 1983, in press).

R W LACEY is Professor of Clinical Microbiology, University of Leeds. His previous appointments include: Lecturer and Reader, Department of Microbiology, University of Bristol, from 1968 to 1974, and Consultant in Infectious Diseases, East Anglian Regional Health Authority, King's Lynn. In 1976, he was Visiting Professor, Department of Genetics, University of Sao Paulo, Brazil. In the past, Professor Lacey has been involved in studies of antibiotic resistance with a view to establishing optimum use of antibiotics, with particular reference to gene transfer in *Staphylococcus aureus*, resistance to trimethoprim and sulphonamides. Currently, he is engaged in work on prophage carriage in *S. aureus*; comparative clinical trials of antibiotic to avoid resistance, and the interaction of antimicrobial agents with skin fatty acids. Among his publications are: 'Antibiotic resistance plasmids of *Staphylococcus aureus* and their clinical importance' (*Bact Rev* 1975; 39:

1–32); 'Evidence for two mechanisms of plasmid transfer in mixed cultures of *Staphylococcus aureus*' (*J Gen Microbiol* 1980; 119: 423–435); and 'Do sulphonamide-trimethoprim combinations select less resistance to trimethoprim than the use of trimethoprim alone?' (*J Gen Microbiol* 1982; 15: 403–427).

PROFESSOR H P LAMBERT is Professor of Microbial Diseases in the University of London and Consultant Physician at St George's Hospital, London. He trained in medicine at Cambridge and at University College Hospital, London. His special interests are respiratory and gastrointestinal infections, and the development of rational policies for the use of antimicrobial drugs. He is the author, with L P Garrod & F O'Grady, of *Antibiotic and chemotherapy*, 5th edn (Edinburgh: Churchill Livingstone, 1981); and, with W E Farrar, of *Infectious diseases illustrated* (Oxford: Pergamon, 1982).

DR A H LINTON is currently Head of the Department of Microbiology, University of Bristol and Reader in Veterinary Bacteriology. After three years in public health bacteriology, he was appointed to the teaching staff of the university with primary responsibility for teaching microbiology to veterinary students. He holds the degrees of PhD and DSc of the University of Bristol and is a Fellow of the Royal College of Pathologists. His major research interests are concerned with the epidemiology of salmonellosis and R plasmids in animals and their environment, and their public health importance. He has published about 70 papers. Three of the more important are: with J F Timoney & M Hinton, 'The ecology of chloramphenicol-resistance in *Salmonella typhimurium* and *Escherichia coli* in calves with endemic *Salmonella* infection' (*J Appl Bact* 1981; 50: 115–129); with J F Timoney, 'Experimental ecological studies on 42 plasmids in the intestines and faeces of the calf' (*J Appl Bact* 1982; 52: 417–424); and 'Has Swann failed?' (*Vet Rec* 1981; 108: 328–331). In addition, he has published two books on microbiology. His work is supported by grants from the ARC, MAFF and various pharmaceutical companies within the UK and USA. Dr Linton is currently a member of the Veterinary Products Committee and a consultant to the World Health Organization, the EEC and BVA on problems of antibiotic resistance and salmonellosis.

DR A A MEDEIROS is Associate Professor of Medicine at Brown University, Providence RI, USA, and is Director of the Division of Infectious Diseases and the Clinical Microbiology Laboratory of the Miriam Hospital. He obtained his MD degree from Georgetown University and completed his training in internal medicine, infectious diseases and clinical microbiology at the Peter Bent Brigham Hospital in Boston, under the mentorship of Professor Thomas F O'Brien. His primary interest is the characterization and distribution of β-lactamases and their role in determining resistance to β-lactam antibiotics. His recent papers include: with R W Hedges & G A Jacoby, 'Spread of a "pseudomonas-specific" beta-lactamase to plasmids of enterobacteria' (*J Bacteriol* 1982; 149: 700–707); with T F O'Brien *et al.*, 'Molecular epidemiology of antibiotic resistance in salmonella from animals and humans in the United States' (*New Engl J Med* 1982; 307: 1–6); and, with R Marre & W L Pasculle, 'Characterization of the beta-lactamases of six species of legronella' (*J Bacteriol* 1982; 151: 216–221).

PROFESSOR D A MITCHISON is the Honorary Director of the Medical Research Council's Unit for Laboratory Studies of Tuberculosis and Director of the Department of Bacteriology at the Royal Postgraduate Medical School, London. His main work has been on the bacteriology, chemotherapy and latterly the immunology of tuberculosis. He is responsible for laboratory aspects of studies on treatment and epidemiology carried out in association with the Medical Research Council's Tuberculosis and Chest Diseases Unit in Britain, East Africa, India, Hong Kong, Singapore, Algeria and Czechoslovakia; the two units together form the WHO Collaborating Centre for Tuberculosis Chemotherapy and its Application. A major interest during the past decade has been the development of short-course chemotherapy of tuberculosis. In addition, projects of his unit include a study on the reasons for breakdown of minimal inactive tuberculosis in Hong Kong, and the immunological changes accompanying BCG vaccination in Britain and South India. Recent publications include 'Treatment of tuberculosis', a summary of the Mitchell Lecture at the Royal College of Physicians (*J R Coll Physicians Lond* 1980; 14: 91–99); with Jean Dickinson, 'Experimental models to explain the high sterilizing activity of rifampicin in the chemotherapy of tuberculosis' (*Am Rev Respir Dis* 1981; 123: 367–371); with A R M Coates, 'Monoclonal antibodies in bacteriology' (in: A J McMichael & J W Fabre, eds. Monoclonal antibodies in clinical medicine. 1982; 301–310). He has been awarded the Weber Parkes Medal by the Royal College of Physicians and the Sir Robert Philip Medal by the Chest, Heart and Stroke Association. He is recognized as an expert on tuberculosis by the World Health Organization and has participated in the formulation of the 9th Report of the WHO Expert Committee on Tuberculosis, in a recent review of tuberculosis control by WHO and the International Union Against Tuberculosis, and in the setting up of a new WHO research programme (IMMTUB) on the immunology of tuberculosis.

IAN PHILLIPS has been Professor of Medical Microbiology at St Thomas's Hospital Medical School since April 1974. He spent his pre-clinical years at St John's College, Cambridge, and moved to St Thomas' in 1958, where he graduated in 1961. He remained there until 1966, when he moved to Makerere University, Uganda as a lecturer in medical microbiology. In 1969 he returned to St Thomas', where he took up the post of Senior Lecturer in Microbiology; in 1972 he became Reader and, two years later, Professor of Microbiology. In addition, Professor Phillips is the Civilian Consultant in Microbiology to the RAF, Editor of the Journal of Antimicrobial Chemotherapy and Sub-Dean for Admissions, St Thomas's Hospital Medical School. In 1966 he obtained the MD degree from the University of London, followed by membership of the Royal College of Pathologists in 1969. Professor Phillips became a Fellow of the Royal College of Pathologists in 1981, and of the Royal College of Physicians in 1983. Professor Phillips' main research interests cover *Pseudomonas aeruginosa*, gonococci, antibiotics and anaerobes. His publications include both books and papers on these and other topics. He is joint editor of *The therapeutic use of antibiotics in hospitals* (Livingstone), of *Infection with non-sporing anaerobic bacteria* (Churchill Livingstone), of *Laboratory methods in antimicrobial chemotherapy* (Churchill Livingstone), and is one of the authors of *Microbial disease; The use of the laboratories in diagnosis, therapy and control* (Arnold) as well as General Editor of the Edward Arnold series *Current Topics in Infection.*

DR P E REYNOLDS is a lecturer in the Department of Biochemistry at the University of Cambridge and Senior Tutor of Magdalene College. His whole career has been spent in Cambridge where he graduated and then carried out research under Professor Ernest Gale. After receiving his doctorate in 1964, he held a Royal Society Research Fellowship and then became a member of staff in the Sub-Department of Chemical Microbiology. Dr Reynolds carried out research on bacterial cell wall synthesis and the action of antibiotics on this process (including vancomycin and bacitracin) before concentrating on β-lactams, an interest stimulated by a period of sabbatical leave spent in the laboratories of Professor Ghuysen at Liege. His present research includes the elucidation of the roles and activities of penicillin-binding proteins and of the mechanisms of intrinsic resistance to β-lactam antibiotics. His published work includes: with E F Gale, E Cundliffe, M H Richmond & M J Waring 'The molecular basis of antibiotic action' 2nd edn.; with H A Chase & J B Ward, 'Purification and characterisation of the penicillin-binding protein that is the lethal target of penicillin' (*Eur J Biochem* 1978; 88: 275–285); and, with H A Chase, 'β-Lactam binding proteins: identification as lethal targets and probes of β-lactam accessibility' (in: M Saltman & G D Shockman, eds. '*β-Lactam antibiotics: Mode of action, new developments and future prospects*' Academic Press, 1981).

DR B ROWE is a consultant medical microbiologist in the Public Health Laboratory Service and is Director of the Division of Enteric Pathogens at the Central Public Health Laboratory, Colindale, London. He graduated in Natural Sciences at St Catharine's College, Cambridge and studied medicine at University College Hospital Medical School, London, qualifying in 1960. After clinical appointments in medicine and pathology, he served in the Royal Army Medical Corps as a pathologist until 1968. During this time he was microbiologist to the Army Personnel Research Committee team which was investigating travellers' diarrhoea in the Middle East. Following army service, he joined the staff of the Salmonella Reference Laboratory at Colindale. He succeeded Dr Joan Taylor as Director in 1970, and in 1978 became Director of the new Division. He is Chairman of the World Health Organization Global Scientific Working Group on Bacterial Enteric Infections and has been a Consultant to WHO Headquarters, Geneva and to several Regional Offices. His main interests are concerned with the epidemiology, pathogenicity mechanisms and drug resistance of intestinal bacteria.

DR J R SAUNDERS has been a lecturer in the Department of Microbiology, University of Liverpool since 1975. He graduated in microbiology at the University of Bristol in 1970 and subsequently obtained his PhD degree at Bristol in 1973 after working with Dr John Grinsted on R plasmids from *Pseudomonas.* Between 1973 and 1975 he was Postdoctoral Research Assistant to Professor Mark Richmond at Bristol, working on the molecular nature of resistance plasmids in *Haemophilus.* After moving to Liverpool his interests have concerned antibiotic resistance in the gonococcus, the mechanism of transformation of bacteria by plasmid DNA and the genetic basis of virulence in gonococci and klebsiellae. His published work includes: 'Human impact on microbial evolution' (In: J A Bishop & L M Cook, eds. *Genetic responses to man-made change*, Academic Press, 1981; 249–294); with F Flett & G O Humphreys, 'Intraspecific and intergeneric mobilization of nonconjugative R plasmids by a 24.5 megadalton conjugative plasmid of *Neisseria gonorrhoeae*' (*J Gen Microbiol* 1981; 125: 123–129); and, with A Docherty & G O Humphreys, Transformation of bacteria by plasmid DNA' (In: M H Richmond, P M Bennett and J Grinsted, eds. *Plasmid technology*, Academic Press, 1983, in press).

DR KEVIN SHANNON has been a lecturer in the Department of Microbiology, St Thomas's Hospital Medical School, London since 1979. He graduated in microbiology from the University of London, subsequently did postgraduate work at University College London and obtained his PhD degree in 1975. From 1974–77 he was Research Fellow, and from 1977–79 Assistant Lecturer, at St Thomas's Hospital Medical School. Dr Shannon has been an Assistant Editor of the *Journal of Antimicrobial Chemotherapy* since 1981 and became a Member of the Royal College of Pathologists in 1982. His main research interests concern the mechanisms of bacterial resistance to aminoglycoside and 3-lactam antibiotics. His publications include: with J Armitage & R J Rowbury, 'A change in cell diameter associated with an outer membrane lesion in a temperature-sensitive cell division mutant of *Salmonella typhimurium* (*Ann Microbiol* (*Inst Pasteur*) 1974; 125B: 233–248); with I Phillips & B A King, 'Aminoglycoside resistance among Enterobacteriaceae and *Acinetobacter* species' (*J Antimicrob Chemother* 1978; 4: 131–142); and, with I Phillips, 'Mechanisms of resistance to aminoglycosides in clinical isolates' (*J Antimicrob Chemother* 1982; 9: 91–102).

PROFESSOR W V SHAW has held (since 1971) the Chair of Biochemistry which was established in the University of Leicester in connection with the foundation of its School of Medicine. He graduated in Chemistry (1955) from Williams College, Massachusetts and received the MD degree of Columbia University's College of Physicians and Surgeons, New York, in 1959. After serving as Intern and Assistant Resident in Medicine in Presbyterian Hospital, New York, he served as Clinical Associate at the National Heart Institute (NIH) and studied microbial biochemistry with Dr E R Stadtman. His studies of microbial resistance to antibiotics began in 1966 when he was Assistant Professor of Medicine at Columbia University. He was later Associate Professor of Medicine and Biochemistry and Chief of Infectious Diseases at the University of Miami, Florida, before spending two years (1972–74) as Visiting Scientist at the MRC Laboratory of Molecular Biology in Cambridge. Professor Shaw's primary research interest is microbial physiology and, in particular, the molecular biology and enzymology of chloramphenicol resistance (*CRC Crit Rev Biochem* 1983; 14: 1–46). He has been a member of the Medical Research Council of the United Kingdom and is now Chairman of the Science Council of Celltech Ltd, the British biotechnology company.

J T SMITH is Professor and Head of the Microbiology Section of the Department of Pharmaceutics, The School of Pharmacy, University of London. Previously, at Guy's Hospital Medical School, he was Senior Lecturer in Bacteriology. He moved to the School of Pharmacy in 1968 as Reader and took up his present appointment in 1974. His research interests include the modes of action of antibiotics and chemotherapeutic agents, biochemical mechanisms of bacterial resistance to antibiotics, and the genetics of transferable antibiotic resistance in gram-negative bacteria isolated from clinical infections. Publications include: with R W Hedges, N Datta & P Kontomichalou, 'Molecular specificities of R-factor-determined β-lactamases: correlation with plasmid compatibility' (*J Bacteriol* 1974; 117: 56–62; with G C Crumplin & J M Midgley, 'Mechanisms of action of nalidixic acid and its congeners' (*Topics in Antibiotic Chemistry* 1980; 3: 11–38; and, with D F Broad, 'Classification of trimethoprim-resistant dihydrofolate reductases mediated by R-plasmids using isoelectric focusing' (*Eur J Biochem* 1982; 125: 617–622). He presented a paper by invitation on 'The biochemistry of plasmid resistance mechanisms' in 1971 at The Royal Society Meeting on Bacterial Plasmids: their genetic and ecological importance. Professor Smith was elected a Fellow of the Pharmaceutical Society in 1982.

DR R B SYKES is Vice President for Biological Sciences at the Squibb Institute for Medical Research, Princeton NJ. He moved to Squibb from Glaxo in 1977 to be Assistant Director of Microbial Biochemistry. Dr Sykes graduated in Microbiology (1969) from Queen Elizabeth College, University of London and obtained a PhD degree (1972) in Microbiology from the University of Bristol. After graduating, Dr Sykes went to work for Glaxo Research, Greenford where he was involved in antibiotic research. His main scientific interests have been in the study of β-lactamases. Publications include: with M H Richmond, 'The β-lactamases of gram-negative bacteria and their possible physiological role' (in: A H Rose & D W Tempest, eds. *Advances in microbial physiology* 9. New York: Academic Press, 1973: 31–88); with M Matthew, 'The β-lactamases of gram-negative bacteria and their role in resistance to β-lactam antibiotics' (*J Antimicrob Chemother* 1967; 2: 115–157); and, with C M Cimarusti, D P Bonner *et al*, 'Monocyclic β-lactam antibiotics produced by bacteria, (*Nature* 1981; 291: 482–491).

DR E J THRELFALL is a Principal Microbiologist in the Division of Enteric Pathogens at the Central Public Health Laboratory, Colindale, London. He graduated from University College, Bangor, Wales in 1966 and obtained a PhD in 1969 from the University of Leicester. Since then he has been engaged in studying transferable antibiotic resistance plasmids in enteric bacteria. His recent publications include: with L R Ward & B Rowe, 'The use of phage-typing and plasmid characterization in studying the epidemiology of multiresistant *Salmonella typhimurium*; and, with J A Frost & G A Willshaw, 'Methods of studying transferable resistance to antibiotics *in vitro*' (in: A D Russell & L B Quessell, eds. *Antibiotics: assessment of antimicrobial activity and resistance*. 1983).

PROFESSOR B WEISBLUM is Professor in the Department of Pharmacology at the University of Wisconsin Medical School in Madison, which he joined in 1964. Following completion of his medical studies at the State University of New York in Brooklyn in 1961, he went on to obtain post-doctoral training in molecular genetics and biochemistry prior to assuming his present appointment at the University of Wisconsin. His current research interest is in the area of the molecular biology of antibiotic action and resistance, with emphasis on regulatory mechanisms involved in the control of antibiotic resistance, both in pathogenic bacteria and in antibiotic-producing organisms. He has also contributed to the area of cytogenetics where his studies of fluorescence properties of DNA-acridine complexes first provided a rational basis for specific cytologic banding patterns obtained with fluorescent dyes.

INDEX

A

Acetyltransferases, 30
Acinetobacter, antibiotic resistance in, 73, 93
Adenine methylase structural gene, 48
Adenyltransferases, 30
Amikacin, resistance to, 32
Aminoglycoside-aminocyclitols, 62
Aminoglycosides, modification, 62
—modifying enzymes, 28–31
—reduced uptake, 31
—resistance to, 28–35
——in clinical isolates, 32
——counteraction, 98
—structure, 29
AMYES S G, *see* SMITH J T, 42
Antibiotic-producing organisms, defence against self-intoxication, 61–67
Antibiotic resistance, chemical inhibition, 97
——chromosomally specified, 54
——counteracting agents, 96–101
——due to chromosomal mutations, 15
——from decreased drug accumulation, 11–17
——genetic determinants, 54–56
——genetic transfer, 56
——impact on therapy, 102–106
——in sexually-transmitted diseases, 104
——inducible, 47–53
——β-lactamase action, 18–27
——molecular model for translational attenuation control, 49
——plasmid-determined, 54, 56
——regulation, negative feedback components in, 51
Antibiotic-resistant bacteria in animal husbandry, 91–95
Antibiotic target site resistance, 3–10, 63
Antibiotics, hydrophilic, exclusion by *Ps. aeruginosa* outer membrane, 11
——gram-negative bacterial resistance to, 11
—use, control methods, 105
Antifolate chemotherapeutic agents, plasmid-mediated, bacterial resistance to, 42–46

B

Bacteria, antibiotic resistance, genetics and evolution, 54–60
———inducible, 47–53
———introduction to symposium, 1
—conjugation, 56
—gram-negative, antibiotic-resistant, 11
—R plasmid incidence in, 58
—resistance genes, origins, 59
—transduction, 58
—transformation, 58
Bacterial infection, antibiotic-resistant, control, 105
———impact on therapy, 102–106
Biographical notes on contributors, 107
BONNER D P, *see* SYKES R B, 96

C

Capreomycin, resistance of *Strep. capreolus* to, 61
Cephalosporins, resistance to, chemical inhibition, 98

Chloramphenicol

Chloramphenicol acetyltransferase, 36
——expression of genes for, 39
——variants, 37
—bacterial resistance to, 36–41
—chemistry and properties, 36
—clinical considerations, 40
—*E. coli* resistance to, 36
—resistance by enzymic acetylation, 36
——counteraction, 99
——non-enzymic, 40
—therapeutic efficiency, 40
CHOPRA I: Antibiotic resistance resulting from decreased drug accumulation, 11–17
Chromosome mutations, antibiotic resistance due to, 15, 54
Contributors, biographical notes on, 107
CUNDLIFFE E: Self defence in antibiotic-producing organisms, 61–67

D

DATTA N: Antibiotic resistance in bacteria. Introduction to symposium, 1
Dihydrofolate reductase, plasmid-mediated, 44
——trimethoprim-resistant, 43, 44
DNA gyrase, target of replication inhibitors, 5

E

Enterobacter, antibiotic resistance in, 73
Enzyme inhibitors, 97
Enzymes, antibiotic-modifying, 61, 62
Erythromycin, induction of MLS resistance and inhibition of protein synthesis are inseparable problems of, 48
—resistance to, 8
——in bacteria, inducible, 47–53
——in *E. coli*, 7
——in *Staph. aureus*, 79
—self-defence of *S. erythraeus* against, 63
Escherichia coli, ampicillin-resistant, β-lactamase types in clinical isolates, 22
——antibiotic resistance in, 7, 73
——distribution in clinical isolates, 22

F

Food poisoning, antibiotic resistance in, 68

G

Gastrointestinal infections, antibiotic-resistant, treatment, 103
Gentamicin resistance in salmonella infections, 70
—structure, 29
Gonorrhoea, antibiotic-resistant, treatment, 103
Gram-negative aerobic bacilli, drug resistance in, 68–76

H

Haemophilus influenzae infections, treatment, 103
Hospital infection, antibiotic-resistant, treatment, 104
——control methods, 105

K

Kanamycin, *E. coli* resistance to, 7
—structure, 29
Kasugamycin, resistance to, 8
Klebsiella, antibiotic resistance in, 73, 93

L

LACEY R W: Antibiotic resistance in *Staphylococcus aureus* and streptococci, 77–83
β-lactam antibiotics, 96
——novel, resistance to, counteraction, 98
———contribution of β-lactamase, 24
———in *Staph. aureus*, 78
——target, 3
β-lactamases, 18–27
—chromosomally-determined, 23
—classification, 18
—contribution to β-lactam antibiotic resistance, 24
—identification, 18
—inhibitors, 97
—novel, 20
—plasmid-determined, 19
—TEM types, 18, 19, 20
—transposon-determined, 21
LAMBERT H P: Impact of bacterial resistance to antibiotics on therapy, 102–106
Lincosamide antibiotics, bacterial resistance to, 47–52
LINTON A H: Antibiotic-resistant bacteria in animal husbandry, 91–99

M

Macrolide antibiotics, bacterial resistance to, 47–52
MEDEIROS A A: β-lactamases, 18–27
Meningitis, drug-resistant, treatment, 102
Methicillin resistance in *Staph. aureus*, 78
MITCHISON D A: Drug resistance in mycobacteria, 84–90
MLS antibiotics, bacterial resistance to, inducibility, 47–53
Mycobacteria, drug resistance in, 84–90
Mycobacterium tuberculosis, drug sensitivity testing in, 87
Mycoplasma pneumoniae infections, treatment, 103

N

Neomycin B, structure, 29
Netilmicin, resistance to, 32

O

Otitis media, acute, antibiotic-resistant, treatment, 103

P

Penicillin resistance, counteraction, 97
Penicillinase, inhibitors, 96
—production by staphylococci, 80
PHILLIPS I & SHANNON K: Aminoglycoside resistance, 28–35
Phosphotransferases, 28

Plasmid pE194: model system and its mutants, 48
Plasmid-mediated antibiotic resistance, 12, 36, 54, 56
——resistance to antifolate agents, 42–46
Plasmids in bacterial population, 58
—staphylococcal, 77, 78
Pneumococci, antibiotic resistance in, 81
Pneumonia, antibiotic-resistant, treatment, 103
Proteins, penicillin-binding, 3, 4
Proteus, antibiotic resistance in, 73, 93
Pseudomonas, antibiotic resistance in, 73, 93
Pyridone carboxylic acids, resistance to, counteraction, 99

R

Respiratory infections, drug-resistant, treatment, 102
REYNOLDS P E: Resistance of the antibiotic target site, 3–10
Ribosome, target of translation inhibitors, 7
Rifampicin, interference with RNA polymerase reaction, 6
—resistant *E. coli* mutants, 6
Rifamycins, resistance to, counteraction, 99
RNA methylation, ribosomal, and MLS resistance in bacteria, 48
—polymerase, target of transcription inhibitors, 6
—ribosomal, alterations causing antibiotic resistance, 8
ROWE B & THRELFALL E J: Drug resistance in gram-negative aerobic bacilli, 68–76

S

Salmonella infection, antibiotic resistance in, 68–72, 92
——treatment, 103
SAUNDERS J R: Genetics and evolution of antibiotic resistance, 54–60
Serratia, antibiotic resistance in, 73
SHANNON K, *see* PHILLIPS I, 28
SHAW, W V: Bacterial resistance to chloramphenicol, 36–41
Shigellosis, antibiotic-resistant, 68–72
——treatment, 103
Sinusitis, acute, antibiotic-resistant, treatment, 103
SMITH J T & AMYES S G B: Bacterial resistance to antifolate chemotherapeutic agents mediated by plasmids, 42–46
Spectinomycin, *E. coli* resistance, 7
—structure, 29
Staphylococcus aureus, antibiotic-resistant, 77–81, 91
——in, relationship to virulence, 79
——DNA distribution in, 77
——β-lactam resistance in, 78
——macrolide resistance in, 79
Streptococci, antibiotic resistance in, 81
———origins, 82
Streptogramin type-B antibiotics, bacterial resistance to, 47–52
Streptomycetes, self-defence against antibiotic products, 62, 63, 64
Streptomycin, resistance of streptomycin-producing strains of *Streptomyces* to, 62
—ribosomal protein resistance, 7
—structure, 29

Streptovaricin, interference with RNA polymerase reaction, 6
Sulphonamides, resistance to, plasmid-mediated, 45
SYKES R B & BONNER D P: Counteracting antibiotic resistance: new drugs, 96–101

T

Tetracyclines, resistance to, counteraction, 99
——plasmid-mediated, 12
Tetrahydrofolic acid biosynthetic pathway in mammals and bacteria, 42
Thiostrepton, bacterial resistance to, 8
—self-defence of *S. azureus* against, 63
THRELFALL E J, *see* ROWE B, 68
Throat infection, drug-resistant, treatment, 102
Tn*3*, transposition system, 55
Tobramycin, structure, 29
Transposons, antibiotic resistance due to, 55
Trimethoprim, dihydrofolate reductase resistance, 43, 44
—resistance in salmonella infections, 70
Tuberculosis, drug-resistant, 84–90
——prognostic significance, 86
—drug sensitivity testing in, 87

V

Vibrio cholerae, antibiotic resistance in, 73
Viomycin, resistance of *Strep. vinaceus* to, 61

W

WEISBLUM B: Inducible erythromycin resistance in bacteria, 47–53

The Journal of Medical Microbiology

■An international journal publishing original work and significant review articles on all aspects of medical, dental and veterinary microbiology

■This journal enjoys a high reputation throughout the world

■Now increased to six bi-monthly issues (in two volumes), giving earlier publication and more extensive coverage of the field

EDITORIAL BOARD

Professor J. G. Collee (Chairman)
Professor B. I. Duerden
Dr M. T. Parker
Professor H. Stern

R. Blowers / N. Datta / R. R. Davies / H. W. K. Fell / R. Freeman / J. V. T. Gostling / D. Greenwood / H. R. Ingham / P. A. Jenkins / R. H. Leach / D. C. Old / R. Parton / N. W. Preston / J. M. Rutter / G. R. Smith / D. C. E. Speller / M. Sussman / D. C. Turk / J. Widdowson

Papers published in 1983 (abbreviated titles)

How macrophages kill tubercle bacilli / Multi-typing scheme for *P. mirabilis* and *P. vulgaris* / Virological course of *Herpes zoster* / Phagocytosis of *Tripanosoma brucei rhodesiense* by peritoneal macrophages: scanning electronmicroscopy / Relatedness of chloramphenicol resistance plasmids in epidemiologically unrelated strains of pathogenic *E. coli* / Characteristics of motile curved rods in vaginal secretions / Importance of classical and alternative complement pathways in serum bactericidal activity against *E. coli* / Pathogenicity of *Mycobacterium avium* and related mycobacteria / Role of DNA and bacteriophage in *campyolobacter* auto-agglutination / Iron deficiency in experimentally induced oral candidosis in the rat / Low intraphagolysosomal pH and antimicrobial activity of antibiotics against ingested staphylococci

Volume 19 (1983) included papers from the following countries –
Australia, Denmark, Eire, Finland, India, Italy, The Netherlands, New Zealand, Nigeria, Norway, Sweden, United Kingdom, USA, West Germany

●1984   VOLUMES 17 & 18   BI-MONTHLY
SUBSCRIPTION £65.00 / $125.00

ORDER FORM

Churchill Livingstone journals are available from your usual subscription agent or from the following address:
Churchill Livingstone Journals, Subscription Dept., Longman Group Ltd., Fourth Avenue, Harlow, Essex CM19 5AA, U.K.

☐Please send me a sample copy of The Journal of Medical Microbiology

☐Cheque enclosed for subscription to The Journal of Medical Microbiology Volumes 17 & 18 (ISSN 0022-2615)
OR
Please charge my
Access/Eurocard/Barclaycard/Visa/American Express/Diners Club Account

My credit card number is | | | | | | | | | | | | | | | | | |

Signature..   Name (please print)..

Address (please print) ....

Churchill Livingstone ⛴